The Official *Autism* 101 Manual

Created and Compiled by Karen L. Simmons
Edited by Jonathan Alderson

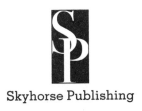

Skyhorse Publishing

Skyhorse Publishing books may be purchased in bulk at special discounts for sales promotion, corporate gifts, fund-raising, or educational purposes. Special editions can also be created to specifications. For details, contact the Special Sales Department, Skyhorse Publishing, 307 West 36th Street, 11th Floor, New York, NY 10018

Skyhorse® and Skyhorse Publishing® are registered trademarks of Skyhorse Publishing, Inc.®, a Delaware corporation.

Visit our website at www.skyhorsepublishing.com.

10 9 8 7 6 5 4 3 2 1

Library of Congress Cataloging-in-Publication Data is available on file.

Jacket design by Rain Saukas
Jacket photograph: iStockphoto

Print ISBN: 978-1-5107-2253-8
Ebook ISBN: 978-1-5107-2255-2

Printed in United States of America

CONTENTS

CHAPTER 6. HELPING CHILDREN
WITH ASD GAIN SOCIAL SKILLS

CHAPTER 7. POSITIVE TOOLS TO BUILD SELF-ESTEEM

CHAPTER 8. EXCEPTIONAL INTELLIGENCE
AND MEASURING IQ

CHAPTER 9. GUIDING ADOLESCENCE AND ADULTS
WITH AUTISM

DEDICATION TO THE REAL STARS OF AUTISM

I dedicate this resource first and foremost to my children, Kimberly, Matthew, Christina, Jonathan, Stephen, and Alex. They are all my favorites! This book sets out to share the wealth of information and resources I found and used to help my two special needs children, Jonathan and Alex. Though there have been many challenges over the years, I wouldn't have my children any other way. They are who they are—whole, loving, and complete—exactly as they are. Jonny's humor and wit make me laugh. His ability to focus and concentrate enables him to hone in on what he enjoys most while offering him hope for the future. Alex's persistence will carry him far in life and certainly keeps us all on our toes! So much for growing old quickly!

I also dedicate this resource to all of Jonny and Alex's peers with Attention Deficit Hyperactivity Disorder (ADHD) or autism. You are the real shining stars of autism, and you offer a unique perspective that enriches the fabric of humankind. I like to say we must all "discover the awesome in autism," and this is what Autism Today is all about. In fact, many leading individuals may have had high functioning autism, including Albert Einstein, Marie Curie, and Thomas Jefferson, to mention a few. Our world is much better because of your contributions.

A great big thank-you goes out to all the wonderful authors and presenters who have contributed to this resource. Your commitment and perseverance in discovering help for this special group of people is what is moving the entire field forward. One of my goals is to facilitate the change of views and attitudes that people have about autism around the world. It is important to help people see that autism is a unique condition, with many symptoms that can be overcome through intervention, rather than as a negative affliction, as it was viewed in days past. Regardless of our circumstances, we can choose to see peace within it. By doing so, the quality of everyone's lives will become more positive and loving. The person with autism is in your life for a reason. Perhaps this person is there to teach you love, patience, and understanding. If you are the person with autism, you also have your lessons to learn. Maybe they are to accept yourself, explore your strengths, and learn to love and laugh more easily. No matter what we are all here to experience, I challenge each and every one of you to look into your hearts and ponder what you are here to learn and then seek to fulfill your true gifts and strengths.

THANK YOU FOR BEING YOU!
—Karen L. Simmons, Founder, CEO Autism Today

INTRODUCTION: WHY THIS BOOK?

Note: Further information and links for the authors and contributors in *The Official Autism 101 Manual* can be found at www.autismtoday.com.

Since the release of *Autism 101* in 2008, a "first of its kind" publication that received the Independent Publishers Gold Medal Award in the Medicine category, so much has changed in the world of autism. In this revised edition, starting at the core, Dr. Janine Flanagan discusses the very definition of this diagnosis, redefined in the latest version of the DSM 5, in which Asperger's is no longer a recognized disorder.

Over the past decade, newsflashes abound: Researchers at the Hospital for Sick Children in Toronto, Canada, using one of the world's largest supercomputers have identified several hundred genes associated with the epigenetics of autism. And in 2014 results from a 17-year-long study were published being the first to conclude that as many as 9 percent of participants diagnosed with ASD had developed past the fundamental challenges associated with autism and no longer qualified for the diagnosis.[1] It is now hard to deny that recovery, at least from the diagnosis, is possible.

From advances in biomedical and nutritional medicine as discussed by Julie Matthews to new research driving innovative interventions such as Jonathan Alderson's Multi-Treatment program and Arnie Gotfryd's MaxiMind Learning Program, and the proliferation of iPad apps specifically designed for autism treatment, the autism field has evolved.

---

1 Anderson DK1, Liang JW, Lord C., *Predicting young adult outcome among more and less cognitively able individuals with autism spectrum disorders.* Journal of Child Psychology and Psychiatry. 2014 May; 55(5): 485–94.

As the mother of a wonderfully unique son diagnosed with autism, I know first-hand the importance of staying abreast of the most up-to-date information I can find. Through my work at Autism Today, my mission has always been to empower parents with evidence-based information that leads to enhanced development of their children.

Especially with the incidence of autism continuing to skyrocket every year for the past two decades, now more than ever, the purpose of this book is to provide parents, family members, educators, professionals, and people on the autism spectrum with new insights, new directions, new hope, and the resources to get there.

We also received a great deal of feedback from our members wanting the Canadian perspective alongside American resources, since our countries are so similar yet unique in their own way. For example, the Friend-2Friend program based in Vancouver, British Columbia, in Canada was inspired by and derived from San Francisco State University Professor Pamela Wolfberg's renowned IPG-model for socialization. From programs to research, we can benefit a great deal by learning and collaborating with one another.

As a parent of a child with autism, author, and educator, I have hosted many conferences with world-class speakers across North America and attended other conferences gathering a great deal of information. I have hosted 67 conferences across North America and was the exclusive Canadian Distributor for Future Horizons across Canada and became familiar with many autism resources during that time in the autism field and learned a wealth of information to share with the autism world as a result.

Wherever I go, I am asked to recommend resources for behavior, social skills, communication, and sensory issues. Throughout this book, I will be doing just that, from my own personal experience, and from the recommendation of many Autism Today members. I feel my unique perspective can help many parents, educators, and professionals find what they are seeking without having to sort through the massive amounts of information online and elsewhere. Time is of the essence when caring for a person on the spectrum, so don't get stuck in denial, misled by misinformation like the myths of autism, or lost in endless hours Googling for help. Your valuable time is always best invested in time with your children. This book was conceived to afford you this priority.

I hope this book helps each and every one of you tremendously.

—Karen L. Simmons, Founder, CEO Autism Today

WHAT IS AUTISM SPECTRUM DISORDER?

WHAT IS AUTISM?

Autism Spectrum Disorder (ASD) is a neurodevelopmental disorder characterized by impaired social communication skills and restrictive, repetitive patterns of behavior and interests with unusual sensory responses.[1] ASD is heterogeneous in its causes, underlying neurobiology, and clinical presentation.[2] ASD comprises a continuum of signs and symptoms that may fluctuate and change over time as a result of the natural history, a child's age, interventions, or combinations of all of these.

The prevalence of these disorders is estimated to be 1 in 68.[3] Advances in autism research and genetic sequencing have identified the biological vulnerability to ASD,[4,5] but its etiology is felt to be heterogeneous with environmental factors and potential gene-by-environment interactions. With this in mind, the recurrence risk in families with at least one child with ASD is between 10–19 percent.[6–8]

Early Diagnosis and Best Outcomes

Early diagnosis and intervention can have a significantly positive impact on the developmental outcomes of children with ASD.[9,10] Between one and two years of age, the brain is refining its neural connections and pruning excess (unused) synapses to operate more efficiently.[11] This process is largely dependent on input from the environment.[12] Identifying developmental differences during this critical window of time and intervening effectively can affect the brain connections in a positive way and optimize prognosis.

Both research and parental reports tell us that symptoms and atypical behaviors are detectable at very young ages.[13,14] The earliest signs and symptoms of ASD that can be used for early identification in clinical practice are becoming more recognized and are highly replicated in research findings. These include reduced levels of social attention (e.g., reduced response to name) and social communication (e.g., reduced joint attention), increased repetitive behavior with objects (e.g., tapping, spinning), abnormal visual attention, abnormal body movements, and temperament dysregulation. The search for underlying bio-markers as well as findings from neuroimaging and neurophysiology studies is promising and may lead to earlier ways to identify ASD.[15–18]

The utility of screening for ASD to facilitate early intervention is supported; however, this must be linked to a timely referral for a more thorough evaluation. The American Academy of Pediatrics has recommended screening for ASD at 18 and 24 months of age using standardized screening tools.[19] The M-CHAT-R/F (Modified Checklist for Autism in Toddlers, Revised with Follow-up)[20] targets ASD-specific behaviors, and the Communication and Symbolic behavior Scales Infant/Toddler Checklist[21] targets a broader range of delays. Adopting screening programs for children at this age may help to optimize the developmental course and potential outcomes in the children identified early. Screening programs for even younger children is under study.

After screening and further evaluation, risk-positive children should have prompt access to the right interventions with proven efficacy to achieve best outcomes. Current best practice interventions should include a combination of developmental and behavioral approaches.[22] Parent involvement is essential at every stage along the way. Studies comparing existing intervention models are few, and a greater understanding of the active components of effective interventions will help to better tailor them to children, providing better outcomes.

Outcome

Outcomes for ASD are variable, as many factors are involved. Some of these include symptoms severity, cognitive and language levels, comorbid medical conditions, or behavioral challenges. Early access to diagnosis and intervention is key. Cultural beliefs, family dynamics and engagement, and socioeconomic circumstances, health disparities ultimately affect outcomes. These and other barriers need to be understood and overcome to ensure optimal outcomes.

References

1. American Psychiatric Association. Diagnostic and Statistical Manual of Mental Health Disorders: DSM-5. 5th ed. Washington, DC: American Psychiatric Association; 2013

2. Early Identification and Interventions for Autism Spectrum Disorder: Executive Summary. Pediatrics. Vol 136, Supplement, October 2015. L Zwaigenbaum, M Bauman, et al.

3. Autism and Developmental Disabilities Monitoring Network Surveillance Year 2008 Principal Investigators, Centers for Disease Control and Prevention—Prevalence of autism spectrum disorders—Autism and Developmental Disabilities Monitoring Network, 14 sites, United States, 2008. MMWR Surveill Summ. 2012;61(3):1–19pmid:22456193

4. Jiang YH, Yuen RK, Jin X, et al.—Detection of clinically relevant genetic variants in autism spectrum disorder by whole-genome sequencing. Am J Hum Genet. 2013;93(2):249–263pmid:23849776

5. Carter MT, Scherer SW—Autism spectrum disorder in the genetics clinic: a review. Clin Genet. 2013;83(5):399–407pmid:23425232

6. Constantino JN, Zhang Y, Frazier T, Abbacchi AM, Law P—Sibling recurrence and the genetic epidemiology of autism. Am J Psychiatry. 2010;167(11):1349–1356pmid:20889652

7. Ozonoff S, Young GS, Carter A, et al.—Recurrence risk for autism spectrum disorders: a Baby Siblings Research Consortium study. Pediatrics. 2011;128(3).

8. Grønborg TK, Schendel DE, Parner ET—Recurrence of autism spectrum disorders in full—and halfsiblings and trends over time: a population-based cohort study. JAMA Pediatr. 13;167(10):947–953pmid:23959427

9. Dawson G, Rogers S, Munson J, et al.—Randomized, controlled trial of an intervention for toddlers with autism: the Early Start Denver Model. Pediatrics. 2010;125(1).

10. Kasari C, Gulsrud AC, Wong C, Kwon S, Locke J—Randomized controlled caregiver mediated joint engagement intervention for toddlers with autism. J Autism Dev Disord. 2010;40(9):1045–1056pmid:20145986

11. Huttenlocher PR—Synaptic density in human frontal cortex—developmental changes and effects of aging. Brain Res. 1979;163(2):195–205pmid:427544

12. Quartz SR, Sejnowski TJ—The neural basis of cognitive development: a constructivist manifesto. Behav Brain Sci. 1997;20(4):537–556, discussion 556–596pmid:10097006

13. Zwaigenbaum L, Bryson S, Lord C, et al.—Clinical assessment and management of toddlers with suspected autism spectrum disorder: insights from studies of high-risk infants. Pediatrics. 2009;123(5):1383–1391pmid:19403506

14. Zwaigenbaum L, Bryson S, Garon N—Early identification of autism spectrum disorders. Behav Brain Res. 2013;251:133–146pmid:23588272

15. Dinstein I, Pierce K, Eyler L, et al.—Disrupted neural synchronization in toddlers with autism. Neuron. 2011;70(6):1218–1225pmid:21689606

16. Wolff JJ, Gu H, Gerig G, et al., IBIS Network—Differences in white matter fiber tract development present from 6 to 24 months in infants with autism. Am J Psychiatry. 2012;169(6):589–600pmid:22362397

17. Voos AC, Pelphrey KA, Tirrell J, et al.—Neural mechanisms of improvements in social motivationafter pivotal response treatment: two case studies. J Autism Dev Disord. 2013;43(1):1–10pmid:23104615

18. Elsabbagh M, Mercure E, Hudry K, et al., BASIS Team—Infant neural sensitivity to dynamic eye gaze is associated with later emerging autism. Curr Biol. 2012;22(4):338–342pmid:22285033

19. Myers SM, Johnson CP, American Academy of Pediatrics Council on Children With Disabilities—Management of children with autism spectrum disorders. Pediatrics. 2007;120(5):1162–1182

20. Robins DL, Casagrande K, Barton M, Chen CM, Dumont-Mathieu T, Fein D—Validation of the Modified Checklist for Autism in Toddlers, Revised with Follow-Up (M-CHAT-R/F). Pediatrics. 2014; 133(1): 3745pmid:24366990

21. Wetherby AM, Brosnan-Maddox S, Peace V, Newton L—Validation of

the Infant-Toddler Checklist as a broadband screener for autism spectrum disorders from 9 to 24 months of age. Autism. 2008;12(5):487–511pmid:18805944

22. Zwaigenbaum L, Bauman ML, Stone WL, et al.—Early identification of autism spectrum disorder: recommendations for practice and research. Pediatrics. 2015;136

Dr. Janine Flanagan, MD, FRCPC, is a developmental pediatrician in Toronto, Ontario, Canada. She is the director of the Child Development Clinic at St. Joseph's Health Centre and has been practising in the field of Autism for over 18 years. She is crossappointed at The Hospital for Sick Children in Toronto and Assistant Professor of Pediatrics at the University of Toronto. She is passionate about teaching the new generation of health care providers about Autism Spectrum Disorders (ASDs) and has written numerous articles for parenting journals, media, hospital-based websites and has also published in prestigious pediatric journals in the field of Autism and Development. She looks forward to helping families understand ASDs in order to empower them to become strong advocates for their children.

WHAT ABOUT ASPERGER'S?

As of 2013 with the new DSM-5, professionals diagnosing children with suspected autism are placing them on the Autism Spectrum. They are no longer using terms like Asperger's Disorder, PDD-NOS, or High Functioning Autism (HFA). Why? These terms have been confusing for service providers, parents, and, more important, diagnosticians. In one clinic, a doctor may diagnose a child with Asperger's, and in another clinic, a doctor may diagnose a similar set of behaviors as HFA. Yet, another professional, such as a psychologist or developmental pediatrician, might call it something different again because the diagnostic criteria and terminology were not clear and allowed for overlap.

Today, researchers and clinicians have a better understanding of the causes of Autism. Genetic and epigenetic (gene-environment interaction) research using the human genome has led researchers to believe that the wide range of autistic symptoms (including challenges formerly called HFA and Asperger's) come from the same genetic roots and consequently are better described as a spectrum of disorders.

This is similar to other disorders in medicine that are now also conceived as spectrum disorders (e.g., Fetal Alcohol Spectrum Disorder, or FASD) Autism Spectrum Disorder encompasses disorders previously referred to as "infantile autism, childhood autism, Kanner's autism, high-functioning autism, atypical autism, pervasive developmental disorder not otherwise specified, childhood disintegrative disorder, and Asperger's disorder" (DSM-5, 2013).[1]

Individuals placed on the spectrum are classified as mild, moderate, and severe and assigned a severity level 1, 2, or 3, which corresponds to the level of recommended support needed (i.e., 1 = requiring support; 2 = requiring substantial support; and 3 = requiring very substantial support). Other specifiers are used to better describe the symptomatology. These include "with or without accompanying intellectual impairment," "with or without accompanying language delay," and "associated with a known medical or genetic condition or environmental factor" (e.g., Fragile X, epilepsy, low birth weight). Additional neurodevelopmental, behavioral, or mental conditions should also be noted (e.g., DCD, ADHD, Tourette's). We believe this is a clearer and better way to understand and diagnose Autism.

References

1.   American Psychiatric Association. Diagnostic and Statistical Manual of Mental Health Disorders: DSM-5. 5th ed. Washington, DC: American Psychiatric Association; 2013

Additional sources:

Yuen, R. K. C., Merico, D., Cao, H., Pellecchia, G., Alipanahi, B., Thiruvahindrapuram, B., Scherer, S. W. (2016)—Genome-wide characteristics of *de novo* mutations in autism. *NPJ Genomic Medicine*, 1, 16027–1–16027–10. http://doi.org/10.1038/npjgenmed.2016.27

Dr. Janine Flanagan, MD, FRCPC, is a developmental pediatrician in Toronto, Ontario, Canada. She is the director of the Child Development Clinic at St. Joseph's Health Centre and has been practising in the field of Autism for over 18 years. She is crossappointed at The Hospital for Sick Children in Toronto and Assistant Professor of Pediatrics at the University of Toronto. She is passionate about teaching the new generation of health care providers about Autism Spectrum Disorders (ASDs) and has written numerous articles for parenting journals, media, hospital-based websites, and has also published in prestigious pediatric journals in the field of Autism and Development. She looks forward to helping families understand ASDs in order to empower them to become strong advocates for their children.

ABOUT AUTISM

Note: The following article is a reproduction of information from *The Autism Speaks 100 Day Kit for Newly Diagnosed Families of Young Children*. The kit was created specifically for families of children ages 4 and under to make the best possible use of the 100 days following their child's diagnosis of autism. Anyone can download the 100 Day Kit for free at www.autismspeaks.org/family-services/tool-kits/100-day-kit

Why Was My Child Diagnosed with Autism? And What Does It Mean?

Your child has been diagnosed with autism spectrum disorder, and you have asked for help. This is an important turning point in a long journey. For some families, it may be the point when, after a long search for answers, you now have a name for something you didn't know what to call, but you knew existed.

Perhaps you suspected autism but held out hope that an evaluation would prove otherwise. Many families report mixed feelings of sadness and relief when their child is diagnosed. You may feel completely overwhelmed. You may also feel relieved to know that the concerns you have had for your child are valid. Whatever it is you feel, know that thousands of parents share this journey. You are not alone. There is reason to hope. There is help. Now that you have the diagnosis, the question is, where do you go from here? The Autism Speaks 100 Day Kit was created to help you make the best possible use of the next 100 days in the life of your child. It contains information and advice collected from trusted and respected experts on autism and parents like you.

Why Does My Child Need a Diagnosis of Autism?

Parents are usually the first to notice the early signs of autism. You probably noticed that your child was developing differently from his or her peers. The differences may have existed from birth or may have become more noticeable later. Sometimes, the differences are severe and obvious to everyone. In other cases, they are more subtle and are first recognized by a daycare provider or preschool teacher. Those differences, the symptoms of autism, have led thousands of parents like you to seek answers that have resulted in a diagnosis of autism. You may wonder: *Why does my child need a diagnosis of autism?* That's a fair question to ask—especially when right now, no one is able to offer you a cure. Autism Speaks is dedicated to funding global biomedical research into the causes, prevention, treatments, and a possible cure for autism. Great strides have been made, and the current state of progress is a far cry from the time when parents were given no hope for their children. Some of the most brilliant minds of our time have turned their attention toward this disorder.

It is important to remember that your child is the same unique, lovable, wonderful person he or she was before the diagnosis.

There are, however, several reasons why having a diagnosis is important for your child. A thorough and detailed diagnosis provides important information about your child's behavior and development. It can help create a roadmap for treatment by identifying your child's specific strengths and challenges and providing useful information about which needs and skills should be targeted for effective intervention. A diagnosis is often required to access autism-specific services through early intervention programs or your local school district.

How is Autism Diagnosed?

Presently, we don't have a medical test that can diagnose autism. As the symptoms of autism vary, so do the routes to obtaining a diagnosis. You may have raised questions with your pediatrician. Some children are identified as having developmental delays before obtaining a diagnosis of autism and may already receive some Early Intervention or **Special Education services.** Unfortunately, parents' concerns are sometimes not taken seriously by their doctor, and as a result, a diagnosis is delayed. Autism Speaks and other autism-related organizations are working hard to educate parents and physicians, so that children with autism are identified as early as possible.

Your child may have been diagnosed by a **developmental pediatrician, a neurologist, a psychiatrist, or a psychologist.** In some cases, a team of specialists may have evaluated your child and provided recommendations for treatment. The team may have included an audiologist to rule out hearing loss, a speech & language therapist to determine language skills and needs, and an occupational therapist to evaluate physical and motor skills. A multidisciplinary evaluation is important for diagnosing autism and other challenges that often accompany autism, such as delays in motor skills. If your child has not been evaluated by a multidisciplinary team, you will want to make sure further evaluations are conducted so that you can learn as much as possible about your child's individual strengths and needs.

Once you have received a formal diagnosis, it is important to make sure that you ask for a comprehensive report that includes the diagnosis in writing, as well as recommendations for treatment. The doctor may not be able to provide this for you at the appointment, as it may take some time to compile, but be sure to follow up and pick up.

For more information, visit the Autism Speaks Autism Treatment Network at www.autismspeaks.org/atn.

What is Autism?

Autism spectrum disorder (ASD) and autism are both general terms for a group of complex disorders of brain development. These disorders are characterized, in varying degrees, by difficulties in social interaction, verbal and nonverbal communication, and repetitive behaviors. With the May 2013 publication of the fifth edition of the *American Psychiatric Association's Diagnostic and Statistical Manual of Mental Disorders* (commonly referred to as the DSM-5), all autism disorders were merged into one umbrella diagnosis of ASD. Previously, they were recognized as distinct subtypes, including autistic disorder, childhood disintegrative disorder, pervasive developmental disorder-not otherwise specified (PDD-NOS), and Asperger's Syndrome. The DSM is the main diagnostic reference used by mental health professionals and insurance providers in the United States.

You may also hear the terms Classic Autism or Kanner's Autism (named after the first psychiatrist to describe autism) used to describe the most severe form of the disorder. Under the current DSM-5, the diagnosis of autism requires that at least six developmental and behavioral characteristics are observed, that problems are present before the age of three, and that there is no evidence of certain other conditions that are similar.

There are two domains where people with ASD must show persistent deficits:

1. *Persistent social communication and social interaction*
2. *Restricted and repetitive patterns of behavior*

More specifically, people with ASD must demonstrate (either in the past or in the present) deficits in social-emotional reciprocity, deficits in nonverbal communicative behaviors used for social interaction; and deficits in developing, maintaining, and understanding relationships. In addition, they must show at least two types of repetitive patterns of behavior, including stereotyped or repetitive motor movements, insistence on sameness or inflexible adherence to routines, highly restricted, fixated interests, hyper- or hyporeactivity to sensory input, or unusual interest in sensory aspects of the environment. Symptoms can be currently present or reported in past history. In addition to the diagnosis, each person evaluated will also be described in terms of any known genetic cause (e.g., Fragile X syndrome, Rett syndrome), level of language and intellectual disability, and presence of medical conditions such as seizures, anxiety, depression, and/or gastrointestinal (GI) problems.

The DSM-5 has an additional category called Social Communication Disorder (SCD). This allows for a diagnosis of disabilities in social communication, without the presence of repetitive behavior. SCD is a new diagnosis, and much more research and information is needed. There are currently few guidelines for the treatment of SCD. Until such guidelines become available, treatments that target social communication, including many autism-specific interventions, should be provided to individuals with SCD.

To read the whole DSM-5 criteria, please visit www.autismspeaks.org/dsm-5.

How Common is Autism?

Autism statistics from the U.S. Centers for Disease Control and Prevention (CDC) released in March 2014 identify around 1 in 68 American children as on the autism spectrum—a tenfold increase in prevalence in 40 years. Careful research shows that this increase is only partly explained by improved diagnosis and awareness. Studies also show that autism is four to five times more common among boys than girls. An estimated 1 out of 42 boys and 1 in 189 girls are diagnosed with autism in the United States. ASD affects over 2 million individuals in the U.S. and tens of millions worldwide. Moreover, government autism statistics suggest that prevalence rates have increased 10 percent to 17 percent annually in recent years. There is no established explanation for this continuing increase, although improved diagnosis and environmental influences are two reasons often considered.

What Causes Autism?

Not long ago, the answer to this question would have been "we have no idea." Research is now delivering the answers. First and foremost, we now know that there is no one cause of autism, just as there is no one type of autism. Over the last five years, scientists have identified a number of rare gene changes or mutations associated with autism. Research has identified more than 100 autism risk genes. In around 15 percent of cases, a specific genetic cause of a person's autism can be identified. However, most cases involve a complex and variable combination of genetic risk and environmental factors that influence early brain development.

In other words, in the presence of a genetic predisposition to autism, a number of nongenetic or environmental influences further increase a child's risk. The clearest evidence of these environmental risk factors involves events before and during birth. They include advanced parental age at time of conception (both mom and dad), maternal illness during pregnancy, extreme prematurity, very low birth weight, and certain difficulties during birth, particularly those involving periods of oxygen deprivation to the baby's brain. Mothers exposed to high levels of pesticides and air pollution may also be at higher risk of having a child with ASD. It is important to keep in mind that these factors, by themselves, do not cause autism. Rather, in combination with genetic risk factors, they appear to modestly increase risk.

A small but growing body of research suggests that autism risk is lower among children whose mothers took prenatal vitamins (containing folic acid) in the months before and after conception. Increasingly, researchers are looking at the role of the immune system in autism. Autism Speaks is working to increase awareness and investigation of these and other issues where further research has the potential to improve the lives of those who struggle with autism.

While the causes of autism are complex, it is abundantly clear that it is not caused by bad parenting. Dr. Leo Kanner, the psychiatrist who first described autism as a unique condition in 1943, believed that it was caused by cold, unloving mothers. Bruno Bettelheim, a renowned professor of child development, perpetuated this misinterpretation of autism.

Their promotion of the idea that unloving mothers caused their children's autism created a generation of parents who carried the tremendous burden of guilt for their child's disability. In the 1960s and 70s, Dr. Bernard Rimland, the father of a son with autism who later founded the Autism Society of America and the Autism Research Institute, helped the medical community understand that autism is a biological disorder and is not caused by cold parents.

More Information about Symptoms of Autism

Autism affects the way an individual perceives the world and makes communication and social interaction difficult. Autism spectrum disorders (ASD) are characterized by social-interaction difficulties, communication challenges, and a tendency to engage in repetitive behaviors. However, symptoms and their severity vary widely across these three core areas. Taken together, they may result in relatively mild challenges for someone on the high functioning end of the autism spectrum. For others, symptoms may be more severe, as when repetitive behaviors and lack of spoken language interfere with everyday life.

It is sometimes said that if you know one person with autism, you know one person with autism.

While autism is usually a lifelong condition, all children and adults benefit from interventions, or therapies, that can reduce symptoms and increase skills and abilities. Although it is best to begin intervention as soon as possible, the benefits of therapy can continue throughout life. The long-term outcome is highly variable. A small percentage of children lose their diagnosis over time, while others remain severely affected. Many have normal cognitive skills, despite challenges in social and language abilities. Many individuals with autism develop speech and learn to communicate with others. Early intervention can make extraordinary differences in your child's development. How your child is functioning now may be very different from how he or she will function later on in life.

The following information on the social symptoms, communication disorders, and repetitive behaviors associated with autism is partially taken from the National Institute of Mental Health (NIMH) website.

Social symptoms

Typically developing infants are social by nature. They gaze at faces, turn toward voices, grasp a finger, and even smile by 2 to 3 months of age. By contrast, most children who develop autism have difficulty engaging in the give-and-take of everyday human interactions. By 8 to 10 months of age, many infants who go on to develop autism are showing some symptoms, such as failure to respond to their names, reduced interest in people, and delayed babbling. By toddlerhood, many children with autism have difficulty playing social games, don't imitate the actions of others, and prefer to play alone. They may fail to seek comfort or respond to parents' displays of anger or affection in typical ways.

Research suggests that children with autism are attached to their parents. However, the way they express this attachment can be unusual. To parents, it may seem as if their child is disconnected. Both children and adults with autism also tend to have difficulty interpreting what others are thinking and feeling. Subtle social cues such as a smile, wave, or grimace may convey little meaning. To a person who misses these social cues, a statement like "Come here!" may mean the same thing, regardless of whether the speaker is smiling and extending her arms for a hug or frowning and planting her fists on her hips. Without the ability to interpret gestures and facial expressions, the social world can seem bewildering.

Many people with autism have similar difficulty seeing things from another person's perspective. Most five-year-olds understand that other people have different thoughts, feelings, and goals than they have. A person with autism may lack such understanding. This, in turn, can interfere with the ability to predict or understand another person's actions. It is common—but not universal—for those with autism to have difficulty regulating emotions. This can take the form of seemingly "immature" behavior such as crying or having outbursts in inappropriate situations. It can also lead to disruptive and physically aggressive behavior. The tendency to "lose control" may be particularly pronounced in unfamiliar, overwhelming, or frustrating situations. Frustration can also result in self-injurious behaviors such as head banging, hair pulling or self-biting.

Fortunately, children with autism can be taught how to socially interact, use gestures, and recognize facial expressions. Also, there are many strategies that can be used to help the child with autism deal with frustration so that he or she doesn't have to resort to challenging behaviors. We will discuss this later.

Communication difficulties

Young children with autism tend to be delayed in babbling, speaking, and learning to use gestures. Some infants who later develop autism coo and babble during the first few months of life before losing these communicative behaviors. Others experience significant language delays and don't begin to speak until much later. With therapy, however, most people with autism do learn to use spoken language, and all can learn to communicate.

Many nonverbal or nearly nonverbal children and adults learn to use communication systems such as pictures, sign language, electronic word processors, or even speech-generating devices.

When language begins to develop, people with autism may use speech in unusual ways. Some have difficulty combining words into meaningful sentences. They may speak only single words or repeat the same phrase over and over. Some go through a stage where they repeat what they hear verbatim (echolalia).

Many parents assume difficulties expressing language automatically mean their child isn't able to understand the language of others, but this is not always the case. It is important to distinguish between expressive language and receptive language. Children with difficulties in expressive language are often unable to express what they are thinking through language, whereas children with difficulties in receptive language are often unable to understand what others are saying. Therefore, the fact that your child may seem unable to express him- or herself through language does not necessarily mean he or she is unable to comprehend the language of others. Be sure to talk to your doctor or look for signs that your child is able to interpret language, as this important distinction will affect the way you communicate with him or her.

It is essential to understand the importance of pragmatics when looking to improve and expand upon your child's communication skills. Pragmatics are social rules for using language in a meaningful context or conversation. While it is important that your child learn how to communicate through words or sentences, it is also key to emphasize both when and where the specific message should be conveyed. Challenges in pragmatics are a common feature of spoken language difficulties in children with autism. These challenges may become more apparent as your child gets older.

Some mildly affected children exhibit only slight delays in language or even develop precocious language and unusually large vocabularies—yet have difficulty sustaining a conversation. Some children and adults with autism tend to carry on monologues on a favorite subject, giving others little chance to comment. In other words, the ordinary "give-and-take" of conversation proves difficult. Some children with ASD with superior language skills tend to speak like little professors, failing to pick up on the "kid-speak" that's common among their peers.

Another common difficulty is the inability to understand body language, tone of voice, and expressions that aren't meant to be taken literally. For example, even an adult with autism might interpret a sarcastic "Oh, that's just great!" as meaning it really is great.

Conversely, individuals affected by autism may not exhibit typical body language. Facial expressions, movements, and gestures may not match what they are saying. Their tone of voice may fail to reflect their feelings. Some use a high-pitched, sing-song, or flat, robot-like voice. This can make it difficult for others to know what they want and need. This failed communication, in turn, can lead to frustration and inappropriate behavior (such as screaming or grabbing) on the part of the person with autism.

Fortunately, there are proven methods for helping children and adults with autism learn better ways to express their needs. As the person with autism learns to communicate what he or she wants, challenging behaviors often subside.

Children with autism often have difficulty letting others know what they want or need until they are taught how to communicate through speech, gestures, or other means.

Repetitive behaviors

Unusual repetitive behaviors and/or a tendency to engage in a restricted range of activities are another core symptom of autism. Common repetitive behaviors include hand-flapping; rocking, jumping and twirling; arranging and rearranging objects; and repeating sounds, words, or phrases. Sometimes the repetitive behavior is self-stimulating, such as wiggling fingers in front of the eyes.

The tendency to engage in a restricted range of activities can be seen in the way that many children with autism play with toys. Some spend hours lining up toys in a specific way instead of using them for pretend play. Similarly, some adults are preoccupied with having household or other objects in a fixed order or place. It can prove extremely upsetting if someone or something disrupts the order. Along these lines, many children and adults with autism need and demand extreme consistency in their environment and daily routine. Slight changes can be extremely stressful and lead to outbursts.

Repetitive behaviors can take the form of intense preoccupations or obsessions. These extreme interests can prove all the more unusual for their content (e.g., fans, vacuum cleaners, or toilets) or depth of knowledge (e.g., knowing and repeating astonishingly detailed information about Thomas the Tank Engine or astronomy). Older children and adults with autism may develop tremendous interest in numbers, symbols, dates, or science topics.

Many children with autism need and demand absolute consistency in their environment.

Unique Abilities that May Accompany Autism

Along with the challenges that autism involves, you may have noticed that your child also exhibits areas of strength. Although not all children have special talents, it is not uncommon for individuals with autism to have exceptional skills in math, music, art, and reading, among others. These areas of expertise can provide great satisfaction and pride for the child with autism. If possible, incorporate your child's areas of expertise into his or her everyday activities and use them whenever possible as a way for him or her to learn and excel.

The following is adapted from Sally Ozonoff, Geraldine Dawson, and James McPartland's A Parent's Guide to Asperger's Syndrome and High-Functioning Autism.

"How Can My Child Have Autism When He Seems So Smart?"

From *Does My Child Have Autism?* by Wendy Stone

Right now you might be thinking about all the things your child with autism learned at a much younger age than other children you know. And yes, you are right: there are also things that children with autism learn on their own much faster than their typically developing peers or siblings. For example, they can be very good at learning to pick out their favorite DVD from a stack, even when it's not in its case. They may learn at a very young age how to operate the remote controls to the TV and DVD player so that they can rewind their videos to their favorite parts (or fast-forward through the parts they don't like). They can be very creative in figuring out ways to climb up on the counter to reach a cabinet that has their favorite cereal or even how to use the key to unlock the dead bolt on the back door so they can go outside to play on the swing. Clearly, these are not behaviors that you would even think about trying to teach a two-year-old child. And yet some children with autism somehow manage to acquire these skills on their own. How can we understand this inconsistency between the things children with autism do and don't learn? How can a child who can't put different shapes into a shape sorter learn to turn on the TV and DVD player, put a DVD in, and push the play button? How can a child who can't understand a simple direction like "get your coat" figure out how to unlock a door to get outside?

What accounts for this unique learning style? In a word: motivation. We all pay attention better to the things that interest us, so we become much more proficient at learning them. Understanding what is motivating to your child (all children are different) will be one of the keys to increasing their learning and their skills. Your child's special talents may be part of his or her unique and inherent learning style and nature.

Just as individuals with autism have a variety of difficulties, they also have some distinctive strengths. Some of the strengths that individuals with autism have may include:

- *Ability to understand concrete concepts, rules, and sequences*
- *Strong long term memory skills*
- *Math skills*
- *Computer skills*
- *Musical ability*
- *Artistic ability*
- *Ability to think in a visual way*
- *Ability to decode written language at an early age (This ability is called Hyperlexia—some children with autism can decode written language earlier than they can comprehend written language.)*
- *Honesty—sometimes to a fault*
- *Ability to be extremely focused—if they are working on a preferred activity*
- *Excellent sense of direction*

Physical and Medical Issues that May Accompany Autism

Seizure disorders

Seizure Disorder, also called epilepsy, occurs in as many as one third of individuals with autism spectrum disorder. Epilepsy is a brain disorder marked by recurring seizures or convulsions. Experts propose that some of the brain abnormalities that are associated with autism may contribute to seizures. These abnormalities can cause changes in brain activity by disrupting neurons in the brain. Neurons are cells in the brain that process and transmit information and send signals to the rest of the body. Overloads or disturbances in the activity of these neurons can result in imbalances that cause seizures.

Epilepsy is more common in children who also have cognitive deficits. Some researchers have suggested that seizure disorder is more common when the child has shown a regression or loss of skills. There are different types and subtypes of seizures, and a child with autism may experience more than one type. The easiest to recognize are large "grand mal" (or toniclonic) seizures. Others include "petit mal" (or absence) seizures and subclinical seizures, which may only be apparent in an EEG (electroencephalogram). It is not clear whether subclinical seizures have effects on language, cognition, and behavior. The seizures associated with autism usually start either early in childhood or during adolescence but may occur at any time. If you are concerned that your child may be having seizures, you should see a neurologist. The neurologist may order tests that may include an EEG, an MRI (Magnetic Resonance Imaging), a CT (Computed Axial Tomography), and a CBC (Complete Blood Count). Children and adults with epilepsy are typically treated with anticonvulsants or seizure medicines to reduce or eliminate occurrences. If your child has epilepsy, you will work closely with a neurologist to find the medicine (or combination of medicines) that works the best with the fewest side effects and to learn the best ways to ensure your child's safety during a seizure.

Genetic disorders

Some children with autism have an identifiable genetic condition that affects brain development. These genetic disorders include Fragile X syndrome, Angelman syndrome, tuberous sclerosis, chromosome 15 duplication syndrome, and other single-gene and chromosomal disorders. While further study is needed, single gene disorders appear to affect 15 percent to 20 percent of those with ASD. Some of these syndromes have characteristic features or family histories, the presence of which may prompt your doctor to refer your child to a geneticist or neurologist for further testing. The results can help increase awareness of associated medical issues and guide treatment and life planning.

Gastrointestinal (GI) disorders

Many parents report gastrointestinal (GI) problems in their children with autism. The exact prevalence of gastrointestinal problems such as gastritis, chronic constipation, colitis, and esophagitis in individuals with autism is unknown. Surveys have suggested that between 46 percent and 85 percent of children with autism have problems such as chronic constipation or diarrhea. One study identified a history of gastrointestinal symptoms (such as abnormal pattern of bowel movements, frequent constipation, frequent vomiting, and frequent abdominal pain) in 70 percent of the children with autism. If your child has similar symptoms, you will want to consult a gastroenterologist, preferably one who works with people with autism. Your child's physician may be able to help you find an appropriate specialist. Pain caused by GI issues is sometimes recognized because of a change in a child's behavior, such as an increase in self-soothing behaviors like rocking or outbursts of aggression or self-injury. Bear in mind that your child may not have the language skills to communicate the pain caused by GI issues. Treating GI problems may result in improvement in your child's behavior. Anecdotal evidence suggests that some children may be helped by dietary intervention for GI issues, including the elimination of dairy and gluten containing foods. (*For more information, see Gluten Free Casein Free diet in the treatment section of this kit.*) As with any treatment, it is best to consult your child's physician to develop a comprehensive plan. In January 2010, Autism Speaks initiated a campaign to inform pediatricians about the diagnosis and treatment of GI problems associated with autism.

For additional information from the Official Journal of American Academy of Pediatrics, go to: pediatrics.aappublications.org/cgi/ content/full/125/Supplement_1/S1.

For information that can be shared with your child's doctor, go to: autismspeaks.org/press/ gastrointestinal_treatment_guidelines.php.

Sleep dysfunction

Is your child having trouble getting to sleep or sleeping through the night? Sleep problems are common in children and adolescents with autism. Having a child with sleep problems can affect the whole family. It can also have an impact on the ability of your child to benefit from therapy. Sometimes sleep issues may be caused by medical issues such as obstructive sleep apnea or gastroesophageal reflux, and addressing the medical issues may solve the problem. In other cases, when there is no medical cause, sleep issues may be managed with behavioral interventions including "sleep-hygiene" measures, such as limiting the amount of sleep during the day and establishing regular bedtime routines. There is some evidence of abnormality of melatonin regulation in children with autism. While melatonin may be effective for improving the ability of children with autism to fall asleep, more research is needed. Melatonin or sleep aids of any kind should not be given without first consulting with your child's physician.

Sensory Integration Dysfunction

Many children with autism experience unusual responses to sensory stimuli or input. These responses are due to difficulty in processing and integrating sensory information. Vision, hearing, touch, smell, taste, the sense of movement (vestibular system), and the sense of position (proprioception) can all be affected. This means that while information is sensed normally, it may be perceived much differently. Sometimes stimuli that seem "normal" to others can be experienced as painful, unpleasant, or confusing by a child with Sensory Integration Dysfunction (SID), the clinical term for this characteristic. (SID may also be called Sensory Processing Disorder or Sensory Integration Disorder.) SIDs can involve hypersensitivity (also known as sensory defensiveness) or hyposensitivity. An example of hypersensitivity would be an inability to tolerate wearing clothing, being touched, or being in a room with normal lighting. Hyposensitivity might be apparent in a child's increased tolerance for pain or a constant need for sensory stimulation. Treatment for Sensory Integration Dysfunction is usually addressed with occupational therapy and/or sensory integration therapy.

Pica

Pica is an eating disorder involving eating things that are not food. Children between 18 and 24 months of age often eat nonfood items, but this is typically a normal part of development. Some children with autism and other developmental disabilities persist beyond the developmentally typical time frame and continue to eat items such as dirt, clay, chalk, or paint chips. Children showing signs of persistent mouthing of fingers or objects, including toys, should be tested for elevated blood levels of lead, especially if there is a known potential for environmental exposure to lead. You should speak to your doctor about these concerns so he or she can help you with treatment. Your child's doctor will help you to assess if your child needs a behavioral intervention or if it is something that can be managed at home.

Mental health

Oftentimes a child diagnosed with ASD may receive an additional diagnosis such as Attention Deficit Hyperactivity Disorder (ADHD). ADHD and anxiety are quite common and addressing these diagnoses properly can help your child make great strides.

Recent studies suggest that 1 in 5 children on the autism spectrum also has ADHD and 30 percent struggle with an anxiety disorder such as social phobia, separation anxiety, panic disorder, and specific phobias. The classic symptoms of ADHD include chronic problems with inattention, impulsivity, and hyperactivity. However, these or similar symptoms can likewise result from autism. For this reason, it is important that evaluation be made by someone with expertise in both disorders. A recent study found that just 1 in 10 children with autism and ADHD was receiving medication to relieve the ADHD symptoms.

In regards to anxiety, children with autism express anxiety or nervousness in many of the same ways as typically developing children. Understandably, many individuals with ASD have trouble communicating how they feel. Outward manifestations may be the best clues. In fact, some experts suspect that outward symptoms of anxiety—such as sweating and acting out—may be especially prominent among those with ASD. This can include a racing heart, muscular tensions, and stomachaches. It is important for your child to be evaluated by a professional who has expertise in both autism and anxiety so he or she can provide the best treatment options for your child.

AUTISM THROUGH MY EYES

My son, Jonathan, is 25 now. When he was first diagnosed we were told the same story that many parents hear: "Your son has autism and we don't know what his life will be like. He may never be able to function in society and could end up in an institution." Today, my son is a very productive, intelligent young man that drives and has a job. And the fact that he spends many hours on the snowy roads of Edmonton, Alberta, Canada managing well amongst aggressive drivers demonstrates his ability to function at a high level. He has a long life ahead of him, and we feel positive about his future. Parents will gain hope for their children by reading his unique perspective and insight on his condition of autism written in his own words.

–Karen L. Simmons, Founder, CEO Autism Today

My name is Jonathan, and I'm a guy with Asperger's Syndrome; or at least, I used to be. The diagnosis shifted, and now I'm classified as a guy with autism. I know roughly that it's a condition that affects people's social skills. I've lived with it my entire life, and yet I'm always finding out new things that drive me that don't drive other people quite the same way. You're probably reading this because someone you know is autistic, or perhaps you've read the book *Little Rainman*, a book written by my mom, about me, for my teachers, siblings, and family.

First when mom got the diagnosis she thought I was just really super smart. She didn't think anything was different about me from my other siblings. In fact she thought I was going to end up like Albert Einstein since I could read at the age of two, and it turned out that I was "hyperlexic." This is when children can read at an early age but are not actually understanding what they are reading. I even went to my big brother's "show and tell" for fourth grade because Matt was super proud of me.

I guess the clearest early memory I have of being different was not really needing, or wanting, to play with the other kids at school. I don't really seek contact with people, but that's OK. It wasn't unpleasant or anything, it just wasn't a huge drive for me. Later, though, I had quite a lot of people telling me things I felt weren't true. For a while I didn't know if I should even believe them! It's OK to listen to friendly advice from people, as long as they're not just heaping it on, or telling you what you want to hear.

I used to be very naive about certain things. Every kid was, right? Maybe. There was this one time I walked home by myself without telling anyone. Everyone was horrified, and Mom even called the police to search for me! I didn't realize there'd be any danger at all! Of course, my parents made very sure to teach me that people might not have my best interests at heart. Mom said she had to teach me how to lie. I guess what I found out later was that my siblings had already picked up lying and that it hadn't occurred to me. I told a story about having to go pee to my teacher in first grade. My aide told me, "A little birdie told me you didn't want to go out to play because you had to pee, that's not true Jonny!" At that time I said, "Whaaaaaaa I didn't know Mrs S. had feathers." I didn't get why everyone started laughing about that.

Early in grade school . . . thanks to Mom, I had lots of help before, during, and after school. She made sure I had the proper support whenever she could though she was gone a lot to conferences. Sometimes I would go with her. This is how I met Temple Grandin. Mom and I had quite a bit of questions for her, and she'd always oblige.

Mom and Dad signed me up for football with Dave E. He said if he could be a coach and still be in a wheelchair, then I was qualified to play football. I got picked on, had to put on that heavy costume, and the ill-fitting mouth-guard, and the jersey that caught on everything, and had to run around the field, and push things, and get tackled by the biggest kid on the team. I swear he was five years older than everyone else. I really didn't like it, but Mom wouldn't let me drop out. She made me go because I agreed to do it in the first place, after being told I couldn't leave until I did. Anyway I got through that year and some of the kids were really proud of me yet some were still jerks. One time during a game, I was body-checked off of my feet, but tucked into a roll, stood up and kept going! Exciting stuff. Still, it wasn't really my bag, so I didn't sign up again next year.

I really didn't like grades 7 to 9. People would gang up on me quite a bit, and the teachers weren't around that much so they didn't really see what was going on. My brothers and sisters actually gave me quite a bit of support with this. This one kid liked to pick on me after school, and even hit me a couple of times. I'm not too proud of this, but I waited until I was behind him getting off the bus and kicked him in the back. Then I ran like hell!

Socially it was a little better for me at high school. There were a couple of people who were jerks, but I learned ways to avoid dealing with them. There were some friends I made there. They were oddballs, but we could deal with that. I also picked up a habit of listening to music. Cell phones could hold music (maybe 50 MP3s max), but atmospheric and ambient music kept me company for the rest of high school.

As I grew older, I began to have doubts about what I was passionate about, my ability to keep my mind set on stuff, what my identity really meant in the big scheme of things . . . I kind of got lost in my own head for a while when I was by myself. The fact that I didn't feel like I identified with many people my age, combined with a very short attention span for things that didn't interest me such as schoolwork, meant that I kind of coasted through school, and that I spent quite a bit of time talking to the guidance counselor.

Between semesters, Mom got me to talk at a couple of her conferences. I was pretty nervous to begin with, and end with, and between every word; but everybody stood up and applauded when I finished. I didn't feel like I deserved all of the praise, but Dad still uses that as an example of why I should have been a public speaker.

I learned that I craved direction and purpose, and Dad was so busy managing his actual office, he couldn't invent ways to have me contribute to the effort. I did learn a bit of web design, but as I was unmotivated, I mostly just sat in an empty office reading articles online. If I was to find purpose, I'd have to hunt it down myself.

As I progressed from high school to a technical college, I realized that I wasn't motivated to do schoolwork at all! The habits I made in high school really hampered my learning in college. I found my self-doubt crushing me at every opportunity! I actually think I made my algebra teacher cry! Cornelia B., I'm so sorry. May your next class pay more attention than mine. This would eventually spiral into something of a depression, where I became self-loathing, hypersensitive to criticism, and timid. I did actually get my diploma though! Some pain is worth it.

Mom and I did a couple more conferences this time and met up again with Temple Grandin.

I ended up asking her about my self-confidence, and she replied that getting a job might do something for that. What she probably had in mind was that I'd find my own profession like she did.

Education had become a nightmare for me, so I stepped away and moved to Lake Tahoe to assist my mom's webmaster. That was a fun job and I learned quite a bit more about web design. That was the first time I lived outside of the house and in another country to boot. It was nice, living by myself, setting my own boundaries, paying my own bills. I didn't own a car and they didn't have public transit, so I hiked to the grocery store. That was pretty good for me, in my opinion.

Upon returning from Lake Tahoe I began an internship at a local doctor's office. Our personalities sort of didn't mix so I didn't want to stay. The office was a frantic mess, we would routinely misplace patient data overnight somehow, and part of our job was basically being a criticism vent for the doctor. Still, the pay was pretty good for my first real job. But what I really gained was knowledge: I learned how to deal with aggressive patients, how to speak confidently on the phone, and I had gained back a lot of my shattered self-confidence.

Between shifts I spoke to a therapist about what I've been feeling. What he told me was that everyone had these kinds of feelings such as self-doubt about themselves at one point or another. Furthermore, he showed me how my family had been trying to help me, to sympathize with me. I realized that back then, I pushed them away, because I thought that being autistic, they wouldn't understand the pain. Not really. I've learned to let people in more, since then.

I decided with my therapist's help, and the help of my family, I would strive to understand myself and how I relate to others. Here's what I know:

- **Autism is a very wide spectrum.** You can have a nonverbal child as well as a very articulate child. Many people with autism become overstimulated by their surroundings. From what I've read, and experienced, autistic people are more likely to have other mental conditions as well. Even though they have a lot of different things going on, they also have a lot in common—difficulty with social skills and abstract thinking are very difficult for them. None of this means that your child is unable to learn; far from it. It's very possible they're aware of the difficulties they have, but can't explain them in terms that make sense to you!

- **Nonverbal communication can be important,** especially to nonverbal children, or for children with poor handwriting. In Junior high I was given this antiquated protolaptop thing called an AlphaSmart. Basically a keyboard attached to a teeny screen. I learned that I could type what I meant to say very easily when I could backtrack and correct something that seemed wrong to me. I'd use it for homework assignments, and gradually I'd see people understanding what I'd typed, instead of me blurting out the first thing that got past my mental word filter.

- **Autistic people are often very literal!** What I mean by that is that they won't understand idioms, metaphors, implied messages, etc. So, if you were to tell the following corny joke "Why is 6 afraid of 7? Because 7 ate (8) 9!" to a person with autism, they would not understand because the joke relies on homonyms, which is hard for them. Since they're very literal, they'll make observations out loud and unfiltered, accidentally offending people. For example, one might say, "Over there, next to the fat guy" or "This is really boring. Why are we reading this?" No social-sensitivity filter. The teachers loved me for this. (Actually, they didn't!)

- **Autistic people may be more internalized.** I can only speak from my experience, but often I wouldn't trust what other people said about me, choosing instead to rely on my own observations. The idea being, I guess, that people might lie to me to boost my ego, or tear it down. I eventually learned that closing myself off from external criticism will leave me ungrounded in terms of how I act, compared to anyone else. I also learned that not everyone is dishonest, and there are ways to convince anyone to really give you an honest critique, without being harsh, or pulling punches. It's very important, to me at least, that I maintain a healthy level of skepticism, but that I don't let it consume my feelings.

- **Social cues.** Winks, eye rolls, looking at your cell phone when someone's talking to you. Body language, crossed arms, delays in speech. A lot of people take these cues for granted, as if they're taught by instinct. Autistic people may not pick up on these, and take what you say at face value. If they see you shrugging your shoulders or rolling your eyes, for example, they might not know what that means, or notice.

- **Direction:** The thing I remember being asked most by my guidance counselor, my mom, my therapist, and basically everyone in my family: "What do you want to do?" Some autistic individuals appreciate clear, concise directions, with little room for misunderstanding. This is a skill that takes time to develop, as you won't always be sure how what you say will be interpreted.

- **Momentum-based motivation:** I find that completing simple, easy tasks gets me into a mindset of completing anything I can, for as long as I can. The upshot of this is that once I start something, it's very hard to get me to stop. This isn't always a good thing, when you need to stop for things like sleeping, and eating. Also, when I stop, it's sometimes hard to start again. But if I can plan my day right, I can avoid distractions and get projects done faster.

- **Emotional control / overstimulation:** Music helped me quite a bit when I felt like I couldn't express myself, or if I needed to get into a certain mood, or if I needed to be by myself in an environment with too many people. If you don't know what bands you'd like to listen to, there's plenty of online services that do mood-based playlists. One other thing that helped, and still helps, me to relax is to take a long bath. It seems to settle me right down especially after being around too many people, or a stressful day. I can dip my ears below the water, and it's like you can turn all the noise off.

Where I am now?

In conclusion: I feel like I've gained quite a bit of control over the direction of my life, and I've learned how to deal with people despite being autistic. I've gained some independence, and I'm even able to help my family at the same time. I'm glad I had a lot of support, especially from my family. I'm playing around with plenty of new technologies, including the library's 3-D Printer. But of course there's always more to learn and do.

—Jonathan Sicoli

2

HISTORICAL PERSPECTIVES ON AUTISM

HOW AUTISM HAS BEEN UNDERSTOOD (1911–2016)

It would be an understatement to say that a wide range of hypotheses are used to account for autism-related disorders. Historically, the disorders have been understood mainly through psychoanalytical, neurobiological, genetic, and executive function approaches. There have, however, also been combinations of unrelated approaches.

HISTORICAL DEFINITION OF AUTISM

Bleuler defined the concept of autism in 1911, believing it was not a separate condition, but one of the secondary effects of schizophrenia.

Thirty-two years later, in 1943, Leo Kanner described autism as a rare psychiatric disorder with onset before age two-and-a-half years of age. Kanner's definition and his subsequent description of its main distinguishing characteristics made autism a medical entity (Kozloff, 1998). As a new psychiatric medical diagnosis, the practitioners of the day offered as treatment psychoanalytic forms of therapy.

By the late 1950s, current thinking about autism was changing. In 1959, for example, Bender characterized autism not as an inborn impairment of the central nervous system, but as a defensive reaction to one—a disorder whose basis is an inability to shield self from unbearable anxiety. A year later, C.E. Benda wrote that the autistic child is "not mentally retarded in the ordinary sense of the word, but rather is a child with an inadequate form of mentation which manifests itself in the inability to handle symbolic forms and assume an abstract attitude."

During the mid-1960s, understanding of autism continued to shift. In 1964, Bernard Rimland published a biogenic theory of autism: "The basis of the autism syndrome is the child's impaired ability to relate new stimuli to remembered experience. Hence, the child does not use speech to communicate because he cannot symbolize or abstract from concrete particulars. And he is unresponsive to his parents because he does not associate them with previous pleasurable experiences." Rimland thought that the underlying cause of autism was an impairment in the brain's reticular formation—the part of the brain believed by many to link sensory input and prior content.

During the 1960s and into the 1970s, researchers offered biogenic explanations of autism—theories focusing on biochemical and metabolic anomalies in people with autism, or on the role in the development of autism of various problems of the central nervous system. Autism was beginning to be viewed as a neurological disorder. This viewpoint is still very much with us. Speaking at the 1999 National Conference of Autism, James Ball referred to autism as a complex developmental disability resulting from a neurological disorder that affects the functioning of the brain.

That year, clinical practice guidelines on autism published by New York State referred to it as a part of a clinical spectrum of pervasive developmental disorders: *"Autism is a neurobehavioral syndrome caused by dysfunction in the central nervous system, which leads to disordered development."*

Beginning in the mid-1960s and carrying forward through the 1980s to 2000, researchers have turned to genetics, searching for the genetic error, perhaps inherited, underlying the development of autism. The roles of several candidate genes are being studied. In the 1990s, other approaches to autism were described, including the executive functions approach, the hypothesis that autism results from early life brain damage, the theory that autism is the result of neuroimmune dysfunction, and that it is the result of autistic enterocolotitis, which may be linked with the measles, mumps, and rubella vaccination.

Resources and links—You can reach Dr. Kaplan at US Autism and Asperger's Association by calling 1-888-9AUTISM or by writing drlkaplan@usautism .org.

Editor's Addendum: Autism in History 2000–2016

By Jonathan Alderson, Ed.M.

Since the new millennium, our understanding of ASD has profited from remarkable advances in genetic research. In 2003, the Human Genome Project (HGP) was declared complete, and for the first time in human history scientists identified the entire human DNA sequence. Leveraging this game-changing data to investigate autism, Dr. Stephen Scherer and Dr. Ryan Yuen at The Hospital for Sick Children in Toronto, Ontario, Canada used one of the world's largest supercomputers, in conjunction with Google, BGI-Shenzhen (China), and with major funding from Autism Speaks, to analyze the whole genomes of 200 families. These 600 fully sequenced genomes came from MSSNG (pronounced "missing"), the world's largest collection of autism genomes and a collaborative effort of Autism Speaks and The Hospital for Sick Children (SickKids) in Toronto. The Autism Speaks MSSNG project has made this invaluable resource of the genomes of families with autism an open source and available to collaborating researchers around the world who are searching for the causes of and treatments for autism.

Many other researchers in medicine and human biology have concentrated on understanding ASD. In 2015, Dr. Derrick MacFabe, Director of the Kilee Patchell-Evans Autism Research Group, was invited to present his ground-breaking findings at the renowned Nobel Forum Symposium. Dr. MacFabe's focus on the gut-brain connection has produced top-tier scientific research that confirms organic byproducts, short chain fatty acids produced by intestinal bacteria that can act as "epigenetic modulators" affecting many of the genes that Dr. Scherer at SickKids in Toronto has associated with autism. Pieces of the puzzle are being connected by these pioneers. It should also be noted that more than at any other time in history, hundreds of millions of dollars are being invested in autism research by governments and by private donors including seriously dedicated individuals like David Patchell-Evans, founder and CEO of GoodLife Fitness and cofoundere of the Kilee Patchell-Evans Autism Research Group, who has donated more than five million dollars to the research team, named after his daughter, a young adult with autism.

More recently, in 2016, Dr. Evdokia Anagnostou and her team at Holland Bloorview Research Institute in Toronto have been investigating the possible beneficial effects of intranasal oxytocin on anxiety and social-receptivity in people diagnosed with autism. Pharmacological research and drug treatments for autistic symptoms is advancing in part because of new genetic information and understanding.

Since 2000, the update in diagnostic criteria of autism has been another important and major shift in the field of autism. The Diagnostic and Statistical Manual-Fifth Edition (DSM-5) was released in 2013, delivering revisions to the criteria needed for a diagnosis of what is now called Autism Spectrum Disorder. Previously, the DSM-IV (4) included Autism as one of several Pervasive Developmental Disorders (PDD) including Asperger's. In the fifth revision, these PDDs were all combined under one umbrella-term Autism Spectrum Disorder. A diagnosing physician can add a severity level qualifier such as "moderate" or "severe" to distinguish along the spectrum and to determine the kinds and amounts of funding and supports a child can receive.

Perhaps the biggest debate that this redefining of autism triggered was the removal of Asperger's as a separate diagnosis. The ramifications of this for the thousands of children and adults formerly diagnosed with Asperger's are yet to be seen. Questions and concerns about access to services, recognition of disability, and all those who identify as and have formed "Aspie" communities are left to find their own way.

The field of autism treatment has seen a shift in the "style" of ABA services from a heavy emphasis and adherence to the more rigid Discrete Trial Training (DTT) toward programs emphasizing broader generalization, more socialization, and playfulness, like Natural Environment Training (NET), Pivotal Response Training (PRT), and Positive behavior Support. ABA-based strategies for Autism Spectrum Disorder continue to be the most researched, available, and commonly used treatments for autism globally. This has been in part supported by the growing number of professionals accredited with the BCBA training and certification.

Outside of the ABA realm, a growing number of multidiscplinary autism treatment centers have opened since 2000. Recognizing that most families choose to "blend" a variety of therapies and professional services including speech therapy and occupational therapy along with behavioral intervention, among others, centers in which these services are closely located under one roof and are well coordinated have gained popularity. The Pacific Autism Family Centre in Vancouver, Canada, and Integrated Services for Autism and Neurodevelopmental Disorders (ISAND) in Toronto, Canada, are two examples of this trend. Building on the multidisciplinary concept, the Integrated Multi-Treatment Intervention (IMTI) is an approach that takes into account the order and timing of blending various approaches into highly customized treatment programs for individual children. (Disclosure Note: This author is the Founder/ Director of the IMTI program). Although there is a dearth of research on integrating different approaches and services, anecdotal evidence of significant improvements in development suggests multidisciplinary models may be a next evolution in autism treatment.

On this note, in July 2014, another evolution in the field of autism was printed in the *New York Times* when it reported the results of a study by Dr. Deborah Fein of the University of Connecticut along with a second study by the well-regarded Dr. Catherine Lord, who found that about 9 percent of people diagnosed with autism will at some point no longer meet the diagnostic criteria. Autism has for decades been considered, and remains to date, an incurable lifelong disorder. The notion of recovery has been dismissed vehemently as impossible, false hope and explained away as misdiagnosis. Truly, this "recovery" research, along with epigenetic and biomedical research, and newly emerging models of integrated treatments, are all challenging the status quo and pushing us all to challenge our belief and to hopefully see even more possibility for positive life outcomes of all those with ASD whom we love and for whom want the very best.

References

1. Press, New York, 1998.
2. Smith N., Tsimpli I.: The Mind of the Savant: Language, Learning and Modularity. Oxford, Blackwell, 1995.

3. Viscott D.: A musical idiot-savant. Psychiatry 1970; 33:494–515.

4. Phillips A.: Talented Imbeciles. 1930 Psychological Clinics 18:246–255.

5. Clark T.: The Application of Savant and Splinter Skills in the Autistic Population Through Curriculum Design: A Longitudinal Multiple-Replication Study. Unpublished Doctoral Thesis, The University of South Wales, School of Education Studies.

6. Donnelly J.A., Altman R.: The Autistic Savant: Recognizing and serving the gifted student with autism. Roeper Review 1994; 16:252–255.

7. Ockelford A.: Sound Moves: Music in the education of children and young people who are visually impaired and have learning disabilities. London, Royal Institute for the Blind, 1988.

8. Rancer S.: Perfect Pitch and Relative Pitch: How to identify & test for the phenomena: a guide for music teachers, music therapists and parents. Self-published. SusanRMT@aol.com.

9. Grandin T.: Thinking in Pictures And Other Reports From My Life With Autism. Vintage Books, New York, 1995.

10. Grandin T.: Animals in Translation: Using the Mysteries of Autism to Decode Animal Behavior. Scribner, New York, 2005.

11. Grandin T., Duffy K.: Developing Talents: Careers for Individuals with Asperger's Syndrome and High Functioning Autism. Autism Asperger's Publishing Company, Shawnee Mission, KS 2004.

12. Conturo, T., Nicolas E., Cull T., Akbudak E., Snyder A.Z., Shimony J.S., McKinstry R.C., Burton, H., Raichle E.: Tracking neuronal fiber pathways in the living human brain. Proc. Natl. Acad. Sci 1999; 10422–101427.

Contributing Author Lawrence P. Kaplan, Ph.D., Health Administration and Research with an emphasis in autism spectrum disorders, Kennedy-Western University—Dr. Kaplan is the Executive Director of US Autism and Asperger's Association, Inc., a national association dedicated to enhancing the quality of life of individuals and their families/caregivers touched by autism spectrum disorders by providing educational and family support through conferences/seminars and published and electronic mediums. Dr. Kaplan is the author of *Diagnosis Autism: Now What? 10 Steps to Improve Treatment Outcomes.*

Jonathan Alderson, Ed.M., is an autism treatment specialist and founder of the innovative Integrated Multi-Treatment Intervention Program (www. IMTI.ca). A graduate of Harvard University, with experience as a Curriculum Specialist Coordinator with Teach for America, he trained at the Autism Treatment Center of America in Massachusetts and worked as Administrator and senior family trainer in their Son-Rise Program. He has worked with over 3000 children and families. Now based in Toronto, he is a contributor for the Huffington Post, a member of the Seneca College behavioral Sciences Advisory Committee, and Cochair of the Young Professionals for Autism Speaks Canada Advisory Board. He has lectured on his multidisciplinary approach to autism treatment throughout Canada, the USA, England, Ireland, Holland, Spain, Australia, Israel, and Mexico. He is the author of *Challenging the Myths of Autism,* which has inspired educators and parents to consider a radical reframing of how we think about and treat people diagnosed with autism. His book has been honored with the Mom's Choice Gold Award, the American Non-Fiction Authors' Association Silver award, and the 2012 International Book Award for Best Parent-Resource.

MOVING PAST HISTORICAL STEREOTYPES OF AUTISM

The medical pathologist focuses the microscope to sharpen his view on the odd-looking cells. Using a special stain to color them, with a closer look, he positively identifies adenocarcinoma. There's no mystery or guess work. The cells meet the globally accepted characteristics of this well-defined type of cancer. Within a few hours, the family is called into the doctor's office for the devastating news. At the same time, he is able to give them clear treatment options, answer their questions, and explain the statistical probability of beating it.

In a different part of the hospital, a less certain diagnosis is being made with an even less certain course of treatment. Unlike the pathologist staring straight at the cancer cells, autism is not a cell we can see. We can't measure it like insulin in blood for diabetes or as a biomarker in urine. Autism doesn't have a certain temperature like a fever or a specific blood pressure. Instead, autism is made up of a group of behavioral symptoms that the doctor observes and then decides, subjectively, if they look "autistic enough." It's not uncommon for parents to get two different opinions about the severity of their child's autism or even if it's autism at all.

One boy is already falling well behind his peers. He can speak but doesn't have conversations, and he doesn't play with toys typically the way his peers do. He lines up any objects he finds in rows, and if someone moves them, he tantrums as if his world has been destroyed. The psychiatrist is looking for a specific yet broad set of behaviors (or absence of typically present behavior) that may add up to the necessary group of symptoms for a diagnosis. It's a complex process. Typically, a diagnosing physician or psychologist has a fairly limited time to observe a young three-year-old's range of behaviors. In some cases, an hour or less. They follow well-defined definitions from the DSM-5 and use standardized screening assessments like the M-CHAT-R (Modified Checklist for Autism in Toddlers Revised). Some of the best physicians I know will take up to as many as three hours and will work in tandem with a team including speech therapist and physical therapist. Even with this rigor, the diagnosis of autism is behavioral and subjective.

At the end of the diagnostic process, the psychiatrist writes down Autism Spectrum Disorder (ASD) on a form followed by "moderate" in parentheses. She says she can't predict how far the boy will develop. The prognosis of ASD is uncertain. The parents are devastated. She offers support and hands them a list of resources with phone numbers to call to get their son on waiting lists for services as soon as possible. As they leave, a thousand questions flood their minds.

Unlike cancer, autism is still an enigma. What causes it? How is it treated? Despite promising new research in epigenetics, there is no consensus. What's more, the criteria for diagnosing autism have changed over time and are still being debated to this day. In other words, there still isn't global consensus about what autism even is.

The unsolved nature of autism and lack of consensus has provided the perfect environment for a Wild West of theories, treatments, and ultimately for myths to exist, unchallenged.

For example, is the incidence of autism on the rise? Autism affects as many as 1 child in 45. There are an estimated over 200,000 children with the disorder in Canada alone. More children will be diagnosed this year with autism than AIDS, cancer, and diabetes combined. Rates of diagnosis have gone up dramatically, over the past ten years especially. This fact alone is a widely debated issue. Some say the increase is due to the definition of autism being broadened to include more kids with milder forms of autism who, in the past, would have been labeled with PDD or Asperger's. Others believe rates have increased because of vaccines or because the environment is getting more toxic. There is so little consensus, entire books are written for and against each of these theories, packed with "science," some more credible than others, and real-life anecdotes to support their compelling side of the argument. Again, the vacuum created by the lack of certain knowledge about autism has been filled by some truths, some half-truths, and some untruths.

Another example of lack of consensus leading to myths is the autism-vaccine link. This is hands-down one of *the* most debated and contentious issues. The arguments aren't explained well in the media, and so headlines like "Vaccines cause autism" have triggered more fear than good. Some researchers like Dr. Andrew Wakfield have proposed that the measles virus in the Measles, Mumps, and Rubella (MMR) vaccine finds its way into the intestines and causes an inflamed bowel disease similar to Crohn's Disease. According to the theory, the inflammation causes leaks of proteins back into the blood that affect the brain, causing autism. As chronicled by Paul Offit, in *Autism's False Profits,* Wakefield's research has now been harshly criticized and discredited most importantly by his own medical community. Offit and others call Wakefield's MMR theory a damaging myth. Indeed, a main thrust for me behind igniting the conversation about the myths of autism is witnessing the negative impacts they can have on this vulnerable population and their families.

However, as enigmatic as autism itself, there are often two or three sides to most theories concerning autism. In *Evidence of Harm, New York Times* reporter David Kirby presents compelling reports and data that vilify drug companies and supports Dr. Wakefield's vaccine-autism link. (Recently, Wakefiled authored his comprehensive self-defense *Callous Disregard*.) Sadly, parents, who need the most direction and support, are left to sort through mountains of conflicting information while children's health is at stake. The number of children getting the MMR has decreased, and, as a direct result, the number of children infected with the measles virus has increased. Outbreaks of measles have resurfaced in underimmunized communities (putting children at risk for brain injury and even death), demonstrating the stakes are high of sorting myth from truth.

Most parents, more than anyone, are desperate to understand what caused their child's autism. Thankfully the "Refrigerator Mother" theory once promoted by Bruno Bettelheim, who claimed unloving cold-hearted parents caused their child to retreat into autism, was completely discredited and shamed out of his career. Recently, there has been a flurry of genetic studies, and over 100 genes have been identified that, through interactions with the environment (Epigenetics), might make a child more susceptible to developing symptoms. However, even the most advanced genetic studies have only been able to find links that account for less than 20 percent of the population. There are still no certain answers for parents searching for the cause.

While experts cannot agree on what causes autism, there's also no consensus on exactly how to treat it. By far, the most widely promoted and researched approach is applied behavioral analysis in behavioral therapy. But since children diagnosed with autism have multiple learning and behavior challenges, there is no one treatment or therapy that can deal with all of their needs. As a result, there has been a huge wide-open market for almost any type of service or product to apply itself to treating autism. Treatments on offer range from swimming with dolphins to infrared saunas, cod liver oil, intensive desk-work drills, skin brushing regimes, mineral clay baths, dance classes, video games, and pet dogs. The number of options available that parents have to choose from is overwhelming. Some of these are evidence-based on science. Others seem more fiction than fact.

As fad theories and bogus treatments come and go, there is a group of characterizations about people with autism that has unfortunately endured. Through the din of debates about genes and vaccines, I think we sometimes forget that we are talking about real people, a population with a very wide-range of strengths and challenges and personalities.

How we talk about people with autism and how we characterize them impact how we treat them.

- The belief that autistic children can't share affection with others has led therapist to use hug or holding therapy where children are held tightly, often against their will, for hours at a time. Screaming and trying to escape, some have been held down by several adults who believe they can force a healthier bond to form.
- The belief that the majority of autistic children are mentally retarded led to thousands being placed in mental institutions and pushed aside in special-education classrooms. Low expectations and condescending attitudes resulted in less opportunity for children with autism to learn, participate, and be included fully with others.
- The belief that people diagnosed with autism don't have imagination blinds us from seeing their different kinds of

creativity and unique thinking capacities. Unusual interests, play, and behavior are judged as inappropriate, instead of as creative and valued, and are shut down.

These perennial inaccurate descriptions, among many others, are what I call the myths of autism. In my book *Challenging the Myths of Autism* (Harper-Collins, 2011), I examine the origin, history, and the evidence that reframes each of seven common descriptors of people with autism. It's true that each is rooted in some observable evidence in some individuals with autism. However, there are many different and equally plausible interpretations.

Over 25 years I have worked with hundreds of families and spent hundreds of hours in therapy sessions with children diagnosed across the autism spectrum. The more children I meet, the more diversity I see. The autism described in books, on TV, and in the media is an averaged caricature that doesn't match what I witness in reality. Why, then, do certain character trait descriptions persist as myths? How do they influence research, policy, treatment, and our personal relations with people with autism?

In the same way that bogus treatments can mislead parents and give false hope, these caricatures of people with autism mislead parents, therapists, and the general public to underestimate the potential of children with autism. They inhibit us from recognizing the unlimited possibilities for interaction with each unique person with autism. *What we believe about a person with autism is the lens through which we greet and interact with them.*

In our education and interactions with these special people, could we put aside definitions and celebrate uniqueness? Choosing to see possibility can lead to hope and can reinvigorate patience and acceptance. A young mother who is told that "if an autistic child doesn't learn to speak before the age of five he will likely never talk" loses hope. Fear and anxiety become her focus. Impatience and judgment manifest. By the time the child reaches the age of five, if he is not yet talking, the mother is now less likely to hear her child's speech-like sounds, and even less likely to interpret any she does hear as attempts to communicate. The myth has become fact. However, there is hope. Much hope. Examples of children who learned to speak after the five-year barrier and those who learned alternate modes of communication break the myth.

Challenging the Myths of Autism reveals much more of this hope. It provokes an examination of our beliefs and helps us see more possibilities in people with autism. In fact, the discussion has already been ignited. Many parents and professionals are forces of change, participating in "awareness" events, talking differently about autism, and helping to write a new more hopeful and inclusive history of autism.

Jonathan Alderson, Ed.M., is an autism treatment specialist and founder of the innovative Integrated Multi-Treatment Intervention Program (www. IMTI.ca). A graduate of Harvard University, with experience as a Curriculum Specialist Coordinator with Teach for America, he trained at the Autism Treatment Center of America in Massachusetts and worked as Administrator and senior family trainer in their Son-Rise Program. He has worked with over 3000 children and families. Now based in Toronto, he is a contributor for the Huffington Post, a member of the Seneca College behavioral Sciences Advisory Committee, and Cochair of the Young Professionals for Autism Speaks Canada Advisory Board. He has lectured on his multidisciplinary approach to autism treatment throughout Canada, the USA, England, Ireland, Holland, Spain, Australia, Israel, and Mexico. He is the author of *Challenging the Myths of Autism,* which has inspired educators and parents to consider a radical reframing of how we think about and treat people diagnosed with autism. His book has been honored with the Mom's Choice Gold Award, the American Non-Fiction Authors' Association Silver award, and the 2012 International Book Award for Best Parent-Resource.

3

EMOTIONALLY COPING WITH A CHILD'S DIAGNOSIS

AFTER THE DIAGNOSIS:
A PARENT'S PERSPECTIVE

When my sister-in-law, Anna, first told me that my son displayed signs of autism, my initial defensive response was "Well, your daughter also shows some signs." Her daughter was the same age as my son, and to prove her wrong, I dragged my son Jonathan kicking, screaming, and dropping to the ground in the middle of the streets, to the Glenrose Hospital for an assessment. We sat through hours, days, and months of test after test to determine what was wrong with him. Of course, in my mind there was nothing wrong with him. He was just more prone to temper tantrums and spinning around in circles than other kids were. And besides, he was bright. My husband and I discovered Jonathan's astute and precocious ability to read at the age of two-and-a-half-years-old, when he read the side a truck repeatedly shouting out, "R-E-C-Y-C-L-E . . . re-sy-cl . . ."

When the doctor finally called us in for the test results, I went by myself, as my husband was always working. He explained, "Your son has PDD-NOS, a form of what could turn out to be autism. Bring him back in a year so we can see how he's doing." A year? A flipping year?! What was I supposed to do in the meantime?

I was doing my best to swallow my own denial and do whatever I could for my son, but it wasn't easy. I had to bite the bullet and tell Anna that she might have been right, even though we wouldn't really know about an autism diagnosis from the doctor for another year. Talk about eating crow! But she was supportive and said, "No way! You can't wait a year. You have to get him into early intervention right away," as she had heard a lady on the radio talk about the importance of getting help as soon after diagnosis as possible. The thought of my two-and-a-half-year-old Jonathan flapping his hands in the air still at 20 years old motivated me to get on track. I reluctantly agreed to follow her advice and took him to a different doctor who managed to get Jonathan into a treatment program.

That was the best decision I could have made for my son. Telling my husband that our son might have autism was one of the hardest things I had ever done. "No way does my son have autism" were the words that spilled out of his mouth. He held onto that attitude for years. Rooted deep in his Italian culture was the notion that having a child with special needs implied there was something wrong with his manhood.

For years, our son's diagnosis was a bone of contention between us. If I were to even bring up the "A" word, it was a problem. It wasn't until Jonathan was in his early teens that my husband decided he would try bringing Jonathan to work with him for the day, as he had with our other children. When they returned from work the first day my husband asked, as if he had noticed for the first time, "did you know that he just sat in the corner all day reading and spinning around?" Of course, this was his first full day one-on-one experience, and in a work environment. Hubby started to see that our son was different. Getting myself through denial was one thing; getting my husband and our surrounding relatives through it, was entirely something different.

Culturally, many of us are taught to believe that being different is being weak. We have been taught that needing help or intervention for care and for behavioral challenges is something to be embarrassed about. Instead, we must learn to accept our children's unique differences and stand up as strong advocates for our children. We can teach our children that thinking and acting differently doesn't mean they are weak or "less than." We can also work to make autism a diagnosis with hope attached to it. It's work, but starting small as I did and then reaching out further made my experiences with Jonathan and our family empowering for him and me.

Jonathan turned out just fine. At the age of 25, after lots of intervention throughout his school years, the rest of the family eventually accepted and understood his uniqueness. And after having written many books, the first of which was *Little Rainman: Autism Through the Eyes of a Child*, and then starting the Autism Today organization, providing lots of autism information with the help of my speakers and attendees from over 65 conferences . . . they all finally got it! When I reflect on the journey, I admit it was a challenge to stay on the path, and I sincerely applaud anyone and everyone who can overcome this most important step of acceptance (versus denial) as soon as they can. The best long-term outcomes start with acceptance first, followed by immediate action at an early age. Jonathan now drives a car, has gone to college, and is quite proud of himself. And we, of course, are very proud of him, too.

The work we did as a family was not small. The work required to raise a child with autism is enormous. The work to gain acceptance for your child from the rest of the world can seem overwhelming. But the benefits are spectacular. The diagnosis is just the first step. The road ahead, step-by-step, can be a wonderful odyssey, and the sooner you embrace your child's unique world, the sooner you can help others do the same. Once the diagnosis is official, there are so many things to do, but the most important thing is acceptance. Jonathan needed acceptance from me, from his family, and from his community.

Stick with it, parents. Trust that when you prioritize love and acceptance of your child, you will advocate for your child and make decisions for them from a clearer, more centred, and energized place. Feeling guilty, being in denial, and staying depressed drain your energy and limits your ability to really give your best. I crossed this bridge. I believe that you can, too. Temple Grandin, to this day, says that my book *Little Rainman: Autism Through the Eyes of a Child* is still the best book of its kind. It illustrates autism in a simple way that teachers and parents can quickly understand. I wrote the book on the bathroom floor at 11 at night when the kids were all sleeping, and it was created by my burning desire to help teachers, parents, and others understand my son.

—Karen L. Simmons, Founder, CEO Autism Today

Karen L. Simmons is the celebrated founder and CEO of Autism Today, an internationally acclaimed resource for autism and all special needs. She is the mother of six children, including one with autism and another with ADHD. She is also the author of four other books, including Chicken Soup For The Soul, Children With Special Needs, along with Mark Victor Hansen and Jack Canfield. Her mission is to celebrate every child's gifts and talents, and by doing so, she has become a highly recognized authority on autism and special needs.

THE DIFFERENCE BETWEEN
HEAVEN AND EARTH

Note: This article was originally published in *Postcards from the Road Less Traveled*, Autism/Asperger's Digest, (www.autismdigest.com), May-June 2005

"The difference between heaven and earth is not so much altitude but attitude."
     —Ken Keys Jr, *The Power of Unconditional Love* (1993)

Mother's Day and Father's Day aren't big events in our house. My husband years ago declared himself allergic to Hallmark-induced holidays. It's enough for me to be a mother on Mother's Day. Although the challenges of raising atypical children can seem staggering, it has been my privilege to have them as mine and to love them unconditionally. It has taught me profound lessons about how excruciating it can be to keep that kind of love in the crosshairs at all times. You, too? Rising above and firmly pushing aside our own fears, disappointments, expectations, and lost dreams can seem like a mission of overwhelming enormity. Your child's limitations become your limitations—the places you can't take him, the social settings he can't handle, the people he can't relate to, the food he won't eat. Yeah, it can be a long list.

It takes great courage to admit that you are scared, feel cheated, heartsick, depleted. Wanting out of that matrix and not knowing how to start. Here's how you start: by knowing you can do this. It's already in you. In the beginning, as I contemplated what Bryce and my family's lives would be like with autism in our midst, I could not deny the fact that *it could be so much worse*. All around me were people who had confronted just that. Close friends had lost their precious two-year-old daughter to a heart defect. It was a life-shattering event, and it was much, much worse than anything autism ever threw at me and my family.

Bryce taught me that happiness does not come from getting what you want, but from wanting what you already have. It is the greatest gift I have ever been given. A friend once asked me: But how do you get there? What do you think is the secret of your success?

It's no secret. It is just this: as much as possible, accept your situation *without bitterness.* Play the cards you drew with grace and optimism. Bitterness can be a formidable foe; overcoming it can be a daily exercise. Some of us make it; some of us don't.

I once spent some time with a father whose mantra was "Because of autism, I can't have a relationship with my son. How do you think I feel knowing that he'll probably end up in prison?" I talked and reasoned and pleaded away the afternoon begging him to see that he was setting up a self-fulfilling prophecy. Couldn't he take one baby step out, imagining a different outcome for his belligerent but very bright child—10 minutes of floor time, coming to school once a month, finding a restaurant only the two of them liked? I think he loved his son, but to the child it no doubt felt conditional, dependent upon a certain kind of behavior, even if there were organic reasons why he could not comply. In the end, they both lost out. This dad could not move beyond his bitterness and grief. Grief is real. But getting stuck in that grief—that is the true tragedy, not the fact that your child has autism.

Directing the focus of autism's difficulties away from yourself and walking with your child in his shoes will liberate both of you. For me, understanding sensory integration propelled me out of my own fears.

I was horrified by the knowledge of what Bryce was living with: his prison of environmental hostility, having no "normal" basis of comparison, never knowing that life can be something other than a bombardment of unpleasant sensations. He was very young, without life experience and without means of communicating his misery. I could not turn away from the raw truth, which was this: if I do not swallow my own anguish and be the one to step up for him, who will?

For some cosmic, not-to-be-understood reason, I was blessed with the serenity to bypass the denial and the anger and the self-pity that frequently come unbidden and unwelcome when we learn our child has a disability. But that is not to say that I don't endure my own bouts with melancholy. I never,

ever fail to be deeply hurt by what I call the "Knife to the Heart" moments. These are the times when the rest of the world seems intent on letting you know that your child is different and apart. Usually there's no conscious malice; it just happens because the "typical" population is steaming about their business in "typical" fashion that doesn't or can't include your child. The offhand child-cruel remark, the birthday party that everyone else is invited to, the snubs on the bus, the questions he asks you as he begins to figure out that he is different. I always thought that if I endured enough of these moments, I would develop scar tissue or the ability to laugh them off. I haven't. But as both my boys move with increasing grace toward maturity and independence, these moments become fewer, more time passes between them, and they become more fleeting. The power I allowed them to have over me has weakened over the years.

Unconditional love requires that you work hard to look beyond what seems like limitations in your child and find the gifts autism has given him. Your daughter doesn't share your passion for skiing, but you can still have fun even if it's just moving the snow from one place to another—like the folks who masterminded the pyramids. Your son won't play the family piano, but his fascination with plumbing is going to save you thousands of dollars!

Loving Bryce unconditionally required making peace with our reduced social opportunities, with the fact that he didn't seem to want conventional friendships, play dates and sleepovers, wasn't interested in the usual after-school activities like soccer or choir. Curiously, I can't say I "missed" these things because he plainly was happy. Our psychologist had once told me, "All children, all people, unfold in their own time. This may just not be his time. His time will come."

And I was determined to let him unfold in his own time. Those times did come as he grew older and played Little League, swam on a swim team, became a rather accomplished actor in community theater, enjoyed Cub Scout activities, read Harry Potter—several years behind the "typical" time line, but just as successfully.

Every day of Bryce's life I have told him that he is the best kid who ever lived, that I am the luckiest mommy who ever lived, that he is great just the way he is. In the beginning, I believed it enough to start saying it, but as time went on a wonderful thing happened. I came to believe it body and soul.

More important, he came to believe it. And because he believes it, he has grown into a young man with remarkable aplomb, self-confidence, empathy, and work ethic—not necessarily the typical hallmarks of autism. He has marvelous self-esteem; he likes himself and is comfortable with who he is. It was contagious.

I began to actively look for things about him to articulate: I told him I was proud of how readily he shared treats and privileges with others, how I admired his devotion to his school work, how much I enjoyed the clever associations he made as he pulled minute details out of movies and related them to his real life. How much I could trust him because he never lied, how nicely he took care of himself with healthy food choices and good hygiene. Think of it as affrmative brainwashing—the more you tell your child he's the greatest, the more both of you are going to believe it.

If you can get to a place where you believe, accept, and put true unconditional love into practice, you will find yourself infused with an incredible energy on behalf of your child. It's that powerful. Without it, you are going to be running this race with a fairly nasty pebble in your shoe. It may be a $100 shoe, but that pebble will ensure that your focus is on the ever more painful wound to your extremity rather than on the span of the road ahead or the beauty of your surroundings. It's a pretty simple choice: let the irritant remain until it cripples you or remove it and head for the horizon.

I actually did get a pretty groovy Mother's Day gift last year, a DVD of my all-time favorite movie, *The Wizard of Oz*. Of course, the lesson of this film is unmistakable. The Scarecrow, Tin Man, and Lion had the brains, heart, and courage they yearned for all along. So do you. Click your heels together three times and believe it.

Contributing Author Ellen Notbohm—Author of *Ten Things Every Child with Autism Wishes You Knew*, winner of iParenting Media's Greatest Products of 2005 Award, and coauthor with Veronica Zysk of *1001 Great Ideas for Teaching and Raising Children with Autism Spectrum Disorders*, winner of Learning Magazine's 2006 Teacher's Choice Award. She is a regular columnist for Autism Asperger's Digest and Children's Voice and is a contributor to numerous magazines and websites. She is the mother of sons with autism and ADHD. Your thoughts and comments are welcome at ellen@thirdvariation.com.

HELPING A PARENT COPE WITH A CHILD'S DIAGNOSIS OF AUTISM

Note: The terms *"parent"* and *"spouse"* are used in this chapter for the sake of simplicity. Their use is not meant to exclude single parents, grandparents, caretakers, guardians, or significant others and partners.

Every 20 minutes, a parent in the United States hears the words: "Your child has autism." Over 48 million parents all over the world have heard these words.

I was one of those parents.

When your child is first diagnosed, you receive a lot of expert advice about which treatments to choose and how to exercise your legal rights to obtain those treatments—all crucial elements in helping to support your child. But what the experts don't tell you is how to support yourself. At the time your child is diagnosed, you're not even thinking about yourself. If you're like most parents, all of your focus and energy goes into helping your child and his or her needs, with little left over for you, your marriage, or your friendships.

The emotional impact of a diagnosis of autism can be devastating. It can be a shock even for parents who suspected there was something wrong with their child in the first place. Our son Jake had some of the classic signs of autism. He reached all of the developmental milestones by age 17 months—he was a happy, healthy, talkative toddler—before we began to notice a decline in his development. Over a period of months, our energetic and vibrant son became a lethargic, disconnected little boy. By age two, Jake stopped speaking entirely. He stopped responding to his name, pointing to objects, and relating even to us, his parents. During the months leading up to Jake's second birthday, I argued with our pediatrician that something wasn't right with our son. He regularly reassured me that Jake was fine. "Boys develop later than girls," he'd say, reminding me that I was a typical first-time mother who worried too much.

When I finally took Jake to another doctor, I thought I'd be relieved to learn that there was a name for Jake's condition. I wasn't. When the doctor told me that Jake had autism, I did what many parents do. I cried for a while and then discovered the door that opened into the world of denial—a lovely place where I didn't have to feel the deep hurt that I'd experienced upon hearing the news of the diagnosis. But my visit was short-lived, and after a week I surfaced, only to find myself plummeting into worlds of anger and then depression that lasted for months. The emotional roller coaster also included other strong feelings often connected to the stages of grieving. It was a long road to reach that last stage of acceptance.

All parents experience and express a range of emotions in response to a child's diagnosis. Because individuals process their feelings in their own ways and in their own time, one parent may remain in the denial stage while the other is struggling with depression. Both parents may get stuck in the anger stage. Coping with a spouse's feelings in addition to your own is not easy. On top of this, the balance in the relationship may change. If one parent chooses to devote all of his or her time to the child with autism, resentment can build on the part of both spouses. Some parents report that they become so involved with their child's life that they lose sight of themselves as individuals.

Keeping a marriage healthy during this time can be a challenge. In addition to the usual day-to-day issues that most married couples face, parents of children with autism find themselves dealing with situations that most parents of typically developing children don't have to deal with—like deciding which treatments are right for a child and determining a child's special education plan. In an attempt to make the right decisions, parents often lose sight of the fact that they are partners on the same team.

If you find yourself still trying to sort out your feelings about your child's diagnosis and the impact of the diagnosis on the rest of your life, you're not alone. Don't lose hope. There are effective techniques to help keep both your marriage and yourself together. In fact, there are ways to create an even stronger bond with your partner and reach a stronger place within yourself.

Through my own experience and through consulting with families of newly diagnosed children with autism, I've learned the following invaluable lessons on how to cope with a child's diagnosis of autism and issues surrounding the diagnosis.

Allow yourself to have your feelings

The beginning is the hardest part. Processing the diagnosis, deciding which treatments to choose, and adjusting to your new life can seem overwhelming. The worst thing that you can do is to hold in your feelings. Allow yourself to grieve. Honor your feelings—don't judge them. People sometimes have this mistaken idea that crying or expressing sadness is a sign of weakness. If you don't allow your feelings to come out, they will remain inside and fester. Anger turned inward can lead to depression. Unexpressed emotions can lead to stress-related physical and psychological ailments. To avoid this, you need to find a way to get your feelings out in a constructive manner. Screaming at your spouse or other children is not constructive; venting your feelings in a therapy session is. Express your feelings in a journal and talk to a friend and/or a therapist.

Don't isolate

Many parents feel that no one can really understand what they're going through and, as a result, shut themselves off from family and friends. As much as a child's diagnosis is a deeply personal experience, it's not healthy to try to handle it all by yourself. Share your feelings with someone—your spouse, best friend, or a therapist. Sometimes parents find that it's easier to self-disclose to a group of strangers who are going through a similar experience and choose to participate in either live or online autism support groups. Do whatever you feel is best for you, but make sure to share your feelings with someone.

Respect your spouses' emotional response—mothers and fathers have different reactions to their child's diagnosis of autism.

Studies show that mothers respond with more depression and guilt to a child's diagnosis than fathers (Gray 2003). Mothers may become consumed with "shoulds," such as "I should have eaten a healthier diet during my pregnancy," or "I should have noticed my child's symptoms earlier." There is considerable evidence that mothers experience the impact of a child's diagnosis far more than fathers (Sharpley, Bitsika, and Efremidis 1997; Seltzer 2001). Mothers also seem to be more open to venting their feelings, while fathers have a tendency to suppress their emotions. As you can imagine, all of this can create enormous stress in a marriage. And while it might be tempting to yell at your spouse for expressing feelings too much or not at all, it is not productive.

To open the lines of communication between you and your partner, psychologists recommend a technique known as "active listening." Active listening involves staying in the moment and listening with no agenda. Instead of formulating your own thoughts or arguments while the other person is speaking, active listening involves focusing on what the other person is saying so that they feel genuinely heard. Don't attack your partner or fall into the blame game. Sometimes, it's helpful to take the other person's point of view.

For example, think about why your spouse might be feeling a certain way. Is his or her denial a self-protection mechanism? Is his or her venting a way to assuage guilt? By taking the other person's perspective, you can be more understanding and compassionate and less resentful. The technique of active listening requires effort, but the payoff can be tremendous. It can help you establish a respectful and loving partnership with your spouse.

Make time for your marriage

Maintaining a strong and solid marriage is not always easy, especially when you have a child with a developmental disorder such as autism. It's up to you to make a conscious effort to work on your relationship, and that includes setting aside time to be with your spouse. Hire a babysitter or enlist the help of a friend or relative to watch your child so that you and your spouse can spend an afternoon or evening together. Go for a walk or out to the movies. It's important to reconnect with your spouse and enjoy time dedicated to just the two of you. Sometimes parents experience feelings of guilt about leaving their child. Your child will be fine without you for a few hours, and those few hours may be crucial to keeping your marriage healthy.

Ask for what you need and want

Often, parents find that they don't want to burden family members and friends with requests for help after their child is diagnosed. They try to do everything themselves, insisting on playing the roles SuperMom or SuperDad. What they don't realize is that it's impossible to do it all—and this is the time when they need to ask for help. In fact, friends and loved ones want to be called upon to help. They often feel just as helpless as parents do after a child is diagnosed. They want to be supportive but don't always know the right things to say or do. So it's up to you, the parent, to tell them. Ask for help—whether it's in the form of childcare, running errands, requesting a shoulder to cry on, or seeking financial help to pay for doctors' appointments and treatments.

Know that you have the power

Even if you may not be in touch with your personal power right now, it's still inside you. You just need to be able to access it. Most parents don't know a lot about autism when their child is diagnosed, which can lead to feelings of powerlessness. To regain a sense of power, it's important to get educated. Remember the adage "knowledge is power." This is the time to educate yourself. Learn about the latest research on autism and different treatments for it. Read books, access information on the Internet, and talk to autism professionals and parents of children with autism, so that you can gain a better understanding of how to help your child and yourself. Educate friends and family, as well. Being informed can lead you to feeling more confident and powerful.

Remember that you are an expert

When parents are constantly surrounded by "expert" advice and opinions from doctors and professionals in the field of autism, they often lose sight of their own expertise. Remember—you know your child better than anyone. Make sure you value your own opinions about your child as highly as those you receive from the experts.

Take ten

You will probably hear friends and loved ones telling you that you should give yourself a break during the day and take some time for yourself. This will make absolutely no sense to you in the beginning, when the autism immersion process first strikes. Most parents find themselves so consumed with helping their children that the notion of taking time out to go to the gym or to dinner with a friend seems preposterous. So here's what I suggest. Take 10 minutes every day to do something that is not autism-related. Take a walk or a drive, or just sit down and drink a cup of tea. I work with parents who cannot bear the thought of taking even 10 minutes a day away from their mission to help their child. So I remind them that this time will actually help their child. Those 10 minutes can help them clear their heads and refocus. A perpetually stressed-out parent cannot effectively help a child. Eventually, you can extend the 10 minutes to longer, but in the beginning, at the very least, take ten.

Remember the basics

Eat, sleep, and take care of yourself. An undernourished or sleep-deprived parent is no good to anyone—including himself or herself! Many parents become so consumed with helping their child that they neglect their own basic needs. They are vigilant about keeping their child's appointments with doctors and specialists but then miss their own. Mothers cancel mammogram appointments and fathers cancel physical exams.

Parents miss out on sleep because they're staying up too late researching or their stress level prevents them from falling asleep or staying asleep. They skip meals because they're racing to bring their child to a speech therapy session.

It's crucial that you, as a parent, maintain your health—for yourself and your family. Keep healthy foods in the house and make time to eat. If your lack of sleep is stress related, try relaxation techniques or natural remedies such as herbal tea before bedtime. Don't do research on autism right before you plan on going to sleep. If your mind is racing, you may have trouble falling asleep. If you find that you are experiencing chronic insomnia, speak with your doctor about medication.

When you can make the time, add in exercise. Exercise can help relieve stress. If you don't have the time to go to the gym, then take a walk. Many parents find themselves spending a lot of time indoors, especially if they are running their child's home treatment program. Make sure to set aside time to go outside. A walk in the park can help to lift your spirits.

Think positive

During this difficult time, it's especially important to surround yourself with people with positive attitudes. They will be your best allies and will offer you the support and guidance you need. Avoid negative friends and family who might not have worked through their own feelings about the diagnosis and may unnecessarily share feelings of anger and fear with you.

Also, be mindful of your own self-talk. What we tell ourselves gets registered in our unconscious and can manifest itself in the way we feel about ourselves. Self-esteem can be adversely affected by negative self-talk. What messages are you sending yourself? Many parents fall into the trap of telling themselves that they are not doing enough for their children or that what they are doing is never good enough. To avoid falling into this trap, give yourself positive affirmations.

Affirmations are statements that are made in the present tense. For example, tell yourself: "I am okay," not "I'm going to be okay," or "I used to be okay." Remind yourself that you're doing the best that you can. Give yourself a pat on the back for the work that you're doing to help your child. Recognize and reward yourself for your efforts.

Try to live in the moment

I purposely use the word "try" in this piece of advice because the notion of living in the moment can often be difficult in this fast-paced, future-focused world in which we live. Sometimes, fears about a child's future can prevent parents from appreciating their child in the present. Parents may get caught up in asking: "What will happen to my child when he or she is five years old, or 12 or an adult?" or focusing on other unknowns such as when their child will speak or learn to relate to others. While it's important to think about and plan for your child's future, you cannot allow it to cloud your vision of where your child is at present. Celebrate your child for who he or she is right now.

You're not alone

As you cope with your child's diagnosis, keep in mind that you are not alone in your journey. Contact other parents who've been through this with their own children. Reach out to your friends and loved ones.

Share your feelings in a support group. Find ways to take care of yourself. You deserve the same love and attention that you are giving your child.

References

1. Gray, D. (2003) Gender and coping: the parents of children with high functioning autism. Social Science and Medicine, 56, pp. 631–642

2. Seltzer, M. et al. (2001) Families of adolescents and adults with autism: uncharted territory. In: International Review of Research in Mental Retardation, L.M. Glidden (ed.) San Diego: Academic Press (Available from the National Autistic Society Information Centre.)

3. Sharpley, C.F., Bitsika, V., and Efremidis, B. (1997) Influence of gender, parental health, and perceived expertise of assistance upon stress, anxiety, and depression among parents of children with autism, Journal of Intellectual and Developmental Disability, 22(1), pp. 19–28.

Contributing Author Karen Siff Exkorn is a consultant who works with families of newly diagnosed children with autism. She is the author of *The Autism Sourcebook: Everything You Need to Know—From a Mother Whose Child Recovered*, published by ReganBooks/HarperCollins in October 2005 with a foreword by Dr. Fred Volkmar, of the Yale Child Study Center.

RELATIONSHIPS ARE EVERYTHING

As a mom, wife, daughter, sister, friend, aunt, and colleague, I know that relationships are everything! We all have many kinds of relationships in our lives, from those with our children, our spouses, students, friends, families, even coworkers . . . relationships are everywhere and mean everything. Relationships are built upon communication, which is also one of the largest deficits that those with autism and special needs children face.

Whether children are able to talk or not, they are still able to communicate. They need us, as caregivers, instructors, parents, siblings, and peers, to help them bridge the relationship between them and the world. Through the power of effective communication mixed with empathy and understanding, we can facilitate and enhance the quality of these relationships.

To paint a picture for you, my son Jonny was in the 4th grade when his class took a field trip to the library to hear a famous author, Andrea Spaulding, talk to the class. She had all the kids sit on the floor while she read them tales from her latest book. When she was done, it was time for questions and answers. The kids eagerly popped their excited hands up into the air to ask questions. After about three questions, there was Jonny's hand frantically waving. I cringed: what could he possibly want to ask? No sooner than Mrs Spaulding called on my son did the words shoot out of his mouth. "Mrs Spaulding?" he said, "I think this is boring!" I knew in my heart that he was just being truthful, but ohhhh the glares I got from the other parents, and of course Mrs. Spaulding. "You know, young man," she scolded, "that was very disrespectful." How could I explain his autism in this desperate situation to everyone who was there? I felt like grabbing his hand and leaving, but I hung in there.

After the moment cleared, and the air seemed to settle down, once again his hand flew in the air. Mrs Spaulding, "What kind of dinosaur is it?" he asked in regard to her book. Thank God! I was so relieved he could also ask something that was appropriate. After the class was dismissed and the library event had come to a close, I took Jonny by the hand to apologize to

Mrs Spaulding, trying to explain to him that while he may have been bored, saying it out loud still probably hurt Mrs Spaulding's feelings. "Oh," he replied and apologized to her. I then explained to Mrs. Spaulding that Jonny had autism and sometimes he understood things quite differently than you or I and this is true whether Jonny is listening to someone read to him or when he's actually reading something because he tends to look through or around the words or the words look distorted when he reads. He didn't mean to hurt her; he was just not used to sitting. It was like a light bulb went off in her head, and she said, "Oh, you're right. I had taught a child with autism once before. I forgot that it could look differently and I wasn't even thinking that could be the issue here. Thank you for reminding me."

I tell you this story because I think it demonstrates how through clear and concise communication, relationships are built. It's virtually impossible to explain Jonny to everyone in the hopes they will understand., but by sharing the importance of understanding and communicating about autism, you can help me to get the message out.

SIMMONS *"SIMPLY AWESOME"* AUTISM RELATIONSHIP TIPS™

I call these ten tips a "take-home toolkit" for parents and professionals to facilitate positive relationship development for those with autism spectrum disorders.

1. **"Get" the label:** We need to get past the label drama by offering a way to help people better understand what's going on and ultimately support differences, not discriminate against them. It's not the label of autism that's the problem, but rather, the fear of the unknown and preconceived notions we associate with the label. We must understand the challenges facing autism, which are first communication and sensory challenges that result in social skill deficits and behavioral challenges.

    For example, because people on the spectrum can be very literal, don't take what they say personally, as I described in the story about Mrs. Spaulding. Also, remember to watch out for areas of concern, for example, bright lights, loud sounds, and possibly uncomfortable clothing, as they may cause discomfort leading to poor social and communication skills, which affect relationships. Understand their lack of ability to process and express themselves. It's not that they don't feel; they just have trouble expressing themselves.

2. **Enhance empathy:** Tune into empathy, not sympathy. Try to put yourself in their shoes and imagine what they may be thinking or feeling, especially since they have difficulties understanding, expressing, and showing emotions, which can be confusing.

3. **Communicate for communities sake:** Help to carefully bridge relationships between peers and those with autism. This is an intuitive process, so be careful of boundaries. Try hooking up with a "peer coach." Reach into who they truly are and help to pull them out. Get them to volunteer, sign up for an acting class, or try to find others who have something in common. By building, nourishing, and enhancing young relationships with peers, employers, family, and community, the fabric of humanity is enhanced.

HOW PARENTS CAN HELP:

After I got Jonny and Stephen into football, it was difficult at first because Jonny was not accepted. He was seen as someone who was different. At the first parent meeting, Coach Dave said, "When the boys are on the field they are mine, when they go home they go back to you parents. Please respect this rule, and the kids will learn respect and discipline." I worked with the Coach to help Jonny fit in. Of course the coach talked and modeled a lot about acceptance, because he too was in a wheelchair. He treated everyone the same and expected the best from everyone. One time, Dave told Jonny to do push-ups. Jonny ran over to me on the sidelines crying because he didn't want to do push-ups. I told him, at the disapproval of the staring parents around me, to do what the coach said. This one thing changed Jonny for life! When Jonny began his practice, he was running behind all the team players as they ran their laps. As the year went on, something happened that caused the team to bond and embrace Jonny for who he was as well as his strengths. He was really a good blocker. The team began running behind Jonny, so that he would be first in line when they ran laps. By the end of the season, the whole team celebrated Jonny at the final pizza party, giving him a great big "hoorah"!

4. **Share the knowledge:** Raise awareness and understanding of autism and the issues surrounding it. Typically, children with autism may have issues around what is safe and what isn't. The literal way of understanding as communicated back through a person with autism can be perceived as being blunt and offensive. Educate peers, teachers, family, and community members that the relationships they build with your child allow them to understand and be understood in return.

5. **Remember, learning styles:** Relationships are built through learning. All people learn in different ways. Whether they process their world through sight, sound, or touch, determines the quality of their communication. Since generally people with autism are visual learners, it is important to communicate with pictures and words.

6. **Scripting for Success:** Relationships rely on solid understanding. People with autism are typically visual. It is useful to write down what you want to communicate, which can be very simple steps at first, so they clearly understand. This can be as simple as explaining the proper way to relate to friends in a director's script. One example was when I took Jonny down to Daphne, Alabama, to visit my mom and dad. Jonny was petrified to get on the plane, so I wrote down what he would do so he could get a visual image in his mind step-by-step in the first person. It went something like this: I will go in a car to the airport. Mom and I will walk through the airport. We will then go through a security gate and on the plane. The plane will go up in the air, fly for a few hours and then land in Alabama. Jonny

grabbed the paper, read it, then threw it down on the floor, shouting, "What if the plane blows up and we have to parachute down?" I guess he watched too many movies about this stuff. I quickly edited his version to add in that they will scan for secret weapons so no one carries any bombs on the plane. After that he got on the plane; no problem.

7. **Understand "the box":** The "box" is the family unit surrounding the person with autism. Many times they either get into denial or have spousal challenges. The outside of the box—teachers, in-laws, and others—don't "live" in it and may not understand the many dynamics. Whether inside or outside the family "box," it's important to understand that the family is a complete entity in itself.

8. **Teamwork works:** Be a team player. While working together for the common goal of helping a person with autism build relationships, be sure to have parents, educators, and professionals on the same page, like Mrs. Spaulding and the coach. It doesn't help the person if the support team can't agree. Sometimes writing out your expectations helps both sides win.

9. **Exude empowerment:** Stand back and empower those with autism to be who they are, not hovering or smothering them. Relationships are also about letting go. It can be hard to let go, however it serves our children the most if you trust them beyond your expectations. They know much more than we give them credit for. This also helps them to build their self-esteem. When they learn to be as independent as possible, all goes well on the positive side.

10. **All about them:** More important than anything. It is all about them, not our egos, personalities, or lack of understanding. We must remember for whom we are investing all this love and energy. It's the children, teens, and adults who have some type of autism spectrum disorder, regardless of severity. Be sure to bring the actual people with autism into planning conversations with parents and professionals as a team player to the best of

your and their abilities. Don't be afraid of what the kids know; be afraid of what you don't know.

Relationships are everything, and building them with and around people with autism is rewarding work.

—Karen L. Simmons, Founder, CEO Autism Today

FAMILY-CENTERED PRACTICE IN ACTION

The term "Family-Centered Practice" (FCP) has been used for decades in many sectors from medical to social services, and education. "Family-Centered" is often used in contrast to the traditional medical model in which the physician determines the course of treatment and makes all of the decisions. A shift in modern medical practice has expanded the role of the patient and families in decision making. This shift has also happened in the field of autism diagnosis and treatment.

As our understanding of the etiology of autism has changed, so too have the suite of therapies on offer. Whereas autism was once framed as a purely psychological disorder whose treatment was directed by psychiatrists and psychologists, it is now understood as a neurodevelopmental disorder requiring more than psychologists counseling mothers. Speech therapy plus occupational therapy plus behavioral therapy is a common equation of treatment. And parents are placed in the role of "program coordinator" and "consumer" as they select which services to use and then schedule and monitor them. To a large extent, professionals have recognized that parents play a key role. The question is, how skilled are they empowering and supporting parents in this role?

Some researchers have focused on this question. There is a decent body of literature that has identified best-practices to involve parents. Beatson (2006) cites eight key elements of family-centered care in Autism Spectrum Disorder (adapted from Shelton TS, Stepanek JS. Excerpts from family-centered care for children needing specialized health and developmental services. Pediatr Nurs 1995;21:362–364):

1. *The family is the constant in the child's life, while service providers come and go.*
2. *Collaboration with families is critical.*

3.   *Professionals must exchange unbiased, complete information with families.*

4.   *Professionals must honor the diversity of families.*

5.   *Professionals must understand the different ways of coping among families and being responsive to such.*

6.   *Family-to-family networking must be encouraged and supported.*

7.   *Policies and systems should be flexible and responsive to the complex issues of children with special needs and their families.*

8.   *In the final analysis, all providers should see children as children and families as families.*[1]

Personally, I see the concept of family-centered practice as a continuum. On one end of the continuum FCP, families are invited to input their opinions into the treatment or education of their children. This is a step beyond the traditional medical model, acknowledging an individual family's ideas, which are sometimes only documented and considered, but ultimately parents are still not the decision makers. On the other end of the continuum, families are active not only in planning services, but also in their implementation. From this view, the family is seen as the agent of change with professionals seen as support-as-needed. Services are embedded within the family context, most often in the home as opposed to a treatment center, and training and supports are provided to the whole family, not just the child.

It goes without saying that a central pillar of FCP is what is called Parent Involvement. While it has long been widely acknowledged in the field that parent involvement is essential (NRC 2001), how agencies and professionals interpret and implement parent involvement is not consistent. Family-Centred Practice is touted by many programs and agencies as their core philosophy. Yet as described above, there is broad range of how family-centered practice can be interpreted. For example, some services allow for family input at meetings just once or twice a year, and this is the full extent of families' involvement. We know that "children whose families are involved in their care have less anxiety, improved health, development, and healing, reduced hospital stays, and enhanced learning."[2] For me, the term Parent Involvement is a reminder that parents are not only an essential partner;

they are the only permanent support for their child. We as service providers are simply there to join them on their journey for a time and do the very best we can to support them to be successful in the future.

It is easy to welcome parent involvement and to behave in family-centered ways when parent-clients agree with the recommendations. However, genuine FCP remains equally inviting of parent involvement, opinions, and choices also when they disagree.

I would love to be able to say, "Gone are the days when professionals told parents what to do because professionals know what is best. . . . Gone are the days when families had to endure treatments that were not right for their child simply because a professional told them to." Sadly, parents are disempowered and put in uncomfortable situations every day. Yesterday, for example, I heard about two parents who sat outside in their car wracked with guilt while a therapist worked on getting their child to sleep, locked in his room screaming for hours until he exhausted himself. The parents didn't feel comfortable with this approach, but because this therapist had not set up their working relationship with the parents at the center, they felt disenfranchised from the process and from decision making. Those hours in the car were painful as they sat feeling torn between what the therapist convinced them was best-practice and what their parent intuition tugged at them to do instead.

Another acute example involved a school using a "time out room" for a child who was being disruptive. He was locked in the padded time out room for more than an hour, screaming and crying to be let out. The staff had been trained by a behavior specialist not to let him out until he calmed down so as not to reinforce the disruptive behavior. The parents and in fact some of the teachers who knew that this child was not yet able to self-regulate to calm down on his own opposed the time out strategy. But in this system, parents were not the decision makers. Their opinions were recorded, but time out was still the only strategy offered by the specialist.

There are countless stories of families enduring the practice of forced physical compliance (i.e., physically forcing a child to sit on command or using force to get a child to do a task) or planned ignoring, even when parents don't agree with the practice.

Usually, parents aren't offered choices. Even when the recommended strategy is well supported in the literature and best-practice, I believe that parents have the right to make the final choices that they feel are best for their child and family. When there are disagreements or differences of opinion on what is the best choice, we need to honor and respect the family context and work flexibly within that context. Service providers need to remain flexible and collaborate with families by presenting program strategies as choices they make rather than rules they follow. Collaborative decisions empower parents to be partners, not bystanders. Collaborative decisions unite parents and professionals to mutually benefit from their expertise. Yes, parents have expertise on their children that Family-Centered Practice leverages to the maximum benefit of the child.

Over and over, our society encourages parents to follow the recommendations of "expert" professionals. Professionals talk about "getting buy in" from the family or "lack of follow-through at home." These types of statements are not family-centered but professional-centered. In fact, our role as professionals should be "empowering families with the knowledge and skills to make the best choices for their children and for the family unit, as a whole."[3]

Family-Centered Practice works well. Last year, we worked with a family that did not want to use "visuals." The consultants recommended using visual supports to help the child communicate. However, the family did not want to use them. But the professionals in this case didn't impose their opinions. Instead, they applied a family-centered approach of empowering the family with as much information about "visuals" as possible and then creating opportunities for the parents to comfortably share their own opinions and decisions. The family felt that visuals would delay the child's language development and make him look different from his peers. In order to understand their perspective, the consultants listened and asked clarifying questions respectfully, as collaborative team members, rather than with an agenda to convince. The consultants explained that visuals are a useful strategy to increase both language understanding and expression and addressed the family's misconceptions around social stigma. Together the team brainstormed ways to show the child that his peers also used visual supports like calendar agendas. Flexible collaboration with the family allowed for solutions within the family context.

Why have I always felt so passionate about active Family Involvement? The answer begins with the very first family I ever worked with. During the second year of my undergraduate degree at the University of Ottawa, I worked in a home-program with a 4-year-old diagnosed with autism. This boy's mother *impacted my perspective permanently.* In the early-90s, very few people knew what autism was. She was pioneering putting together a "home program" before many even existed! She never let anything get in the way of us moving forward. We worked closely together in collaboration and tried many different strategies. She taught me that a parent's voice must be respected and that parents can be amazing collaborative partners. She was a woman full of strength and resilience, and I will be forever grateful for all she taught me.

Since then, I have met many families and continue to see the positive impact of Family-Centered Practice. Parents are their children's first and most important advocate. They are the only adults who will be the constant . . . supporting their child through childhood and well beyond into adulthood. They are their child's voice when the child doesn't have a voice. As professionals, we need to remember that "once you are in a relationship with a child, you are also in a relationship with the child's family."[4] Family-Centered Practice is not just a buzzword. It is a commitment to a daily practice of putting these words and concepts into action.

References

1. Beatson J (2006) "Preparing Speech-Language Pathologists as Family-Centered Practitioners in Assessment and Program Planning for Children with Autism Spectrum Disorder." Seminars in Speech and Language, vol 27, no 1.

2. Beatson J (2006) "Preparing Speech-Language Pathologists as Family-Centered Practitioners in Assessment and Program Planning for Children with Autism Spectrum Disorder." Seminars in Speech and Language, vol 27, no 1.

3. Prizant (2009) "Creating a Culture of Family-Centered Practice for the Autism Community." Straight Talk About Autism; Autism Spectrum Quarterly Summer 2009.

4. Prizant (2009) "Creating a Culture of Family-Centered Practice for the Autism Community." Straight Talk About Autism; Autism Spectrum Quarterly Summer 2009.

Terri Duncan, SLP, is the Founder and Executive Director of Children's Autism Services of Edmonton, Alberta, Canada. In 2004, he founded CASE, which is a family-centered therapy center for younger children. She hosts conferences in Edmonton, bringing in many of the top speakers including Deepak Chopra.

4

FIRST STEPS AFTER DIAGNOSIS

BEGINNING DOWN THE AUTISM PATH: ADVICE FOR PARENTS OF YOUNG CHILDREN WITH AUTISM

Note: This paper is geared toward parents of newly diagnosed autistic children and parents of young autistic children who are not acquainted with many of the basic issues of autism. Our discussion is based on a large body of scientific research. Because of limited time and space, detailed explanations and references are not included.

Although for some parents a diagnosis of autism offers the relief of a label for their child's symptoms, the diagnosis can also be devastating. Many parents can be overwhelmed by fear and grief for the loss of the future they had hoped for their child.

Joining parent support groups may help. However, these strong emotions also motivate parents to find effective help for their children. The diagnosis is important because it can open the doors to many services and help parents learn about treatments that have benefited similar children.

The most important point we want to make is that autistic individuals have the potential to grow and improve. Contrary to what you may hear from outmoded professionals or read in outmoded books, *autism is treatable*. It is important to find effective services, treatments, and education for autistic children as soon as possible. The earlier these children receive appropriate treatment, the better their prognosis. Their progress though life will likely be slower than others, but they can still live happy and productive lives.

What is autism?

Autism is a developmental disability that typically involves delays and impairment in social skills, language, and behavior. Autism is a spectrum disorder, meaning that it affects people differently. Some children may have speech, whereas others may have little or no speech.

Left untreated, many autistic children will not develop effective social skills and may not learn to talk or behave appropriately. Very few individuals recover completely from autism without any intervention. The good news is that there are a wide variety of treatment options that can be very helpful. Some treatments may lead to great improvement, whereas other treatments may have little or no effect. No single treatment helps everyone. A variety of effective treatment options will be discussed below.

Onset of autism: early onset versus regression

"Autism develops sometime during pregnancy and the first three years of life. Some parents report that their child seemed different at birth. These children are referred to as early-onset autism. Other parents report that, from their observations, their child appeared to develop normally up to 2 years or older until developmental delays such as lack of speech development and decreased socialization began to present.

One recent study, conducted by the first author, compared 53 autistic children with 48 typical peers. The parents of the early-onset autism group reported a significant delay in reaching developmental milestones, including age of crawling (two-month delay), sitting up (two-month delay), walking (four to five month delay) and talking (11 month delay or more). Thus, there appeared to be a delay in gross motor skills as well as talking. In contrast, the late-onset autism group reached developmental milestones at the same time as typical children up to a later age."

Speech development

One of the most common questions parents ask is: "Will my child develop speech?"

An analysis of Autism Research Institute's (ARI) data involving 30,145 cases indicated that 9 percent never develop speech. Of those who develop speech, 43 percent begin to talk by the end of their first year, 35 percent begin to talk sometime between their first and second year, and 22 percent begin to talk in their third year and after. A smaller, more recent survey conducted by the first author found that only 12 percent were totally nonverbal by age five. So with appropriate interventions, there is reason to hope that children with autism can learn to talk, at least to some extent.

There are several ways to help autistic children learn to talk, including:

- Teaching speech with sign language: it is easy for parents to learn a few simple signs and use them when talking to their child. This is referred to as "simultaneous communication" or "signed speech." Research suggests that the use of sign language increases the chance of children learning spoken language.
- Teaching with the Picture Exchange Communication System (PECS): This involves pointing to a set of pictures or symbols on a board. As with sign language, it can also be effective in teaching speech.
- Applied Behavior Analysis: This will be discussed further in this section.
- Encouraging child to sing with a video or audio recording.
- Vestibular stimulation, such as swinging on a swing, while teaching speech.

Several nutritional/biomedical approaches have been associated with dramatic improvements in speech production including dimethylglycine (DMG), vitamin B6 with magnesium, and the gluten-/casein-free diet. This will be discussed further in this section.

Genetics of Autism

Genetics appear to play an important role in causing some cases of autism. Several studies have shown that when one identical twin has autism, the cotwin often has autism. In contrast, when one fraternal twin has autism, the cotwin is rarely autistic. Studies trying to identify specific genes associated with autism have been inconclusive. Currently, it appears that over 100 or more genes may be associated with autism. This is in contrast to other disorders, such as Fragile X or Rett's Syndrome, in which single genes have been identified.

A large number of studies have found that autistic individuals often have compromised immune systems. In fact, autism is sometimes described as an autoimmune system disorder. One working hypothesis of autism is that the child's immune system is compromised genetically and/or environmentally (e.g., exposure to chemicals). This may predispose the child to autism. Then, exposure to an (additional) environmental insult may lead to autism.

If parents have a child with autism, there is an increased likelihood, estimated at 5-8 percent, that their future children will also develop autism. Many studies have identifed cognitive disabilities, which sometimes go undetected, in siblings of autistic children. Siblings should be evaluated for possible developmental delays and learning disabilities, such as dyslexia.

Possible environmental causes of autism

Although genetics play an important role in autism, environmental factors are also involved. There is no general consensus on what those environmental factors are at this point in time. Since the word "autism" is only a label for people who have a certain set of symptoms, there are likely to be a number of factors that could cause those symptoms.

Prevalence of autism

There has been a rapid increase in the number of children diagnosed with autism. The most accurate statistics on the prevalence of autism come from California, which has an accurate and systematic centralized reporting system of all diagnoses of autism. The California data show that autism is rising rapidly, from 1 per 2,500 in 1970 to 1 per 45 in 2016. Similar results have been reported for other states by the U.S. Department of Education. Whereas autism once accounted for 3 percent of all developmental disabilities, in California it now accounts for 45 percent of all new developmental disabilities. Other countries report similar increases.

We do not know why there has been a dramatic increase in autism over the past 15 years, but there are several reasonable hypotheses. Since there is more than one cause of autism, there may be more than one reason for the increase. A small portion of the increase of autism where speech is delayed may be due to improved diagnosis and awareness, but the report from California reveals that this only explains a minute part of the increase.

Common cooccurring conditions in Autism

Mental retardation

Although it has been estimated that up to 75 percent of people with autism have mental retardation, research studies have frequently used inappropriate IQ tests, such as verbal tests with nonverbal children and, in some cases, estimating the child's intelligence level without any objective evidence. Parents should request nonverbal intelligence tests that do not require language skills, such as the Test for Nonverbal Intelligence (TONI). Furthermore, regardless of the result, realize that autistic children will develop more skills as they grow older and that appropriate therapies and education can help them reach their true potential. [Editor's Note: Please read more in Jonathan Alderson's article "Measuring IQ and the Myth of Mental Retardation" below.]

Seizures

It is estimated that 25 percent of autistic individuals also develop seizures, some in early childhood and others as they go through puberty. (Changes in hormone levels may trigger seizures.) These seizures can range from mild (e.g., gazing into space for a few seconds) to severe, grand mal seizures.

Many autistic individuals have subclinical seizures that are not easy to notice but can significantly affect mental function. A one- or two-hour EEG may not be able to detect any abnormal activity. So a 24-hour EEG may be necessary. Although drugs can be used to reduce seizure activity, the child's health must be checked regularly because these drugs can be harmful.

There is substantial evidence that certain nutritional supplements, especially vitamin B6 and dimethylglycine (DMG), can provide a safer and more effective alternative to drugs, for many individuals. (Write to the Autism Research Institute for publication P-16 for more information.)

Chronic constipation and/or diarrhea

An analysis of the ARI's autism database of thousands of cases show over 50 percent of autistic children have chronic constipation and/or diarrhea. Diarrhea may actually be due to constipation—i.e., only liquid is able to leak past a constipated stool mass in the intestine. Manual probing often fails to find an impaction. An endoscopy may be the only way to check for this problem. Consultation with a pediatric gastroenterologist is required.

Sleep problems

Many autistic individuals have sleep problems. Night waking may be due to reflux of stomach acid into the esophagus. Placing bricks under the legs at the head of the bed may help keep stomach acid from rising and provide better sleep. Melatonin has been very useful in helping many autistic individuals fall asleep. Other popular interventions include using 5-HTP and implementing a behavior modification program designed to induce sleep. Vigorous exercise will help a child sleep, and other sleep aids are a weighted blanket or tight fitting mummy-type sleeping bag.

Pica

Thirty percent of children with autism have moderate to severe pica. Pica refers to eating nonfood items such as paint, sand, dirt, paper, etc. Pica can expose the child to heavy metal poisoning, especially if there is lead in the paint or in the soil.

Low muscle tone

A study conducted by the first author found that 30 percent of autistic children have moderate to severe loss of muscle tone, and this can limit their gross and fine motor skills. The study found that these children tend to have low potassium levels. Increased consumption of fruit may be helpful.

Sensory sensitivities

Many autistic children have unusual sensitivities to sounds, sights, touch, taste, and smells. High-pitched intermittent sounds, such as fire alarms or school bells, may be painful to autistic children. Scratchy fabrics may also be intolerable, and some children have visual sensitivities. They are troubled by the flickering of fluorescent lights. If the child often has tantrums in large supermarkets, it is possible that he/she has severe sensory oversensitivity. Sensory sensitivities are highly variable in autism, from mild to severe. In some children, the sensitivities are mostly auditory; in others, mostly visual. It is likely that many individuals who remain nonverbal have both auditory and visual processing problems, and sensory input may be scrambled. Even though a pure tone hearing test may imply normal hearing, the child may have difficulty hearing auditory details and hard consonant sounds.

Some children have very high pain thresholds (i.e., be insensitive to pain), whereas others have very low pain thresholds. Interventions designed to help normalize their senses, such as sensory integration, Auditory Integration Training (AIT), and Irlen lenses, will be discussed further in this section.

Medical testing and treatments

Routine medical tests are usually performed by traditional pediatricians, but they rarely reveal problems in autism that can be treated. Genetic testing for Fragile X syndrome can help identify one possible cause, and this testing is typically recommended when there is mental retardation in the family history. Many physicians do not conduct extensive medical testing for autism, because they believe, incorrectly, that the only useful medical treatments are psychiatric medications to reduce seizures and behavioral problems.

Some of the major interventions suggested by the ARI Conference include:

- Nutritional supplements, including certain vitamins, minerals, amino acids, and essential fatty acids
- Special diets *totally* free of gluten (from wheat, barley, rye, and possibly oats) and free of dairy (milk, ice cream, yogurt, etc.)
- Testing for hidden food allergies and avoidance of allergenic foods
- Treatment of intestinal bacterial/yeast overgrowth
- Detoxification of heavy metals

Psychiatric medications

The various topics covered in this overview paper for parents of young autistic children represent, for the most part, a consensus of the views, based on research and personal experience, of all four authors. However, the authors differ in their opinions on the role psychoactive drugs should play. We will present you with the conflicting opinions, so that you can decide for yourself.

In summary, Dr. Grandin has a relatively accepting position on the use of psychiatric medications in autistic children. She feels that it is worthwhile to consider drugs as a viable and useful treatment. Dr. Rimland and Dr. Edelson, on the other hand, are strongly opposed to the use of drugs except as a possible last resort. They feel the risks are great and consistently outweigh the benefits. Dr. Adams has an intermediate view.

Dr. Grandin

There are no psychiatric medications for "autism," but there are many psychiatric medications used for treating specific symptoms often found in autism, such as aggression, self-injury, anxiety, depression, obsessive/compulsive disorders, and ADHD. These medications generally function by altering the level of neurotransmitters (chemical messengers) in the brain. There is no medical test to determine if a particular medication is called for; the decision is based on the psychiatrist's evaluation of the patient's symptoms. This is a "trial and error" approach, as dosages need to be adjusted to suit each person, and one medication may be ineffective or have negative effects while others are helpful.

For some classes of drugs, the doses that successfully reduce symptoms such as aggression or anxiety are much lower for those with autism than for normal people. For the SSRI drugs, such as Prozac (Fluoxetine), Zoloft (Sertraline), and other antidepressants, the best dose may be only one-third of the normal starting dose. Too high a dose may cause agitation or insomnia. If agitation occurs, the dose must be lowered. The low dose principle also applies to all drugs in the atypical or third-generation antipsychotic drug class, such as Risperdal (Risperidone). The effective dose will vary greatly between individuals. Start low and use the lowest effective dose. Other classes of drugs, such as anticonvulsants, will usually require the same doses that are effective in normal individuals.

Psychiatric medications are widely used to treat the symptoms of autism, and they can be beneficial to many older children and adults. However, there are concerns over their use. There is relatively little research on their use for children with autism. There are almost no studies on the long-term effects of their use, especially for the newer medications, and there is a concern that their long-term use in children may affect their development. They treat the symptoms, but not the underlying biomedical causes of autism. One must balance risk and benefit. A drug should have an obvious positive effect to make it worth the risk. In order to observe the effect of a drug, do not start a drug at the same time as you start some other treatment.

Drs. Rimland and Edelson

The ARI Conference recommendations for treating some biological symptoms of autism described above was developed by a group of advanced physicians and scientists (including a number of parents of autistic children) because the treatments offered as standard practice by traditional pediatricians, child psychiatrists and child neurologists is far from satisfactory. For the most part, traditional doctors rely on psychoactive drugs, such as Ritalin, Risperdal, and Prozac. None of these drugs are approved by the FDA for autistic children and, like all drugs, may have serious side effects, including death. ARI doctors rarely use drugs, relying instead primarily on nutritional supplements—safe substances that the human body routinely depends upon to keep the brain and body functioning smoothly and safely.

The Autism Research Institute has collected data from many thousands of parents about their experiences with psychiatric medications and other treatments. In general, parents report that the medications are about equally likely to cause problems or to help, with some being worse than others. This is in contrast to other treatments for which the ARI has collected data, such as nutritional supplements, special diets, and heavy metal detoxification, which were more likely to help and very rarely caused problems. The results of this ongoing collection of parent survey data is available at www.Autism.com.

Here are the parent ratings of three of the most often-used drugs and three of the most often-used nutrients:

Three most-used drugs	Got Worse	No Effect	Got Better	Better: Worse	No. of Cases	Three most-used vitamins	Got Worse	No Effect	Got Better	Better: Worse	No. of Cases
Ritalin	45%	26%	29%	0.7:1	3650	Vit. B6 & Mag.	4%	49%	46%	10:1	5284
Benedryl	24%	51%	25%	1.1:1	2573	DMG	7%	51%	42%	5.7:1	4725
Risperidal	19%	28%	53%	2.8:1	401	Vit. C	2%	58%	39%	16:1	1408

Note: These data pertain only to *behavioral* effects. The drugs, but not the vitamins, often cause significant *physical* problems.

We feel that psychoactive drugs should not be used at all on your children and should be used only as a last resort, not as an initial treatment, on autistic teenagers and adults. ARI has collected information from parents of autistic children on their evaluation of various treatments, including drugs, since 1967.

Some adolescents and adults are helped by antipsychotic drugs, such as Risperdal, or antidepressants, such as Tofranil, but the risk of side effects is significant. Drugs should be the last resort, not the first choice. When psycho-active drugs are used with autistic teenagers or adults, it is often found that a very low dose, perhaps one-fourth or one-fifth of the normal dose, is sufficient.

Dr. Adams

Psychiatric medications are not well tested in young children with autism, especially for long-term use, and often have significant side effects. ARI approaches (nutritional support, diet changes, detoxification) are significantly safer and address core problems rather than symptoms. So, I think ARI approaches should be tried first, especially in young children.

However, there are some children and adults who have benefited from psychiatric medications. So these types of medications are reasonable options to consider after ARI approaches have been tried. In young children, they should be used only very cautiously, and beginning with low doses.

Educational/behavioral approaches

Educational/behavioral therapies are often effective in children with autism, with Applied Behavioral Analysis (ABA) usually being the most researched. These methods can and should be used together with biomedical interventions, as together they offer the best chance for improvement.

Parents, siblings, and friends may play an important role in assisting the development of children with autism. Typical preschool children learn primarily by play, and the importance of play in teaching language and social skills cannot be overemphasized. Ideally, many of the techniques used in Applied Behavior Analysis, sensory integration, and other therapies can be extended throughout the day by family and friends.

Applied Behavior Analysis

Many different behavioral interventions have been developed for children with autism, and most of them fall under the category of Applied Behavioral Analysis (ABA). This approach generally involves therapists who work intensely, one-on-one, with a child for 20 to 40 hours/week. Children are taught skills in a simple step-by-step manner, such as teaching colors one at a time. The sessions usually begin with formal, structured drills, such as learning to point to a color when its name is given. After some time, there is a shift toward generalizing skills to other situations and environments.

A study published by Dr. Ivar Lovaas at UCLA in 1987 involved two years of intensive, 40 hour/week behavioral interventions by trained graduate students working with 19 autistic children ranging from 35 to 41 months of age. Almost half of the children improved so much that they were indistinguishable from typical children, and these children went on to lead fairly normal lives. Of the other half, most had significant improvements, but a few did not improve much.

ABA programs are most effective when started early (before the age of five), but they can also be helpful to older children. They are especially effective in teaching nonverbal children how to talk.

There is general agreement that:

- Behavioral interventions involving one-on-one interactions are usually beneficial, sometimes with very positive results.
- The interventions are most beneficial with the youngest children, but older children can benefit.
- The interventions should involve a substantial amount of time each week, between 20–40 hours, depending on whether the child is in school.
- Prompting should be used as much as necessary to achieve a high level of success, with a gradual fading of prompts.
- Proper training of therapists and ongoing supervision are beneficial. Regular team meetings should be held to maintain consistency between therapists and check for problems.
- Most important, keeping the sessions fun for the children is necessary to maintain their interest and motivation.

- Parents are encouraged to obtain training in ABA, so that they provide it themselves and possibly hire other people to assist. Qualified behavior consultants are often available, and there are often workshops on how to provide ABA therapy.

Sensory integration

Many autistic individuals have sensory problems, which can range from mild to severe. These problems involve either hypersensitivity or hyposensitivity to stimulation. Sensory integration focuses primarily on three senses—vestibular (i.e., motion, balance), tactile (i.e., touch), and proprioception (e.g., joints, ligaments). Many techniques are used to stimulate these senses in order to normalize them.

Speech therapy

This may be beneficial to many autistic children, but often only 1–2 hours/week are available. So it probably has only modest benefit unless integrated with other home and school programs. As mentioned earlier, sign language and PECS may also be very helpful in developing speech. Speech therapists should work on helping the child hear hard consonant sounds such as the "c" in cup. It is often helpful if the therapist stretches out and enunciates the consonant sounds.

Occupational therapy

This can be beneficial for the sensory needs of these children, who often have hyposensitivities and/or hypersensitivities to sound, sight, smell, touch, and taste. This may include sensory integration.

Physical therapy

Often children with autism have limited gross and fine motor skills. So physical therapy can be helpful. This may also include sensory integration.

Auditory interventions

There are several types of auditory interventions. One with significant scientific backing is Berard Auditory Integration Training (called Berard AIT or AIT), which involves listening to processed music for a total of 10 hours (two half-hour sessions per day, over a period of 10–12 days). Many studies support its effectiveness. Research has shown that AIT improves auditory processing, decreases or eliminates sound sensitivity, and reduces behavioral problems in some autistic children.

Other auditory interventions include the Tomatis approach, the Listening Program, and the SAMONAS method. Some empirical evidence supports their efficacy. Information about these programs can be obtained from the Society for Auditory Intervention Techniques' website, www.sait.org.

Computer-based auditory interventions have also received some empirical support. They include Earobics (www.cogconcepts.com) and Fast ForWord (www.fastforword.com). These programs have been shown to help children who have delays in language and have difficulty discriminating between speech sounds. Earobics is much less expensive (less than $100) and appears to be less powerful than the Fast ForWord program (usually over $1,000). Some families use the Earobics program first and then later use Fast ForWord.

Vision training

Many autistic individuals have difficulty attending to their visual environment and/or perceiving themselves in relation to their surroundings. These problems have been associated with a short attention span, being easily distracted, excessive eye movements, difficulty scanning or tracking movements, inability to catch a ball, being cautious when walking up or down stairs, bumping into furniture, and even toe walking. A one- to two-year vision training program involving ambient prism lenses and performing visual-motor exercises can reduce or eliminate many of these problems. Visit www.AutisticVision.com. More information on vision training can be found on the Internet website of the College of Optometrists in Vision Development (www.pavevision.org).

Irlen lenses

Another visual/perceptual program involves wearing Irlen lenses. Irlen lenses are colored (tinted) lenses. Individuals who benefit from these lenses are often hypersensitive to fluorescent lights, bright sunlight or other types of light, or certain colors or color contrasts and/or have difficulty reading printed text. Irlen lenses can reduce sensitivity to these lighting and color problems as well as improve reading skills and increase attention span. See www.Irlen.com.

Relationship Development Intervention (RDI)

This is a method for teaching children how to develop relationships, first with their parents and later with their peers. It directly addresses a core issue in autism, namely, the development of social skills and friendships. Visit www. connectionscenter.com.

Preparing for the future

Temple Grandin

As a person with autism, I want to emphasize the importance of developing the child's talents. Skills are often uneven in autism, and a child may be good at one thing and poor at another. I had talents in drawing, and these talents later developed into a career in designing cattle handling systems for major beef companies. Too often, there is too much emphasis on the deficits and not enough emphasis on the talents.

Abilities in children with autism will vary greatly, and many individuals will function at a lower level than I. However, developing talents and improving skills will benefit all. If a child fixates on trains, use the great motivation of that fixation to motivate learning other skills. For example, use a book about trains to teach reading, use calculating the speed of a train to teach math, and encourage an interest in history by studying the history of the railroads.

Developing friendships

Although young children with autism may seem to prefer to be by themselves, one of the most important issues for older children and adults is the development of friendships with peers. It can take a great deal of time and effort for them to develop the social skills needed to be able to interact successfully with other children, but it is important to start early. In addition, bullying in middle and high school can be a major problem for students with autism. The development of friendships is one of the best ways to prevent this problem.

Friendships can be encouraged informally by inviting other children to the home to play. In school, recess can be a valuable time for teachers to encourage play with other children. Furthermore, time can be set aside in school for formal "play time" between children with autism and volunteer peers—typical children usually think that play time is much more fun than regular school, and it can help develop lasting friendships. This is probably one of the most important issues to include in a student's Individualized Education Program (IEP, or education plan for the child). Children with autism often develop friendships through shared interests, such as computers, school clubs, model airplanes, etc. Encourage activities that the autistic individual can share with others.

State services

Most states will provide some services for children with autism, primarily funded by the federal Medicaid program. Many states have waiting lists for a limited number of slots. The quality of services varies widely state to state. Most states have one set of services for children under three years old (early intervention) and a second set of services for older children and adults. Typical state services for people with autism include respite, habilitation, speech therapy, and occupational therapy. To qualify for services, children or adults must be diagnosed with autism by a licensed psychiatrist or psychologist with training in childhood development. Furthermore, the applicant must meet three of seven functional limitations:

- Self-care
- Receptive and expressive language
- Learning
- Mobility
- Self-direction
- Capacity for independent living
- Economic self-sufficiency

Contact your local ASA chapter to obtain more information about the developmental disabilities services in your community. Once a child is determined to be eligible, he/she may be awarded service hours. Many states have waiting lists for services, but some states provide services to everyone who qualifies. It is then up to the parent to choose a provider agency for each type of service. Speech therapists, occupational therapists, and physical therapists are in high demand, and the state pays only modest rates. Thus, it can be a challenge to find them. Similarly, it can be very challenging to find respite and habilitation providers (for an ABA program), and an even greater challenge to train and retain them. Often parents need to advertise for therapists and then bring them to a provider agency for hiring. Often parents need to hire behavior consultants to train their habilitation (ABA) workers; this is very important and highly recommended if the parents can afford it.

School programs

For children younger than three years old, there are early intervention programs. For children over three years of age, preschool and school programs are available. Parents should contact the local school district for information about local programs. In some cases, a separate program for special needs children may be best, but for higher-functioning children, integration into a regular school setting may be more appropriate, provided that there is enough support (a part- or full-time aide, or other accommodations as needed). It is important that parents work with their child's teacher on an Individual Education Plan (IEP), which outlines in great detail the child's educational program. Additionally, meeting with the child's classmates and/or their parents can be helpful in encouraging other students to interact positively with the autistic child.

In some states, home therapy programs (such as ABA and speech therapy) may be funded by the school district, rather than through the state. However, it may take considerable effort to convince the school district to provide those services. Check with your local ASA chapter and other parents about how services are usually provided in your state.

Special needs trusts

Children who have assets over approximately $2,000 are ineligible to receive state and federal services. They must spend their money first. However, most states allow "special needs trusts" to be set up for children with disabilities. These are irrevocable trusts in which a guardian decides how to spend the money on the child. They are the best way for relatives to leave funds to the child, because these monies do not count against the child when determining their eligibility for government services.

For more information, contact a lawyer who specializes in special needs trusts. In addition to working out the financial details, it is very useful to write up a description of suggestions of how you want your child cared for and/or supported. MetLife also has a special program for children with developmental disabilities.

Long-term prognosis

Today, most adults with autism are either living at home with their parents or living in a group home. Some higher-functioning people live in a supported-living situation, with modest assistance, and a very few are able to live independently. Higher-functioning adults generally are able to work, either in volunteer work, sheltered workshops, or private employment, but many do not. Adults generally are more likely to live independently and are more likely to work. Unfortunately, they often have difficulty finding and then maintaining a job. The major reason for chronic unemployment is not a lack of job skills, but rather their limited social skills. Thus, it is important to encourage appropriate social skills early on, so they are able to live and work independently as much as possible.

Some of the most successful people on the autism spectrum who have good jobs have developed expertise in a specialized skill that often people value. If a person makes himself or herself very good at something, this can help make up for some difficulties with social skills. Good occupation for higher functioning people on the spectrum are architectural drafter, computer programmer, language translator, special educator, librarian, and scientist. It is likely that some brilliant scientists and musicians have a mild form of Asperger's Syndrome (Ledgin, 2002). The individuals who are most successful often have mentor teachers either in high school, college, or at a place of employment. Mentors can help channel interests into careers. Untreated sensory oversensitivity can severely limit a person's ability to tolerate a workplace environment. Eliminating fluorescent lights will often help, but untreated sound sensitivity has caused some individuals on the spectrum to quit good jobs because ringing telephones hurt their ears. Sensory sensitivities can be reduced by auditory integration training, diets, Irlen lenses, conventional psychiatric medications, and vitamin supplementation. Magnesium often helps hypersensitive hearing.

It should also be pointed out that the educational, therapy, and bio-medical options available today are much better than in past decades, and they should be much better in the future. However, it is often up to parents to find those services, determine which are the most appropriate for their child, and ensure that they are properly implemented. Parents are a child's most powerful advocates and teachers. With the right mix of interventions, most children with autism will be able to improve. As we learn more, children with autism will have a better chance to lead happy and fulfilling lives.

National societies

Autism Research Institute

Founded by Bernard Rimland, the parent of an autistic adult, now deceased, who was a leading advocate of research on autism. Publishes a quarterly newsletter summarizing current research on autism and maintains a website full of relevant information about autism. ARI also hosts the biannual ARI Conference, the leading conferences on biomedical treatments for autism.

Visit www.Autism.com.

Autism Society of America

Publishes a newsletter, sends out monthly e-mails, hosts a national meeting, and maintains a good website. Most important, it is the major lobbying body for people with autism, including efforts to increase research on autism and educational opportunities and to generally improve the lives of people with autism. Parents should be encouraged to join and support the ASA.

Call 1-800-3-AUTISM or visit www.autism-society.org.

Families for Early Autism Treatment (FEAT) Provides valuable information regarding Applied Behavior Analysis. Visit www.feat.org.

Suggested reading

Books with an asterisk are available from the Autism Research Institute

(4182 Adams Ave. San Diego, CA 92116 fax: 619-563-6840

www.AutismResearchInstitute.com)

*Facing Autism by Lynn Hamilton. This is one of the first books parents should read. It tells how one mother helped her child recover from autism, and it gives a good overview of testing, treatments, and resources.

*Children with Starving Brains by Jacquelyn McCandless, MD. This is probably the best book on the medical conditions of people with autism and how to treat them. Available from www.amazon.com.

*Biomedical Assessment Options for Children with Autism and Related Problems by Jon Pangborn, Ph.D., and Sidney Baker, MD. Recommended series of tests and treatments for autistic individuals and those with related disorders.

Biological Basis of Autism by William Shaw, Ph.D. Available from

Great Plains Laboratory, (913) 341-8949, www.greatplainslaboratory.com.

Covers many biological issues and treatments, including yeast/bacterial infections and casein-free/ gluten-free diets.

*Let Me Hear Your Voice by Catherine Maurice. A story of how one mother helped her autistic child with ABA.

*Unraveling the Mystery of Autism & PDD: A Mother's Story of Research and Recovery by Karyn Seroussi. Discusses one mother's successful search for interventions for her child, with a focus on wheat-free, dairy-free diets.

*Special Diets for Special Kids by Lisa Lewis. Recipes for wheat-free, dairy-free foods. Available from www.autismndi.com.

*Emergence: Labeled Autistic by Temple Grandin and Margaret M. Scariano (contributor).

*Thinking in Pictures: And Other Reports from My Life With Autism by Temple Grandin.

Relationship Development Intervention with Children, Adolescents, and Adults by Steven E. Gutstein, Ph.D., and Rachelle K. Sheely. An excellent book on developing social skills.

Autism, Handle With Care by Gail Gillingham. This book deals with the sensory issues often seen in people with autism.

Little Rainman by Karen L. Simmons.

Challenging the Myths of Autism by Jonathan Alderson

What to do next?

Take one or more of the following steps:

1. Attend one or more parent support groups: Parents can be a wonderful source of support and information. There are over 200 chapters of the Autism Society of America, over 70 chapters of FEAT, and other informal parent support groups. Consider joining at least one.

2. Contact your state's Developmental Disabilities program and apply for services. Be persistent.

3. Contact your local school district and ask about school programs. See what they have to offer.

4. Find a local physician, preferably one who is familiar with the ARI Conference, and plan a series of medical tests and treatments. Some physicians will be open to medical testing and biomedical treatments, but others will not—find one who is willing to help your child, as opposed to just monitoring the severity of your child's problems. Do not take your child to a physician who does not support you or respect your viewpoint.

5. Attend local and/or national autism conferences.

6. Make sure you still find some time for your other children and spouse/significant other. Having a child with autism can result in many challenges, and you need to be prepared for the long term.

7. Continue trying to learn all you can. **Good luck!**

Contributing Author James B. Adams, Ph.D. (Arizona State University, Tempe, Arizona) is the father of a young girl with autism and has served for several years as the President of the Greater Phoenix Chapter of the Autism Society of America. He is also a Professor of Chemical and Materials Engineering at Arizona State University, where much of his research is focused on finding the biomedical causes of autism and effective treatments for it.

Contributing Author Stephen M. Edelson, Ph.D., Experimental Psychology (Autism Research Institute, San Diego, California), has worked in the field of autism for 25 years. He is the Director of the Center for the Study of Autism in Salem, Oregon, which is affiliated with the Autism Research Institute in San Diego, CA. He is also on the Board of Directors of the Oregon chapter of the Autism Society of America and is on the Society's Professional Advisory Board. His main autism website is www.autism.org.

Temple Grandin, Ph.D. (Colorado State University, Fort Collins, Colorado), is an Associate Professor of Animal Science at Colorado State University and a person with autism. She is the author of *Emergence: Labeled Autistic and Thinking in Pictures* and a designer of livestock handling facilities. Half of the cattle in North America are handled in facilities she has designed. She is a popular speaker at colleges and autism conferences. Her website is www. grandin.com.

The late Bernard Rimland, Ph.D., was the director of the Autism Research Institute (ARI) in San Diego, which he founded in 1967, and the founder of the Autism Society of America, which he founded in 1965. He was also the cofounder of the Defeat Autism Now! (DAN!) Project, which was sponsored by ARI. Dr. Rimland is the author of the prize-winning book *Infantile Autism: The Syndrome and Its Implications for a Neural Theory of Behavior*, which is credited with debunking the "mother-blaming" theories of autism prevalent in the 20th century. He was also the father of an autistic adult.

A PARENT-PHYSICIAN TEAM APPROACH

Note: This section is based on excerpts from *Diagnosis Autism: Now What? 10 Steps to Improve Treatment Outcomes.*

As parents, my wife and I remember our pediatrician explaining that our child would be fine, that he would talk and walk. As our older son and the other twin developed normally, we were advised to be careful not to compare the kids. While it was difficult to refrain from making comparisons, it was obvious that one of the twins was not progressing on the same path as the other boys. This was evident when our son was not walking at 18 months of age, had had episodes when he banged his head on the walls, and was very limited in his development.

While we have met many understanding and helpful healthcare practitioners, we have also experienced many frustrations of the waiting room: completing lengthy medical forms and enduring the embarrassment as our son screamed and ran throughout the halls while we were looked upon as inadequate parents. Visiting experts resulted in responses of "There isn't anything I can do for you."

Even though my wife and I at times have nearly exhausted ourselves during the past 12 years trying to gain assistance for our son, we continue to persevere and maintain patience. We have been extremely fortunate to have met many individuals who have furthered understanding of this complex disorder. And though there are not any cures, organizations have developed rapidly over the last few years that are dedicated to helping all of our children who fall within the spectrum of autism disorders.

A pediatric partnership

It has taken many years for us to develop a pediatric partnership. While it is not entirely perfect and resistance does exist, we are fortunate to have partnered with a wonderful and caring pediatrician. When I bring our son in for an appointment, she is no longer intimidated by the fact that I am holding a stack of books with the most recent information on autism. At times, there is a role reversal, when the patient educates the pediatrician!

The majority of pediatricians are absolutely wonderful for primary care, but it is a mammoth challenge for a pediatrician, or any physician, to be proficient in all aspects of disease. I challenge you, the parent, and the health care practitioner to empower each other. Form partnerships to investigate the best methods to improve care for your child.

The causes of ASD are a complex maze of hypotheses. The abundance of theories has caused many practitioners to either overlook the disorder or proceed extremely slowly in providing referrals to specialized practitioners. What complicates the issues further is that the diagnosis includes various assessment methods. Different evaluations result in a diversity of intervention and treatment protocols that lead to different paths for different individuals. And these paths can change as the child grows.

Pediatricians who evaluate infants during the first years of life should be able to identify relevant abnormal milestone markers. Once the diagnosis is confirmed, case management should be implemented without delay. Physicians need to integrate all of the information they gather and provide effective patient care. This care includes making the parents aware of the risks and benefits of a proposed course of treatment, and fostering an effective dialogue between the healthcare practitioner and parents regarding what action to take. The parents should be just as involved as the physician in the decision-making process.

For example, pediatricians should inform parents of the relevant benefits of vaccinations as well as the possible risks. However, the pediatrician should not simply give the parents this information and ask them for a decision. The parents and pediatrician should engage in a dialogue, where the parents can express concerns and the pediatrician can relate her/his personal experiences and discuss ways to help reduce some of the risks of vaccinations.

If the goal is to ensure a successful outcome for your child, how do you begin? You start the implementation process by following the 10-step program from the book *Diagnosis Autism: Now What? 10 Steps to Improve Treatment Outcomes; A Parent-Physician Team Approach*. The 10 steps apply to partnering with many different types of health care practitioners, not just pediatricians. The following steps occasionally refer to materials found in the book.

Steps to an effective parent-physician team approach

Step1: Monitor and chart your child's development

The first step toward a parent-physician team approach is to provide your doctor with a thorough record of your child's development. Accurate, up-to-date records of your observations and concerns are essential for accurate diagnosis and early intervention treatment. The preparatory tools for your physician meeting and initial appointment include a *Daily Log* and a *School Activity Chart* that allow you to monitor and record your child's development at home and at school. As you chart behaviors and reactions of your child in these two logs, the list of *Common Characteristics of Autism Spectrum Disorders* may be helpful in identifying additional traits.

Step 2: Organize information for physician interview

Two steps prepare you for the first appointment with the physician.

1. Gather essential information, including:
    *   Your complete *Daily Log* and *School Activity Chart*
    *   Health insurance information
    *   Your written expectation of achieving the best outcome for your child, including the use of consultants (e.g., neurologist and speech therapist)
    *   Medical records from all laboratory tests and diagnostic procedures
2. Recognize distractions in and around the clinic.

Step 3: Develop an assessment and evaluation plan

Studies have demonstrated that early intervention improves a child's behaviors, language skills, and cognitive abilities. Using various assessment and evaluation tools may identify areas for additional treatment, increasing the likelihood of successful outcomes. Scales and developmental testing tools commonly used by clinicians are found in the *Assessment, Evaluation, and Testing Tools Chart* of my book.

Step 4: Acquire a knowledge base through research

Acquiring a strong knowledge base on autism spectrum disorders is imperative, and your research should begin before your first meeting with the physician. A considerable amount of material may be obtained from libraries, universities, nonprofit organizations, and friends in similar circumstances. In my book I introduce five key points for Internet research in Step 4. The *Research Resources Chart* lists links and contacts that may help you as you develop an effective parent-physician partnership.

Step 5: Formulate questions for the physician appointment

It is important that you understand the physician's practice policies and know how the clinic's group of physicians will treat your child. Step 5 in my book provides sample *Questions for Physician Interview*.

Step 6: Initiate treatment and program approaches

Interventions can be divided into three main categories: educational, medical, and complementary. Charts in my book include *Educational Therapy, Medical Therapy, Nutritional Supplements Therapy*, and *Dietary Therapy*. According to the *Nelson Textbook of Pediatrics* (2004): "There is compelling evidence that intensive behavioral therapy, beginning before three years of age and targeted toward speech and language development, is successful both in improving capacity and later social functioning." *The Manual of Pediatric Therapeutics* (Graef 1997) supports this. Once the pediatrician has identified the disorder, it is essential to initiate treatment that "consists of a structured program in a supportive special education environment. This includes behavioral treatment for improving social responses and communication, and decreasing inappropriate behaviors; and parent education."

Step 7: Carefully choose your primary physician

One approach is to use a primary care pediatrician for general pediatric visits, and a supplemental practitioner who specializes in autism spectrum disorders. In my book, Step 7 includes recommended options for sourcing a pediatrician and a ARI recommended practitioner, as well as other healthcare practitioners whose skills reflect the healthcare needs for your child with ASD.

Step 8: Respect your doctor/earn your doctor's respect

To create a working relationship with your physician, first, respect your doctor. Then, during your interview, you should strive to earn your doctor's respect. Respect refers to your acknowledgment that the doctor is a well-trained professional and your recognition that you both have the same goal: the best outcome for your child.

Step 9: Listen and be open-minded

Once you have made your case during your initial appointment, it is the physician's turn to talk. If you want to be a better communicator, learn to listen.

Keep your focus on the physician, giving the physician your undivided attention. Try not to be distracted by your surroundings. It helps to have your initial appointment without your child. Step 9 proposes 10 steps leading to effective listening and receiving advice from your physician.

Step 10 : Review, negotiate, and follow through

Now that you have met the pediatrician or other health care practitioners, it is time to evaluate the interview. In order to effectively assess the initial meeting, list the advantages and disadvantages.

Step 10 in my book covers the appointment review, negotiation, and follow-through. There is a list of advantages and disadvantages in the *Interview Worksheet*. The *Negotiation Tips Worksheet* offers suggestions on how to negotiate with your doctor.

To acquire an in-depth knowledge on how to successfully achieve a parent-physician partnership, read the book *Diagnosis Autism: Now What? 10 Steps to Improve Treatment Outcomes; A Parent-Physician Team Approach.*

Resources and links—You can reach Dr. Kaplan at US. Autism and Asperger's Association by calling 1-888-9AUTISM or by writing drlkaplan@usautism .org

Contributing Author Lawrence P. Kaplan, Ph.D., Health Administration and Research with an emphasis in autism spectrum disorders, Kennedy-Western University—Dr. Kaplan is the Executive Director of US Autism and Asperger's Association, Inc., a national association dedicated to enhancing the quality of life of individuals and their families/caregivers touched by autism spectrum disorders by providing educational and family support through conferences/ seminars and published and electronic mediums. Dr. Kaplan is the author of *Diagnosis Autism: Now What? 10 Steps to Improve Treatment Outcomes.*

5

TREATMENTS, THERAPIES & METHODOLOGIES

MEDICATION MANAGEMENT OF AUTISM SPECTRUM DISORDERS

Note: "I would like to sincerely acknowledge my colleague Dr. Keith McAfee, whose article previously published in the first edition of *Autism 101* (2008) served as the basis and template for my article below. I have attempted to update Dr. McAfee's article to reflect important advances in medication since 2008 while keeping in place much of what he originally wrote."

General Principles:

Using medications to help manage behavior in anyone is a difficult decision, and I am often asked to discuss this with patients and their families. No one should even consider using medication unless they think that the patient has a problem, and it is really important to spend time assessing any "difficult behavior" in order to decide if it needs treatment. There are many things that need to be reviewed: when did the behavior start (and why?); what has been done already to help manage it?; is there enough support available?, and so on.

There are **NO** medications that treat the underlying social communication disorder we identify under the heading of ASD, but there are a number of other behavioral conditions that can be present in a patient with ASD and might be treatable with medication. Like anyone else, persons with ASD can have a challenge with attention span, become anxious, can develop tics or seizures, may have trouble sleeping at night, and can have mood disorders or even (very rarely) develop schizophrenia. The most common symptom that presents to our clinic for medical management is tantrums or meltdowns, which may be associated with self-directed or other-directed violent outbursts (often called "aggression," although it usually isn't truly "aggressive"). People who struggle to communicate and tolerate changes poorly have a high risk of becoming frustrated and can hurt themselves or others at these difficult moments. Since most people with ASD are male, and most caregivers are female, physical management difficulties often become a problem in adolescence as boys become bigger and stronger. While we always hope to prevent this (and minimize frustration by increasing communication as much as possible), I am often asked to intervene in a crisis, and it can be very difficult to keep everyone safe until supports and nonmedication interventions are in place.

If a trial of medication is being considered for yourself or your child, these are the things I would encourage everyone to think about and discuss:

1. What specific symptoms are being targeted by medication, and what do we think is the underlying condition?
2. How frequent are these behaviors (there is a difference between very frequent small behaviors and less frequent major outbursts), and how will they be monitored (by whom, using what measurements?).
3. What are the costs and risks of the medication? (Nothing with the power to change behavior in a big way is ever completely "safe," although serious side effects are not common.)
4. How much is the medication likely to change the behavior, and over what time frame?
5. Can we get the patient to take this particular medication? There are very practical issues of taste, texture, pill or capsule size & shape, etc.
6. Who will decide if the medication is working, and if the side effects are acceptable?
7. What is the target dosage of medication, and time frame in which to expect a result?
8. How will all this be discussed (and by whom?) so that a decision about ongoing treatment can be made.

Medications may not work right away but should be helpful within a reasonable time period. Dosages can be adjusted up or down. It is important to remember that a trial of medication is just that, a TRIAL: if things don't work out well (or if they go better than expected), make changes!

One important principle related to all behavioral medication is the balance between "steady state medication" (i.e., something that needs to be taken every day at the same dosage in order to work properly) and "as needed medication" (i.e., extra dosages that can be administered on particularly difficult days but DON'T need to be given every day in order to work).

Specific Symptoms that are often the target of medications:

Seizures: These may be difficult to identify, especially if they are "little ones" (big convulsions are usually pretty hard to miss). Ideally, seizures should be completely stopped in order to let the brain develop, but sometimes the side effects of lots of seizure medication may be worse than the effect of a few seizures. ALL seizure medication has an effect on brain functioning (usually a negative effect), so side effects need to be watched for. Many antiseizure medications can have an effect on other symptoms (e.g., attention span and mood), so they might be used in people without seizures or might be useful even when they don't actually stop the seizures. By adulthood, one third of patients with ASD will have developed epilepsy (repeated seizures).

Tics: Rapid involuntary twitches, jumps, or vocalizations can be seen in patients with Tourette's syndrome, which is more common in patients with ASD than in the general population. They can be made worse by some medications and better by others, although they do not usually require treatment for themselves. Tourette's syndrome is also associated with attention problems, obsessive-compulsive behavior (or fixations), and an increased risk of violent outbursts or "rages."

Attention span: Although there are good treatments to improve attention span, it can be very difficult to tell whether a patient is failing to pay attention because of cognitive limitations, anxiety/fixations, limited social communication, or a primary disorder of attention. The medications that have the best effect on attention span (i.e., the stimulants) often have a very negative effect on anxiety/fixations, sleep, and appetite, so even in patients with a primary disorder of attention, they may have big side effects. Other medications available to increase attention span may be quite difficult to administer (e.g., atomoxetine is quite irritating to the stomach so has to be swallowed as a capsule; guanfacine is available as a patented XR tablet that is not supposed to be cut or chewed).

Obsessive-Compulsive behavior or "fixations": This is commonly seen in many (but not all) patients with ASD and can be very distracting, trigger violent outbursts, or otherwise get in the way of function. Although a few patients with ASD may develop classical Obsessive Compulsive Disorder (defined as a personal discomfort with these fixations and an interest in stopping the compulsive behavior), most people with ASD enjoy their fixations and have no real wish to stop (it is the people supporting them who often have this wish). For this reason, fixations are quite hard to stop in ASD (neither cognitive-behavioral therapy nor medications are particularly effective). When they are associated with other forms of anxiety, however, I do suggest a trial of medication to try to control this behavior.

Anxiety: The emotion attached to the perception of danger is fear, worry, or anxiety. Being kept from a fixation (or subjected to unexpected changes, even minor ones) can provoke extreme anxiety and may then lead to meltdowns or tantrums. The primary treatment for anxiety is avoidance, but not every anxiety-provoking situation can be avoided. Most of us have some rituals or repetitive behaviors that help us manage internal stress, and we see these behaviors prominently in patients with ASD (because of their limited social communication). If stress-related rituals are not harmful to the person themselves, my preference is to accept and/or redirect them.

There are a number of sensory-based interventions that can help anyone self-regulate, and we should make these available to patients with ASD whenever possible. Eventually, a "cognitive-behavioral" approach should be promoted (i.e., self-talk, thinking one's way through), but this requires maturity and teaching. There are several groups of medication that can help reduce anxiety, both in the moment ("as needed") or taken continuously. The most effective "as needed" medications, which are the benzodiazepines or minor tranquilizers, should NOT be used continuously (once they work one time, however, the temptation to use them again and again can be quite high). The best medication for continuous use is an older medication called clomipramine, but this has a small (but possible) chance of serious cardiac side effect. Therefore, the first choice of continuous medication for anxiety is one of the (safer) Serotonin reuptake inhibitors (SRI), such as fluoxetine (Prozac). Although these medications have some value, they are less effective and may cause an increase in activity level as a side effect.

Sleep: None of us can function well on less sleep than we need, and this becomes an even bigger issue when both a child and supervising parent have had a difficult night. There are many, many bad habits that interfere in sleep, ranging from a lack of consistent bedtime to electronic hyperstimulation. We are all a bit more "hypervigilant" in the night (i.e., paying attention to very little noises: humans have always been defenseless when asleep, and those noises may historically have needed our attention). Some of us are "night-owls," while others are wired up to be "larks" (early-morning risers), and the match between a caregiver and the person with ASD may not fit well in their natural sleep pattern. Although a great number of chemicals have "sedation" as a side effect, these are almost always effects that wear off or we get used to with continuous exposure. The only specific "sleep timer" known so far is melatonin, which is the hormone present in our brains that tells us when the sun sets, so giving extra melatonin to a "night owl" can sometimes help them get to sleep more quickly, though big doses of this may actually disturb the internal rhythm of the natural hormone and not everyone is a night owl.

Mood disorders: In children, negative mood or depression is almost always a reaction to their life circumstances and should primarily be addressed by changing those circumstances rather than with medication. Into adolescence and adulthood, a negative mood that is innate or "endogenous" may develop, and this needs to be managed both by paying attention to safety (depression & suicide is a serious life-threatening condition) and with the use of antidepressant medications. Adolescents may also be at risk for unusually elevated mood (or "mania"), sometimes provoked by chemical exposure (street drugs, SRIs or stimulants can all do this) but also as a result of a two-directional or "bipolar" illness.

Hallucinations/Delusions: Persons with ASD are at risk for a thought disorder or psychosis (i.e., schizophrenia), which begins in mid to late adolescence. They are also more likely to be given a wide variety of chemicals (medications, THC, other street drugs) that can all cause hallucinations or delusions, and patients with ASD seem to be more susceptible to these side effects. It is not clear that a patient with ASD who gets hallucinations from their medication (stimulants, antiseizure medications, etc.) is at increased risk for psychosis, since only time will tell, and these events are not well reported or studied.

Violent outbursts (aggression): All of us can have a tantrum or meltdown, and persons with ASD are less likely to recognize/respect personal space under ordinary circumstances. Anxious or fixated people are more likely to become frustrated by small unexpected events or changes, and the usual way that other people prevent bad behavior during a meltdown is by co-regulation using social communicative means. For all these reasons, persons with ASD are at higher risk for bad behavior during a tantrum or meltdown, and this can become quite violent.

Attempts to physically interfere are often not appreciated as "helpful" (even if intended that way), so the violence may be directed at others and therefore interpreted as "aggression." Principles of behavior analysis and the control of reinforcers need to be understood by everyone dealing with bad behavior. The behavioral learning that takes place with even accidental reinforcement is so powerful, however, that sometimes it cannot be unlearned quickly (even if everyone involved knows exactly what they are doing and are doing it really well!). There are a number of medications that can downregulate violent behavior (whatever the provocation, whatever the reinforcers), including alpha-agonists (clonidine or guanfacine) and neuroleptics/major tranquilizers. Long-term studies suggest that the lifetime "risk" of exposure to these fairly powerful (both in effect and side effects) medications in persons with ASD is more than 50 percent.

Medical issues: Patients with ASD may be at increased risk for a number of common medical conditions, and their limited social communication may make some of these harder to identify in at least some of those patients. For example: constipation, dietary intolerances, dental caries, or migraine can all make behavior worse either intermittently or chronically. These need to be considered and can be hard to identify in a patient with limited social communication.

Specific Medication Groups:

SRIs (Serotonin Reuptake Inhibitors)

These include citalopram, escitalopram, fluoxetine, fluvoxamine, paroxetine (this is out of favour), and sertraline. Very useful as an adjunct to mental health therapy for anxiety disorders, these medications may also be of help for OCD and/or depression in adolescence (with very limited evidence of efficacy). Although they are commonly used in patients with ASD, they do have a significant risk of "activation" or mania. A treatment trial should start at a low dosage and slowly increase to a target of 1 mg/kg, stopping the increase when there appears to be a useful effect or if side effects emerge. If sufficiently effective, these medications are safe for long-term use (but should be stopped if ineffective).

SNRIs (serotonin-norepinephrine reuptake inhibitors)

These include venlafaxine, duloxetine and perhaps mirtazapine. These three medications share the advantages of SSRIs in terms of serotonin effects (if any) to improve anxiety and possibly depression but also have norepinephrine effects that might also treat fatigue, lack of motivation, and anhedonia (common symptoms of depression in adults). In young children, combination drugs such as these have very little use; children rarely present with typical adult symptoms of depression. They might be considered for adolescents.

Tricyclic antidepressants (TCAs)

Although no longer first line because of their side effect profiles and potentially dangerous cardiac toxicity, TCAs occasionally can be very helpful in certain situations (e.g., clomipramine for OCD). Used judiciously in 83 select patients, TCAs can work very well. Some physicians would classify TCAs as older versions of SNRIs.

Bupropion

A norepinephrine-dopamine reuptake inhibitor used mainly for depression, but with special effectiveness against anhedonia (lack of motivation and interest) and fatigue, this is also helpful in some patients with ADHD. As mentioned above, young children rarely need medication for depression. Buproprion has a risk of sleep disturbance and seizures, both of which are of concern in patients with ASD.

Stimulants

These include methylphenidate, d-amphetamine and l-amphetamine compounds. Although most patients with ASD do have ADHD as well, they also have a very high risk of anxiety/fixations, are often picky eaters, and frequently sleep poorly. Stimulants are just as effective in improving attention span for patients with ASD as they are for everyone else, but the major side effect is emotional fragility (a common problem already). They may also reduce appetite and interfere in sleep. If used, these medications are usually cleared very rapidly from the body, which means that they either have to be given several times per day or as a "long-acting" preparation. There are various different preparations available, and each person may respond differently.

Atomoxetine

This medication is less effective than the stimulants but less likely to create the emotional fragility seen with stimulants (it may not reduce anxiety, but it does not usually make it worse). Because of its longer duration (usually 24-hour effectiveness), it also avoids the typical "peaks and valleys" of the stimulants. On the other hand, patients who have learned to take their stimulants five days per weeks or to stop on weekends have to remember to take this medication every day (year-round). The major side effect is stomach irritation, so this medication must be given with food (if the patient doesn't eat breakfast, it can be given after the evening meal). It comes as a thick capsule that should not be opened or compounded, so the patient has to be able to swallow a capsule.

Alpha 2 adrenergic agonists

These include clonidine and guanfacine, both of which have some benefit for the impulsive component of ADHD and help with emotional regulation. Clonidine can also help with insomnia, and guanfacine may either be sedative or activating (if sedative, give at bedtime, but if activating, give in the morning and consider using clonidine for the nighttime). The biggest advantage to these medications is their long-term safety, so even if they are not very effective, they might be of some help for violent outbursts. Clonidine is quite short-acting, so it can be used "as needed," but if used continuously, it might need to be given as many as 4–6 times daily. Guanfacine is usually presented as a patented XR tablet, with instructions from the company not to cut or chew this. While it does shorten the activity a little to cut or chew the tablet, the medication itself remains effective however it is delivered.

Atypical neuroleptics (atypical antipsychotics/major tranquilizers)

These are called "atypical" pharmacologically because they are serotonin-dopamine antagonists (rather than dopamine antagonists alone) and clinically because they have a lower risk of causing extrapyramidal symptoms (involuntary movement disorders from these medications) than the older "typical" neuroleptics.

This class includes aripiprazole, clozapine, olanzepine, quetiapine, risperidone, paliperidone, lurasidone, and ziprasidone (clozapine, with its really serious side effect profile, is essentially never used.) These medications represent a very powerful class of medications, having many advantages but just as many serious side effects. They are designed to treat serious psychiatric disorders like psychosis/schizophrenia or major depression, but it has been noticed that they also reduce anxiety, impulsivity, and violent outbursts. Because of their very broad spectrum of effects, these medications have become the most popular and widely-used treatments for patients with ASD, both "as needed" and for continuous use.

It is important to recognize the very serious side-effect profile of atypical neuroleptics and continue to try to find an alternative treatment even if they are started and work really well. The major short-term side effect is excessive sedation or "tranquilization," and although this may present some immediate relief if the patient had a violent outburst, it does present difficulties for ongoing cognitive functioning. In the intermediate term, these medications are all likely to cause a significant increase in appetite. Again, this may be of short-term interest in a person who has previously been very picky, but now the patient has a new fixation, and the result is usually a steady increase in weight, which has serious long-term health (and behavior management) risks. Cholesterol and insulin levels need to be monitored. The most serious side effect of these medications is called "tardive dyskinesia" and involves a movement disorder (dyskinesia) that comes on very slowly (tardive); sometimes this might take many years to appear. The problem, however, is that the movement disorder (Parkinson's disease is similar) can become permanent even if the medication is stopped once it appears. For this reason, the daily dosage of these medications should be reduced whenever possible and any and all alternatives need to be explored.

Lithium

This has well-documented efficacy as a mood stabilizer, but with higher incidence of potentially serious side effects that need careful monitoring (including frequent blood tests). Therefore, not generally a first line agent.

Anxiolytics

Benzodiazepines are very effective on an immediate "as needed" basis to treat anxiety, but their effectiveness almost immediately begins to wear off with continuous or frequent use. This phenomenon is called "tolerance" and is associated with persistence of side effects (which may even increase as the effectiveness reduces). It can be extremely difficult to convince caregivers NOT to use a medication that was "really effective last time," so many physicians are reluctant to even prescribe this medication. In the proper circumstances (e.g., infrequent big events like airplane travel or dental visits), these are very useful.

Anticonvulsants

These include valproic acid, phenobarbital, carbamazepine, lamotrigine, gabapentin, levetiracetam, clobazam, and topiramate. These are certainly indicated if a seizure disorder is present (depending on the kind of seizure, each may help in a different way). They are quite varied in their usefulness for other issues. Gabapentin can help with insomnia (it is actually one of the medications with the least detrimental effect on the sleep cycle). Valproic acid is quite effective for mood instability. Levetiracetam, lamotrigine, and topiramate can all help stabilize mood but may also create a mood disorder. As a general rule, stopping seizures should improve behavior, but if behavior deteriorates on these medications, their use needs to be reconsidered.

Sleep medications

"Sleep hygiene" should always be the first treatment for insomnia, but it is sometimes insufficient and may take some time to work. Trying to manage a patient's difficult bedtime behavior when the caregiver has had a chronic lack of sleep is a big problem, and sometimes medications can be helpful to make an acute change in the patient's behavior. Like the anxiolytics, however, tolerance is an issue with ALL sleep medications. A chronic lack of sleep is a big problem, and sometimes medications can be helpful to make an acute change in the patient's behavior. Like the anxiolytics, however, tolerance is an issue with ALL sleep medications. The dosage should be minimized and the medication used on a "temporary" basis if at all. Some of the above medications (neuroleptics, clonidine, or gabapentin) have sedative side effects, and sometimes these are a convenient addition if that medication is indicated for other reasons already. The only specific medication for sleep is the sleep "timer" melatonin, mentioned in the section on insomnia. There is very little indication of tolerance for melatonin (if it works at all).

Keith Goulden, M.D., graduated in Medicine from the University of Western Ontario in 1980 and interned at the Royal Alexandra Hospital in Edmonton. He trained in Pediatrics and Child Neurology at the IWK Hospital for Children in Halifax, Nova Scotia, and then in Developmental-Behavioral Pediatrics at the Albert Einstein College of Medicine, Bronx, NY.

Keith's career as an academic began at Memorial University of Newfoundland and the Janeway Child Health Centre, the only hospital dedicated to the health needs of children in Newfoundland and Labrador. He has been an Associate Professor of Pediatrics at the University of Alberta for the past 10 years. In 2002, he was appointed Director of the UofA's Division of Neurodevelopmental / Neuromotor Pediatrics and Clinical Director of the Capital Health Authority's Regional Neurodevelopmental Program. He also is a member of the Applied Developmental Neurosciences Group (Faculty of Rehabilitation Medicine, University of Alberta) and of the Canadian Autism Intervention Research Network. He is involved in clinical neurodevelopmental pediatrics in Edmonton at both the Glenrose Rehabilitation Hospital and at regional Level II Clinics, with a particular interest in children with autism and their families.

Keith is a staunch supporter of family-centered approaches to treatment and broad spectrum care that recognizes the whole person. He is a beacon of light to many in his field!

EVALUATING THE EFFECTS OF MEDICATION

When a medication is being evaluated to modify the behavior of a person with autism, one must assess the risks versus the benefits. The benefits of the medication must outweigh the risks. Some medications can damage the nervous system and other internal organs, such as the liver. These risks may be greatest in young children because an immature nervous system may be more sensitive to harmful side effects. A good general principle is that the use of powerful drugs should be avoided in young children when the risk is great. The younger the child, the greater the risk. For example, it would be justified to give a young child Prozac to stop severe self-injury, but it would probably not be justified if the only effect was that it made him slightly calmer. If a medication improved language, its use would probably be recommended.

The brain of a teenager or an adult is fully formed, so that medications pose less risk. Many teenagers and adults with autism may benefit from Prozac or Zoloft. There is a possibility in some cases that if too many drugs are given to young children, they may not work when the child needs them when he becomes a teenager. This may be a problem especially with drugs such as haldol or other neuroleptics. Practical experience has shown that the nutritional supplement DMG is safe for young children.

A medication that works to change behavior should have an obvious and dramatic effect. One of the best ways to evaluate a medication is a blind evaluation. A simple way to do this is to start the medication, and do NOT tell the teacher at school. If the teacher says, "Wow, your son's behavior has improved remarkably," then you know that the medication works. To evaluate a medication, it is important that the other therapies be not changed at the same time. Change only one thing at a time, so that you can see the effect of what you have changed. A new medication cannot be properly evaluated if the child goes to a new school around the same time that the medication is tried.

If a medication does not show enough benefit to outweigh the risk, you should discontinue using it. Medications should work. If the change is not obvious and is not dramatic, it probably is not worth giving the medication. It is also important to start only one medication at a time so that its effects can be evaluated.

Many people with autism are taking too many different medications. If the person has been on a medication for a long time, it must never be abruptly stopped. The dosage should be reduced slowly. If you try a new drug for a few days or weeks and decide you do not like it, you can usually stop it, but it is best to check with your child's doctor.

There are many different brands of medications. For example, Prozac, Paxil, and Zoloft are very similar, but there is just enough difference between them that some people will do better on Prozac and others will do better on Zoloft. If you do not like one, then try another. If you are using a generic, do NOT switch brands. Find a brand that works and stay with it.

People with autism have very sensitive nervous systems. Some individuals may require much lower doses of medications than people with a normal nervous system. This will vary from individual to individual. If some individuals are given too high a dose of either an older tricyclic antidepressant or one of the newer medications, such as Prozac or Zoloft, there may be side effects. Antidepressants have a dosage window. Too little will not work and too much causes side effects. The first sign of too high a dose of an antidepressant is (seen at) early morning awakening. This can usually be corrected by lowering the dose. If the excessive dosing continues, the person will escalate into insomnia, irritability, agitation, and aggression. To determine the correct dose, you must be a good observer. Enough must be given to be effective, but too much can have almost the opposite effect.

Both parents and doctors have reported that when the antidepressant was first given, the person became calmer, and then about two weeks later, he went berserk. This is due to a slow buildup in the system. This is especially a problem with Prozac. The dose must be lowered at the first indication of insomnia. In this article I have not discussed the full range of medications that can be used for autism. The basic principles of assessing risk versus benefit and using a blind evaluation should be used with all types of medications that are used to improve a child's behavior and/or language development.

Resources and links—You can learn more about Dr. Grandin and her work at www.grandin.com.

Contributing Author Temple Grandin, Ph.D., Animal Science, University of Illinois—One of the most world's most accomplished and well-known adults with autism, Dr. Grandin is a prominent speaker and writer on this subject. In her book *Thinking in Pictures*, Dr. Grandin delivers a report from the country of autism. Writing from the dual perspectives of a scientist and an autistic person, she tells us how that country is experienced by its inhabitants and how she managed to breach its boundaries to function in the outside world. What emerges documents an extraordinary human being, one who gracefully and lucidly bridges the gulf between her condition and our own. Dr. Grandin is also a gifted scientist who has designed livestock handling facilities used worldwide and is an Associate Professor of Animal Science at Colorado State University.

BIOLOGICAL TESTING FOR UNDERLYING PATHOLOGIES

Note: The article below is reprinted with permission from the July–August 2004 issue of the *Autism Asperger's Digest*. The publisher, Future Horizons Inc., is a world leader in autism/Asperger's/PDD publications. The article was updated by editor Jonathan Alderson.

Autism Spectrum Disorder is a neurodevelopmental condition that has some etiological basis in genetics with effects on the brain. However, decades of treatment theory and programs have mostly focused on the behaviors associated with autism. Government-funded treatment focuses on alleviating challenging behaviors and teaching more functional ones. Meanwhile, a growing number of researchers and doctors within the field have drawn connections between autistic behavior and dysfunction and possible underlying physiological pathologies (imbalances in nutrition and/or toxins, for example).

Dr. Martha Herbert, M.D., Ph.D., Harvard University medical school professor and researcher, explains these biology behavior links in her book *The Autism Revolution*. She provides peer-reviewed research that supports testing individual children who exhibit symptoms associated with gut dysbiosis including chronic constipation and bloating, insomnia, hyperactivity, chronic fatigue, food allergies, and eczema, among other symptoms. Although no one, including me, is claiming any causal relationship, recent investigations confirm that some people in the ASD population have underlying physiological pathologies that not only are uncomfortable, including pain and irritation, but that may contribute to autistic-like behaviors. Many other doctors have published research and books available for parents that explain the physiology and biology of these links.

Planning treatment programs for individuals with autism spectrum disorders should therefore consider the biomedical component equally systematically and seriously as behavior (language, socialization, self-help skills, etc.). Given the lack of consensus on the underlying biological associations to autistic behavior as well as the wide range of treatment options, parents and medical professionals can be understandably overwhelmed. Which special diet is best for my child? Does my child need an Omega oil supplement? How do I determine which tests are most appropriate for my child or adult with an ASD in light of the vast array of tests available?

The recommendations for testing that follow are based on my (Dr. William Shaw) ten years' experience as a director of The Great Plains Laboratory, a medical laboratory that specializes in biological tests for people on the autism spectrum. My experience with my own 14-year-old stepdaughter, Paulina, diagnosed with severe autism, has also strongly influenced my understanding and work.

Food allergy testing

The most common foods prompting an abnormal reaction in children and adults on the spectrum are cow's milk, cheese, yogurt, wheat, barley, rye, spelt, and soy. We have documented these allergies at The Great Plains Laboratory by testing thousands of blood samples from people on the spectrum from across the world. Multiple articles in the medical journals report similar sensitivities within the ASD population. The recommended test to identify food sensitivities is the comprehensive IgG food allergy test. "Ig" stands for immunoglobulin. This is part of your immune system. There are different types of immunoglobulins that are identified in science by letters including "A," "E," and "G," for example. IgG is the most abundant antibody found in many body fluids.

The incidence of high IgG antibodies to wheat and milk is approximately 90 percent in people on the autistic spectrum. Most individuals with IgG allergy or sensitivity to cow's milk are also allergic to goat's milk. Other common allergies include peanuts, eggs, citrus fruit, corn, sugar, and baking yeast. There are various allergy tests available. So it is very important to check which type of allergy test is being offered. Although helpful in some cases, I have not seen IgE food allergy testing to be as valuable for individuals with ASD. Unfortunately, this is the only kind of food allergy test that most laboratories offer.

Determining whether or not IgG food allergies are present is important. These allergies or sensitivities are associated with reaction to foods with certain white blood cells that release powerful cytokines, protein substances like gamma-interferon that can cause observable behavioral changes and even psychosis. IgG allergies are found in children and adults across the autistic spectrum from severe to moderate and beyond. These abnormalities are also very common in attention deficit disorder.

Wheat and milk restriction has been a successful allergy-restriction treatment for individuals on the spectrum. Prior to initiation of the gluten- and casein-free diet, Paulina spent most of the day screaming, crying, throwing tantrums, and pulling things off the shelves. She could not go to dinner at a restaurant because she was so hyperactive that she would squirm out of her seat and wander around the restaurant. All of these difficult behaviors ceased after implementation of the gluten-free and casein-free diet (as well as an antifungal treatment).

Testing for Celiac disease

Celiac disease, a common disorder of wheat intolerance, has an incidence of about 1:150 among people of European descent. The incidence of this disorder does not appear to be higher in the autistic population than in the general population. Celiac disease can be confirmed by the presence of antibodies to the intestinal enzyme transglutaminase, which is involved in the biochemical processing of gluten.

Inhalant allergy testing

Allergies to things in the air are termed inhalant allergies. In contrast to food allergies, these allergies do need to be tested with IgG or IgE tests. Some of the most common allergies are mold, mildew, pollen, cats, dogs, birds, and dust. One child with autism had a severe behavioral reaction whenever a certain teacher entered the classroom. After testing for inhalant allergies, we found that the child had severe cat allergies. The teacher had several cat pets at home. Cat hair on the teacher's clothes triggered allergic reactions in the child. Since it wasn't reasonable to ask the teacher to get rid of her pets, the child was transferred to a different class, and the severe behavioral reactions ceased.

Testing for yeast

Another very common abnormality in the autistic population is a gastrointestinal overgrowth of Candida. Candida is a member of the yeast family—a type of fungus. Drugs that kill yeast or fungus are called antifungal drugs. The greatest bulk of Candida is present in the intestinal tract, although it may occasionally enter the bloodstream and has been detected in the blood of children with autism by a highly sensitive test called PCR that measures the Candida DNA. There are about a dozen species of Candida, but three of the most common are Candida albicans, Candida parapsilosis, and Candida krusei.

There are many reasons why it is important to control Candida overgrowth. Excessive Candida can disrupt normal digestion and absorption of nutrients into the bloodstream, as well as prevent the production of important vitamins needed for optimal health.

Candida produces many toxic by-products, including gliotoxins, which can impair the immune system. In addition, large portions of a Candida cell wall protein (HWP1) have a structure that is virtually identical to the wheat protein gluten. Because of this similarity, Candida binds to the enzyme transglutaminase, which is present in the intestinal lining. This binding to transglutaminase anchors long strands of the yeast cells to the intestine like ivy vines climbing a brick wall. This anchoring inhibits the yeast from being mechanically dislodged as digested food passes by.

The binding of Candida to transglutaminase also interferes with the normal function of this enzyme in the digestion of gluten. If pieces of the Candida cell wall protein (which is similar to gluten) enter the bloodstream, they may react with one of the blood clotting factors that also has transglutaminase activity, leading to interference in the blood clotting mechanism. These modified proteins may not be recognized by the immune system, which can lead to autoimmune diseases. Last, the Candida cells can also produce digestive enzymes like proteases and phospholipase that actually eat away the intestinal lining, allowing undigested food molecules to pass through into the bloodstream and, as a result, cause more food allergies.

Candida can be detected by culturing the stool on Petri dishes or by measuring the amount of chemicals they produced (yeast fermentation by-products) in the intestinal tract. These by-products are called biomarkers and can be measured in a urine organic acid test (OAT). This urinalysis also checks for inborn errors of metabolism, nutritional deficiencies, and other factors. These chemicals or fermentation products are absorbed from the intestinal tract by the blood vessels that are called the portal veins. These blood vessels carry these fermentation products to the liver, where they are distributed throughout the bloodstream. The blood containing these fermentation products is filtered through the kidney, and they are excreted in the urine.

It is important to know that stool testing can frequently miss the presence of Candida when there are high amounts of antibodies called IgA in the intestine. These IgA antibodies may coat the yeast cells and inhibit their growth enough to prevent them from growing in the Petri dish even though they may still be able to grow enough in the intestine to cause problems. Such a situation can lead to a false negative result. By testing the yeast fermentation products in urine (Organic Acid Test), we can detect the presence of yeast even under the condition of high IgA antibodies.

However, about 10 percent of yeast does not produce the common fermentation products (organic acids), so these won't be detected in an OAT and instead must be detected in the stool (feces). Therefore, for those doctors and families wanting to crossreference and to cover all of the bases, we offer a combination test for both the yeast fermentation products in urine as well as the yeast culture from stool. This combo set then determines the "sensitivity" or susceptibility of the yeast to various drugs and natural antifungal agents. Many yeasts have developed resistance to various antifungal drugs because of the widespread use of these drugs in people with human immunodeficiency virus (HIV) infection. Furthermore, like people with HIV, many people on the autism spectrum have a serious lack of immunity to Candida. One possible reason is that the measles vaccine virus can severely impair the ability of the cellular immune system (Vaccine, Jan. 8, 2001) to control Candida. We have found this same lack of cellular immunity in people with autism. The Great Plains Laboratory expects to have a test for this condition available shortly and a possible treatment, as well.

Alongside the Gluten-Free/Casein-Free diet, reducing or eliminating yeast overgrowth has been one of the more effective methods of reducing some autistic symptoms. Paulina had been on an antifungal treatment (Nystatin) for several years, but her behavior began to deteriorate markedly. Testing showed that her yeast had developed resistance to Nystatin. Therefore, even with Nystatin antifungal treatment, the yeast was increasing, not decreasing. She became extremely hyperactive and uncooperative. She spent much of the time crying and whining, had difficulty sleeping, and pulled things off the table. Based on the Great Plains Labs yeast sensitivity test, we determined that her specific yeast overgrowth would be susceptible to a different drug called Diflucan. Within six hours of starting Diflucan, her normal smiling behavior returned. Unfortunately, with prolonged use, Diflucan can sometimes cause liver damage. So, after an intial yeast die-off, in order to keep the yeast levels low, we implemented a limited and specific carbohydrate diet designed to starve the yeast of the carbohydrates they feed on and grow from. With successful antifungal treatment, parents have reported reduced aggressive and self-harmful behaviors, improved focus and concentration, better sleep, and reduced hyperactivity. Many people don't know that antifungal treatment is often a long-term issue and stops too early before the overgrowth is properly controlled, while others treat yeast overgrowth with antifungal drugs to which the yeast is resistant. It is important that antifungal treatment be done under the supervision of a qualified medical professional. A less expensive microbial organic acid test can be done regularly to make sure that the yeast or harmful bacteria have not returned.

Testing for Clostridia

I once did a collaborative study with Dr. Walter Gattaz, a Research Psychiatrist at the Central Mental Health Institute of Germany, in Mannheim, to evaluate urine samples of patients with schizophrenia. These samples were very valuable, since they were obtained from patients who were at the time drug-free. Thus, any biochemical abnormalities would be due to their disease and not a drug effect. Five of the 12 samples contained a very high concentration of a compound identified as a derivative of the amino acid tyrosine, which is very similar, but not identical, to 3,4-dihydroxyphenylpropionic acid. I have since identified this compound as 3-(3-hydroxyphenyl)-3-hydroxypropionic acid, or HPHPA. This particular compound has been linked to colonization of the intestinal tract with Clostridia bacteria.

How is this associated to autism? HPHPA is found to be much higher in the urine of autistic children than in normal children. People with autism who have high values of this compound may have extremely abnormal or even psychotic behavior.

One child with high amounts of HPHPA in urine kicked out the windows of the family car while being transported to school. Clostridia can be treated with the antibiotics vancomycin, or flagyl. The first patient in a medical study improved after flagyl treatment but then regressed when the drug was discontinued. The same child was retreated with a six-week course of vancomycin. A developmental specialist estimated that the child had gained six months of development after the six-week course of antibiotic. Again, the child regressed after discontinuation. One approach to keeping the pathogenic (disease-causing) bacteria at bay after the antibiotic treatment is to add probiotics (good bacteria) to the intestines. This in effect repopulates the intestines with healthy bacteria that aids in digestion. The use of beneficial bacteria, Lactobacillus acidophilus GG, whose brand name is Culturelle, is very useful in controlling Clostridia species in most cases and can be safely used for years if necessary. This product has about a millionth of a gram of the milk protein casein in each capsule, but such a small amount is unlikely to have a significant effect in most milk-sensitive people.

Testing for HPHPA is included on the Full Organic Acid Test or microbial organic acid test of the Great Plains Laboratory. It is important to be aware that some laboratories incorrectly measure DHPPA as a marker for Clostridia instead of HPHPA. DHPPA is a by-product of chlorogenic acid, a common substance found in beverages and in fruits and vegetables such as apples, pears, tea, coffee, sunflower seeds, carrots, blueberries, cherries, potatoes, tomatoes, eggplant, sweet potatoes, and peaches. In addition, it is a chemical by-product of the good bacteria E-coli and Lactobacillus.

Mercury toxicity

Mercury is a naturally occurring metal found throughout the environment. Mercury can enter the environment from deposits of ore containing mercury due to wind or rain or from the actions of humans. Major sources of mercury that contaminate humans include older dental fillings, which can be as much as 50 percent mercury, and large fish such as tuna and swordfish. Prior to 2000, some vaccines contained trace amounts of the preservative Thimerisol, which is a mercury derivative. However, this has been removed from the MMR vaccine and most other vaccines, for example, with the exception of the influenza shot. There is no research to support that the trace amounts of Thimerisol were at levels high enough to trigger neurotoxicity. It is likely that pathogenic/acute levels of mercury toxicity are acquired by compounding many different sources.

Mercury exists in two major forms, inorganic and organic. Inorganic mercury consists of metallic mercury and inorganic mercury compounds called salts. Metallic mercury is a liquid at room temperature. It is the shiny silver material in thermometers and was once commonly combined with silver as an alloy for dental fillings. Liquid mercury from thermometers can give off vapor if a thermometer breaks, which could then be absorbed through the lungs. Mercury is also used in alkaline batteries. Organic mercury compounds include methylmercury, ethylmercury, and phenylmercury. Methylmercury is produced from inorganic mercury by microorganisms in the environment and perhaps by the microorganisms in the intestinal tract. Methylmercury is extremely toxic. Exposure to three drops of methylmercury to the gloved hands of a researcher was fatal. Mercury exposure should be avoided at all costs.

It is interesting to note that the symptoms of mercury toxicity closely mirror the clinical symptoms of autism. Parents of a child who had developmental delays and a muscle disorder contacted me because the child's tests had revealed high levels of mercury in the hair and in blood. They reported that their child ate salmon or tuna five or six times a week. Although fish are an excellent source of essential fatty acids, most large fish have significant amounts of methylmercury. The FDA has recommended that pregnant women abstain from certain fish high in mercury. Since methylmercury is fat soluble, it might also contaminate supplements derived from fish oils. In addition, mercury was used as an antifungal agent in paint prior to 1992.

Therefore, anyone in an older house needs to be aware that peeling paint or sanding off existing paint could lead to mercury exposure. Mercury in the fillings of pregnant women may be a significant source of exposure to developing infants in utero. Ethyl-mercury has been present as a preservative in contact lens solutions, nasal sprays, and in ear- and eye drops.

Testing for heavy metals

Heavy metals may often have combined/ compound effects, so that exposure to multiple heavy metals at low levels might be just as toxic as exposure to one metal at a high level. Heavy metals found to be elevated in children and adults with autism include uranium, mercury, cadmium, arsenic, lead, aluminum, and antimony. Hair is the easiest sample to collect in most cases and is generally considered one of the best samples for screening for heavy metals, since a heavy metal like mercury may be present in the hair at a level 250 times higher than in the blood. However, the use of hair for heavy metal testing is controversial. The State of New York bans hair testing for heavy metals, while the Environmental Protection Agency (EPA) of the U.S. Government promotes hair screening for mercury as a very useful method. In New York State, tests for heavy metals in blood or urine may have to be used instead of hair.

Summary

Multiple tests can be very useful to pinpoint the most significant biochemical abnormalities to focus treatment on. Each autistic child may experience varying levels of success from treatment based on biomedical testing The tests emphasized in this article have been useful to people with autism of every degree of severity. Parents and treating professionals who want to embark on biomedical testing should firs start with the group of tests discussed in this article. Most tests are covered by insurance, but HMOs generally do not pay unless the physician gets advance approval from a review committee.

The Great Plains Laboratory offers frequent free webinars for parents and professionals to learn more about biological tests, results interpretation, and implications. We are also willing to work in collaboration with medical doctors, pediatricians, licensed naturopathic doctors, and other professionals and to educate them through our printed resources to facilitate a patient's biomedical treatment plan. Private consultations with our medical staff are available.

As concerned parents and professionals, it is vitally important that we be holistic in our approach to treatment and investigate whether or not biomedical/biochemical agents are contributing to autistic symptoms. This, combined with quality behavioral treatment, speech, and occupational therapies and other evidence-based approaches, can work together for maximum benefit.

Dr. William Shaw is the Director of The Great Plains Laboratory (www. greatplainslaboratory.com), which specializes in metabolic and nutritional testing, especially in autism. He is board certified in the fields of Clinical Chemistry and Toxicology by the American Board of Clinical Chemistry. He has supervised large endocrinology, nutritional biochemistry, toxicology, and immunology departments in positions at the Center for Disease Control and Smith Kline Clinical Laboratories in Atlanta, Georgia. He was director of Clinical Chemistry, Endocrinology, and Toxicology at Children's Mercy Hospital, the teaching hospital of the University of Missouri at the Kansas City School of Medicine.

SPECIALIZED DIET AND NUTRITION
FOR CHILDREN WITH AUTISM

Children with autism benefit from nourishing hope. Parents and caregivers can strategically add and remove specific foods from their diet as the first step to improving health and well-being. Certain food substances (most notably gluten and casein) are known to be problematic and should be avoided.[1] Other foods rich in healing nutrients are beneficial when added to children's diets to help balance biochemistry, affect systemic healing, and can provide relief from some autism symptoms. In simple terms, these are the underlying tenets of special diets for the treatment of autistic symptoms.

As an autism nutrition specialist, I encourage you to discover the opportunity to help your child through diet and believe that even the pickiest eaters can make marked improvements. I work with families around the globe as they apply diets as a complement to behavioral therapies and other approaches to their child's treatment plan. Parents, pediatricians, and passionate professionals like me have observed remarkable results. Improvements can include better sleep and cognitive ability, less pain and rashes, a positive change in digestion, and improvement in various behaviors.

The choices you make about what to feed your child have profound impact on proper development and health. Nutrient-dense foods supply the building blocks for neural development. A healthy gastrointestinal (GI or "gut") tract provides the proper environment for good bacteria, proper enzyme function, and the ability to digest and absorb nutrients.

Autism: A Whole Body Disorder

Historically, autism was considered a "mysterious" brain disorder, implying that it begins and ends in the brain. Through the array of common physical symptoms observed and the breakthrough work of the Autism Research Institute, a more appropriate "whole body disorder" perspective of autism has emerged. The brain is affected by the biochemistry generated in the body.

Martha Herbert, M.D., Ph.D., and professor at Harvard University, was one of the first to describe autism this way in her book *The Autism Revolution* (Ballantine, 2013) and refers to the brain as "downstream" from the body's functioning. When we appropriately identify autism as a whole body disorder (i.e., not existing exclusively in the brain), we can comprehend how what happens in the rest of the body and cells affects the brain; and how the food we feed a child affects not only the body, but also biochemistry in the brain.

The Gut-Brain Connection

According to Hippocrates, "All disease begins in the gut." In more recent history, a medical doctor and researcher named Michael Gershon, who spent many years studying the gut-brain connection, said it best with the title of his book, calling the human gut *The Second Brain* (1999, HarperCollins). Understanding that gut and brain are connected helps explain how some symptoms associated with ASD are improved through a diet that supports good digestion/GI health.

The gut breaks down our food so we can have the nutrients needed to support biochemistry and allow the brain to function properly. Like for all humans, nutrient deficiencies and imbalanced biochemistry and digestion play a role in the physical condition of people on the autism spectrum. Research statistics show that common physical conditions that can be comorbid in children with autism include diarrhea, constipation, bloating and GI pain, hypoimmunity leading to frequent infections, sleep disturbance, and inflammation.[2]

Some physiological and behavioral symptoms of autism may stem from, or are exacerbated by, impaired GI function. One research study concluded that "unrecognized gastrointestinal disorders . . . may contribute to the behavioral problems of the nonverbal autistic patients."[3] For example, a condition known as leaky gut can lead to inflammatory (allergy) responses to food particles that are not broken down that "leak" back into the bloodstream from the intestine. The allergic reaction can result in headaches, GI pain, and other symptoms associated with inflammation. Importantly, the leaky gut does not absorb nutrients like vitamins and minerals from food well enough.

The largest part of the immune system is found in the gut. Therefore, when the gut is dysfunctional, the immune system may be compromised too, leading to an inability to fight viruses, yeasts, and other pathogens. Certain amino acids produced by bad (pathogenic) bacteria and yeast in the gut have been shown to be neurotoxic to the brain. Derrick MacFabe, M.D., PhD, Director of the Kilee Patchell-Evans Autism Research Group, identified this gut-brain connection through his groundbreaking research on propionic acid.[4]

The following is a list of common biological imbalances and their negative effects with action steps that can improve some physical conditions associated with autism:

When there is yeast overgrowth in the GI tract, toxic by-products can enter the bloodstream and make their way to the brain, where they can cause symptoms ranging from spaciness, foggy thinking, and drunken behavior.[5]
   Try to

- Remove sugars.
- Remove yeast-containing foods.
- Reduce refined starches and, in some cases, even remove them.
- Add probiotic-rich foods.

When the biochemistry of methylation is not working properly, neurotransmitters cannot be methylated (functioning) as they need to be, increasing the likelihood of anxiety, depression, ADHD, and sleeping issues.[6]
   Try to

- Remove phenolic foods—artificial ingredients, and foods high in natural salicylates, amines, and glutamates.
- Improve methylation and sulfation through supplementation.

Inflammation in the gut and brain can be caused by toxins, food sensitivities, or bad bacteria or yeast in the gut. This can cause pain that triggers behavior such as self-injury, including eye poking and head banging, as well as repetitive behavior.[7]

Try to

- Remove foods that inflame the gut such as gluten, casein, and soy.
- Add foods that are antiinflammatory such as antioxidant and probiotic-rich foods.
- Add foods that supply beneficial bacteria (probiotics) such as nondairy yogurt and raw sauerkraut.

When detoxification is poor, as is common with autism, toxins from food and the environment can build up and act like drugs on the brain (causing irritability, aggression, brain/cellular damage), as with salicylates, artificial ingredients, MSG, mercury, and aluminum.[8]

Try to

- Avoid food additives.
- Avoid toxins in food supply and meal preparation.
- Eat organically.
- Add foods that support the liver.

When digestion is poor and the gut is too permeable (leaky gut), the nutrients that are supposed to get through cannot absorb properly. This leads to nutrient deficiencies, which can affect all cellular function including poor brain function.

Try to

- Increase the quality and digestibility of food.
- Supplement (under direction of a certified professional).
- Sneak in vegetables for picky eaters.
- Juice vegetables and offer homemade bone broths.

Choosing a "Special Diet"

The most successful parents (and children) in my private practice are those who take steps to carefully implement special diets. They believe that calculated food choices can make a difference. As I guide parents, we chart nutrient intake and carefully record improvement in sleep, energy level, behavior, cognitive ability, language, eye contact, aggression, digestive problems, rashes, pain, and more.

There are many so-called "autism diets" to choose from, and deciding how to begin nutritional intervention can seem overwhelming. Ten years ago, it was a simpler choice when the Gluten-Free Casein-Free Diet (GFCF) was the only main option. Eliminating gluten (the protein in wheat) and casein (the protein in dairy) was the primary focus of diet for children with ASD for many years. However, advances in biomedical nutrition research and mom-driven anecdotal data have resulted in a greater variety of dietary options. These days, one has to decide which diet to apply.

Since each diet has its own group of professional and parent advocates, parents whose children did well with a particular diet, who aptly tout it—it is very hard to know which one to try. This happens in the world of weight loss diets, too: people who have success with a particular regime, the Atkins Diet versus the South Beach Diet for example, swear it is the only one that works. How can all of the diets have advocates . . . are they all "the only on that works"? Since each individual adult and child has their own unique health challenges and nutritional needs, different diets are better suited for some than for others. Each child has unique biochemistry, immune qualities, genes, environment assaults, and eating preferences. In a very practical way, it is good that there are different diets to address different biological needs.

As an Autism Nutrition Consultant, I specialize in individualized and customized nutrition intervention focused on improving systemic health and relieving physiological and behavioral symptoms. I help parents choose the best initial diet for their child and then work to customize that diet to further meet their specific needs. In my book, *Nourishing Hope for Autism*, I discuss thirteen different diets that are recommended to address symptoms commonly associated with autism. The top three most frequently recommended diets in my practice are the 1) the Gluten-Free and Casein-Free Diet (GFCF), 2) the Specific Carbohydrate Diet (SCD), and 3) the Body Ecology Diet (BED).

Getting Started

If your child is a candidate for a special diet, before starting any diet that involves restricting certain food groups and ingredients, I strongly recommend that you find a certified nutritional practitioner to work in partnership with you and a medical doctor if possible who can monitor your child's basic vital health indicators. The easiest and most important initial action, no matter which diet you choose, is to remove artificial ingredients and junk food. Artificial ingredients can be toxic and difficult for the liver to break down. They can be associated with hyperactivity, asthma, aggression, irritability, and sleep disturbances. Once you realize the deleterious nature of certain foods, you'll naturally choose to eliminate them from your child's diet.

Picky Eaters

I know what you are thinking: "My child is picky and very inflexible with eating new foods. I'm never going to be able to get him to eat anything other than cereal and chicken nuggets, never mind anything "healthy." I appreciate this concern. I have worked with many very picky eaters in my private practice, many of whom ate only bread and dairy, and others who subsisted on just pancakes and fries. However, there are explanations for why these children are so restrictive in their food choices: primarily cravings.

Opiate-like by-products derived from digestion can have addictive properties and can cause craving for those same foods. Another reason why some children seem to have a strong preference for certain foods is yeast overgrowth. Yeast is a living organism that uses humans as a host and has been shown to omit by-products that trigger the brain to crave carbohydrates, to essentially feed themselves. Children eventually narrow their food choices to include only those that make them "feel better" (in the short term). However, if you can push through the initial withdrawal cravings, several days to a few weeks, children often expand food choices dramatically, and the special diet becomes much easier.

Most of my clients' children eat limited amounts of vegetables, if any. However, it's also very common that once they change the child's diet and their cravings diminish, a child will begin to try vegetables, meat, and fish often the first time. With children who are severely self-restricting and resistant, it takes time to change, but keep at it. Sometimes as occupational therapy or sensory integration begins to address food textures, the child will be more open to new foods.

Until then, get creative and make foods crunchy or smooth based on their preferences. Stagger the changes. Begin to add new food options such as gluten-free pasta before changing the sauce, too. Be aware that a child may have a brand preference because it contains MSG or other additives that can be addictive, making that food seem to taste better. Add enough salt to make your different versions of their favorites more flavorful. Don't go overboard, but don't feel you need to limit salt.

Believe in the possibility of change

I often hear from parents that their children start taking many steps forward once digestive problems like diarrhea and constipation are addressed. Relieved of constant pain and distraction, they can focus better and engage more in school and therapy. Language learning and behavior improve. Another common feedback I hear, with great elation from the parents, is sleep improves, which supports the well-being of the whole family.

I have witnessed children recover from autism with individualized treatment programs that include special diets and supplementation. I encourage every parent to consider if their child is a candidate for a special diet. I believe many are. Believe that change is possible. Even picky eaters' diets can be improved. Patience, persistence, and a belief that your child can change are critical ingredients for success. By envisioning the changes you want, you will take the first steps toward the goals (the mind and body are connected!). Diet alone is not a cure for autism. But in all of my years of practice, I have never seen a child who didn't benefit in some important way from having a more healthy diet. By following the steps outlined in my book *Nourishing Hope for Autism*, and by customizing a diet and supplement plan to address the specific issues associated with the autistic population that a child might suffer from, change will be amplified.

Like you, I am committed to helping children get better. "Nourishing hope" comes from the depths of my heart and is fueled by intense love and devotion. Always have hope.

References

1. Knivsberg AM, Reichelt KL, Nodland M. (2001). Reports on dietary intervention in autistic disorders. Nutritional Neuroscience, 4(1):25–37.
2. Molloy CA, Manning-Courtney P. Prevalence of chronic gastrointestinal symptoms in children with autism and autistic spectrum disorders. Autism. 2003 Jun;7(2):165–71.

3. Horvath K, Papadimitriou JC, Rabsztyn A, Drachenberg C, Tildon JT. Gastrointestinal abnormalities in children with autistic disorder. J Pediatr. 1999 Nov;135(5):559–63.

4. MacFabe DF et al. Neurobiological effects of intraventricular propionic acid in rats: possible role of short chain fatty acids on the pathogenesis and characteristics of autism spectrum disorders. Behav Brain Res 2007:176(1): 149–69.

5. Logan BK, Jones, AW. Endogenous ethanol "auto-brewery syndrome" as a drunk-driving defence challenge. Med Sci Law. 2000 Jul;40(3):206–15.

6. Miller AL. The methylation, neurotransmitter, and antioxidant connections between folate and depression. Altern Med Rev. 2008 Sep;13(3):216–26.

7. Waring RH, Ngong JM, Klovrza L, Green S, Sharp H. Biochemical Parameters in Autistic Children. Dev Brain Dysfunct 1997;10:40–43.

8. Wang HT, Luo B, Huang YN, Zhou KQ, Chen L. Sodium salicylate suppresses serotonin-induced enhancement of GABAergic spontaneous inhibitory postsynaptic currents in rat inferior colliculus in vitro. Hear Res. 2008 Feb;236(1–2):42–51. Epub 2007 Dec 15.

Julie Matthews is a Certified Nutrition Consultant and Founder and President of Nourishing Hope. She is an internationally respected autism diet and nutrition specialist providing intervention guidance backed by extensive scientific research and applied clinical experience. She has been a Defeat Autism Now! Practitioner for over ten years and has helped thousands of children worldwide through public education programs, conferences, private consultation, her blog, website, and Facebook group. Julie serves on the scientific advisory panel of The Autism File, and is an honored member of the National Association of Nutrition Professionals (NANP). Julie is the author of *Nourishing Hope for Autism*, an award-winning guide for parents and clinicians to the fundamentals of autism nutrition and dietary implementation and supplementation. Julie is also the creator of Cooking to Heal™, an autism education and cooking class program offered in cities across the country along with in-home resources. Julie is a graduate of Bauman College and the University of California, Davis. She lives in San Francisco with her family, where she runs her private consultation practice

THE SCERTS MODEL™: A COMPREHENSIVE EDUCATIONAL APPROACH

The SCERTS Model is a comprehensive, multidisciplinary approach to enhancing communication and socioemotional abilities of young children with ASD. The acronym "SCERTS" refers to Social Communication (SC), Emotional Regulation (ER) and Transactional Support (TS), which we believe should be the priorities in a program designed to support the development of children with ASD and their families. In the SCERTS model, it is recognized that the most meaningful learning experiences in childhood occur in everyday activities within the family and at school. Therefore, efforts to support a child's development should occur with a variety of partners (e.g., parents, other caregivers, brothers and sisters, and other children) in everyday routines in a variety of social situations, and not primarily by working with children or "training skills" outside of these natural and more motivating contexts.

The SCERTS framework has been designed to enhance abilities in social communication and emotional regulation by providing transactional supports throughout a child's daily activities and across social partners. The SCERTS model is best implemented as a carefully coordinated multidisciplinary approach that respects and infuses expertise from a variety of disciplines, including regular and special education, speech-language pathology, occupational therapy, psychology, and social work, in a collaborative partnership with parents and family members. The SCERTS Model is designed to have broad application in educational and clinical settings and in everyday activities at home and in the community. The model is applicable for children at different developmental levels, including beginning preverbal communicators through children who are conversational. It is grounded in explicitly stated core values and principles that guide educational efforts.

SCERTS Model statement of core values and guiding principles

1. The development of spontaneous, functional communication abilities and emotional regulatory capacities are of the highest priority in educational and treatment efforts.

2. Principles and research on child development frame assessment and educational efforts. Goals and activities are developmentally appropriate and functional, relative to a child's adaptive abilities and the necessary skills for maximizing enjoyment, success, and independence in daily experiences.

3. All domains of a child's development (e.g., communicative, socioemotional, cognitive, and motor) are interrelated and interdependent. Assessment and educational efforts must address these relationships.

4. All behavior is viewed as purposeful. Functions of behavior may include communication, emotional regulation, and engagement in adaptive skills. For children who display unconventional or problem behaviors, there is an emphasis on determining the function of the behavior and supporting the development of more appropriate ways to accomplish those functions.

5. A child's unique learning profile of strengths and weaknesses plays a critical role in determining appropriate accommodations for facilitating competence in the domains of social communication and emotional regulation.

6. Natural routines across home, school, and community environments provide the educational and treatment contexts for learning, and for the development of positive relationships. Progress is measured with reference to increasing competence and active participation in daily routines.

7. It is the primary responsibility of professionals to establish positive relationships with children and with family members. All children and family members are treated with dignity and respect.

Family members are considered experts about their child. Assessment and educational efforts are viewed as collaborative processes with family members, and principles of family-centered practice are advocated to build consensus with the family and enhance the collaborative process.

Domains of the SCERTS Model:

Social Communication

The social communication domain addresses the overriding goals of helping a child to be an increasingly competent and confident communicator, and an active participant and partner in social activities. This includes communicating and playing with others in everyday activities and deriving joy and pleasure in social relationships with children and adults. In addressing this goal, we believe children must acquire capacities in two major components of social-communicative functioning: joint attention abilities and symbol use. With increasing capacities in joint attention, children become more able to share attention, share emotions, as well as express intentions with social partners in reciprocal interactions. Capacities in joint attention enable children to attend to and respond to the social overtures of others and, ultimately, to become a partner in the complex "dance" of reciprocal social communication. At more advanced levels of ability, the capacity for joint attention supports true social conversation by fostering a child's awareness of a social partner's emotional state, attentional focus, knowledge, and preferences.

With increasing capacities in symbol use, children develop more sophisticated and abstract means of communicating and playing with others. One aspect of symbol use is the means that children use to communicate or "how" children communicate, also referred to as communicative means. Communicative means may include presymbolic behaviors, such as the use of gestures or objects to communicate, or symbolic behaviors, including signs, picture symbol systems, and/or speech ranging in sophistication from single word utterances to complex expressive language used in conversation. Multimodal communication is valued and targeted in the SCERTS Model. Children are more effective communicators when they have a variety of strategies, so that if one strategy does not work (e.g., speech), a child may shift to another (e.g., pictures or gestures). In fact, a high level of communicative competence is defined, in part, by the degree of flexibility a child has available in the means used to communicate, rather than having to rely on only one way to communicate.

We also believe that children are more competent communicators when they are able to communicate for a variety of purposes or functions in everyday activities, such as expressing needs, sharing observations and experiences, expressing emotions, and engaging others in social interactions. Children who communicate for a limited range of functions (e.g., primarily for requesting and labeling) tend to be less socially engaging and less desirable social partners.

With increasing abilities in social communication, a child is better able to participate with shared attention in emotionally satisfying social interactions, which are the foundation for developing relationships with children and caregivers. Research as well as clinical experience has demonstrated that with increased social communication abilities, behavioral difficulties may be prevented or lessened. Put simply, if a child has socially acceptable nonverbal or verbal means to make choices, to protest and to get attention, there is less of a need to express strong emotions or attempt to exert social control through socially undesirable behavior.

Social communication and language abilities also are essential for learning in educational settings and everyday activities and have wide-ranging effects on a child's understanding of daily experiences and growing sense of competence and self-esteem. The great majority of opportunities for learning in childhood occurs through symbolic activities such as language use and pretend play, as well as through nonverbal communication. Therefore, the more competent a child is in language and communication abilities and symbolic play, the more opportunities that child will have for benefiting from learning experiences.

Emotional Regulation

The emotional regulation domain of the SCERTS Model focuses on supporting a child's ability to regulate emotional arousal. Emotional regulation is an essential and core underlying capacity that supports a child's "availability" for learning. In order to be optimally "available," a child must have the capacities and skills: (1) to independently remain organized in the face of potentially stressful events (referred to as self-regulation component), and (2) to seek assistance and/or respond to others' attempts to provide emotional regulatory support (referred to as mutual regulation component), when faced with stressful, overly stimulating, or emotionally dysregulating circumstances. A child must also be able to "recover" from extreme states of emotional dysregulation (referred to as recovery from extreme dysregulation), through mutual and or/self-regulation.

A plan for enhancing capacities for emotional regulation may occur at three different developmental levels and include: (1) sensory- and motor-level strategies, such as providing opportunities for movement or sensory experiences that are organizing or calming; (2) language-level strategies, such as providing information that reduces anxiety or using visual supports to help a child understand expectations for participation in an activity; and (3) when a child is aware of different regulation strategies and can choose the most appropriate strategies. This is referred to as a "metacognitive level." Approaches are individualized and goals are targeted based on assessment of a child's emotional regulation profile and developmental abilities.

Many factors may be the source of emotional dysregulation: physiological, cognitive, sensory, motor, interpersonal, and social. Physiological factors may include illness, allergies, and sleep disturbances. Cognitive factors may include language processing diffculties, memories of negative emotional experiences associated with an activity or place, violations of expectations, and an extreme need to have events occur in a particular sequence or manner.

Sensory factors may include a hyperreactive response bias to sensory input, which may include auditory, visual, tactile, or olfactory stimuli. Motor factors may include motor coordination and motor planning difficulties impeding goal-directed behavior and resulting in frustration. Interpersonal factors may include partners who do not read or who misread a child's signals of dysregulation, and who therefore are not able to respond in a supportive manner.

Social factors may include social activities and social environments that are confusing and anxiety-arousing. Therefore, the ultimate goal of the ER domain of the SCERTS Model is to support a child in adapting to and coping with the inevitable and uniquely individual daily challenges the child will face in maintaining optimal and well-regulated states of arousal most conducive to learning, relating to others, and experiencing positive emotions.

Transactional Support

Transactional support is the third and final domain of the SCERTS model. Most meaningful learning occurs within the social context of everyday activities and within trusting relationships; therefore, transactional support needs to be infused across activities and social partners.

Transactional support includes the following:

1. Interpersonal supports, including the adjustments made by communicative partners in language use, emotional expression, and interactive style that are effective in helping a child with ASD process language, participate in social interaction, experience social activities as emotionally satisfying, and maintain well-regulated states. Interpersonal support also includes support from other children, which provides a child with positive experiences with children who provide good language, social, and play models, leading to the development of positive relationships and friendships.
2. Learning and educational supports, including: the ways settings and activities are arranged to foster social communication and emotional regulation; visual supports for social communication and emotional regulation, which may be implemented in educational settings as well as in everyday activities; and modification and adaptations to academic curricula to support success in learning when a child is less able to succeed within the regular school curriculum.
3. Support to families, including: educational support, such as the sharing of helpful information and resources, or direct instruction in facilitating a child's development; and emotional

support to family members, which is provided to enhance skills for coping and adapting to the challenges of raising a child with ASD.

4. Support among professionals and other service providers, including opportunities for enhancing educational and therapeutic skills, and for providing emotional support, to cope with the challenges of working with children with ASD.

In summary, the ultimate goals of the TS domain of the SCERTS model are to coordinate efforts among all partners in using interpersonal supports, in providing learning experiences with other children leading to the development of meaningful peer relationships, and in providing the necessary learning and educational supports. Additionally, families must be supported with educational resources and emotional support, and professionals and other service providers need to be supported through professional growth opportunities, as well as opportunities to support one another emotionally.

In the SCERTS Model, it is recognized that when professionals and other caregivers begin to work with a child with ASD and with one another, they enter into complex and dynamic relationships with the child, parents, and other caregivers and service providers.

Important qualities of all these relationships that must be nurtured include trust, respect, and empowerment for the child and family to be competent and independent. Furthermore, these relationships must change and evolve over time, as children grow and develop, and as parents become more knowledgeable about ASD, more confident in supporting their child's development and more clear about their priorities for both the child and the family. As parents change and family needs change, professionals must be flexible and responsive to such changes, and respectful of family decisions.

The whole is greater than the sum of the parts

Although we just have discussed SC, ER, and TS as separate entities, they are by no means mutually exclusive in theory, in how children develop, or in educational practice. Here are but a few brief examples we have observed repeatedly in youngsters we have known:

1.   Increased abilities in social communication prevent or lessen behavioral difficulties. Social communicative abilities allow children to seek assistance from others (e.g., requesting help), to express emotions (e.g., communicating anger or fear), and to have social control in socially acceptable ways (e.g., choosing activities). By communicating in these ways, a child's emotional regulation is supported.

2.   When communicative partners sensitively adjust levels of language and social stimulation, or use visual supports in daily activities, a child's ability to process and respond to language and to stay engaged in a social activity with focused attention is enhanced.

3.   If a student is given opportunities to engage in organizing or emotionally regulating movement activities, and is provided with a visual schedule (transactional support) to clarify the transition from a school bus to the classroom in the morning, the student is more likely to be able to participate successfully in social classroom activities rather than needing more "settle-in" time.

The SCERTS model reflects our conviction that by prioritizing social communication, emotional regulation, and transactional support, educators, parents, and clinicians are best able to have a positive impact on a child's development and quality of life. We believe that the focus on these domains is supported by research on core challenges in ASD and priorities and concerns as expressed by parents as well as persons with ASD who have written about and speak about their challenges. We also believe that these capacities are essential for children to succeed academically and to support optimal learning of functional skills, such as self-help and adaptive living skills. Finally, SC, ER, and TS are lifespan abilities.

Our initial work on the SCERTS model has focused primarily on children in the preschool and elementary school years. However, professionals and parents to whom we consult or who have attended seminars on the SCERTS model have provided feedback that it is not a model just for children, but that it is a "lifespan" model and, as such, is relevant for persons from childhood through adulthood. The SCERTS Model manuals include a detailed curriculum-based assessment in the domains of SC, ER, and TS, and numerous reproducible forms for data collections and tracking progress, and for gathering information from parents and other caregivers.

In summary, we believe multiple sources of information, including research on children with ASD and priorities expressed by parents, support the need for an educational model that focuses on social communication and emotional regulation, with the strategic implementation of transactional supports. Furthermore, the very process of enhancing social communication abilities and supporting emotional regulation is an essential part of "connecting" with a child leading to long-term trusting relationships.

References

Prizant, B., Wetherby, A., Rubin, E., Rydell, P., and Laurent, A. (2005). THE SCERTS Model Manual: A Comprehensive Educational Approach. (Volume I Assessment: Volume II Educational Programming). Baltimore, MD: Brookes Publishing www.brookespublishing.com.

Prizant, B. M., Wetherby, A., Rubin, E., Rydell, P., Laurent, A. and Quinn, J. (January, 2003). THE SCERTS Model. Jenison Autism Journal.

Prizant, B.M., Wetherby, A., Rubin, E., Rydell, P., and Laurent, A. (2003). THE SCERTS Model: A family-centered, transactional approach to enhancing communication and socioemotional abilities of young children with ASD. Infants and young children, 16, 296–316 (may be downloaded at International Society for EI website:http://depts.washington.edu/isei/).

Prizant, B.M. (2004). Autism Spectrum Disorders and the SCERTS Model: A Comprehensive Educational Approach. 3 part videotape series. Port Chester, NY: National Professional Resources. (www.nprinc.com) and Paul Brookes Publishing: Baltimore, MD.

Wetherby, A.M. and Prizant, B.M. (eds.) (2000). Autism spectrum disorders: A developmental, transactional perspective. Baltimore, MD: Paul Brookes Publishing Company.

Contributing Author Barry M. Prizant, Ph.D., CCC-SLP—Dr. Prizant is the Director of Childhood Communications Services; an Adjunct Professor at the Center for the Study of Human Development, Brown University; and a Fellow of the American Speech-Language-Hearing Association. He has more than 30 years experience as a clinical scholar, researcher, and consultant to young children with ASD and other communication and socioemotional disabilities and their families. Dr. Prizant has published more than 90 articles and chapters on autism spectrum disorders and children with language and communication disabilities, serves on the advisory board of five professional journals, and has presented more than 500 seminars and presentations nationally and internationally. He is coeditor (with Amy Wetherby, Ph.D.) of the book *Autism Spectrum Disorders: a Developmental, Transactional Perspective.* (2000) Baltimore, MD: Paul Brookes Publishing Company. The SCERTS Model, a new intervention model he has developed with colleagues, is his most recent accomplishment. A videotape series about the SCERTS Model and the *SCERTS Model Manual* by Paul Brookes Publishing Co is currently available. SCERTS Model Collaborators: Amy Wetherby, Ph.D., Emily Rubin, MS, Amy Laurent, OTR/L, Patrick Rydell Ed.D.

WHAT IS ABA?

Behavior Analysis is the scientific study of behavior. Applied Behavior Analysis (ABA) is the application of the principles of learning and motivation from Behavior Analysis, and the procedures and technology derived from those principles, to the solution of problems of social significance. Many decades of research have validated treatments based on ABA.

Over the past 40 years, several thousand published research studies have documented the effectiveness of ABA across a wide range of:

- Populations (children and adults with mental illness, developmental disabilities and learning disorders)
- Interventionists (parents, teachers, and staff)
- Settings (schools, homes, institutions, group homes, hospitals, and business offices), and
- Behaviors (language, social, academic, leisure and functional life skills, aggression, self-injury, oppositional and stereotyped behaviors)

Applied behavior analysis is the process of systematically applying interventions based upon the principles of learning theory to improve socially significant behaviors to a meaningful degree and to demonstrate that the interventions employed are responsible for the improvement in behavior (Baer, Wolf & Risley, 1968; Sulzer-Azaroff & Mayer, 1991).

DISCRETE TRIAL TRAINING

Discrete trial training (DTT) is a particular ABA teaching strategy that enables the learner to acquire complex skills and behaviors by first mastering the subcomponents of the targeted skill. For example, if one wishes to teach a child to request by saying, "I want to play," one might first teach subcomponents of this skill, such as the individual sounds comprising each word of the request, or labeling enjoyable leisure activities as "play." By utilizing teaching techniques based on the principles of behavior analysis, the learner is gradually able to complete all subcomponent skills independently. Once the individual components are acquired, they are linked together to enable mastery of the targeted complex and functional skill. This methodology is highly effective in teaching basic communication, play, motor, and daily living skills.

Initially, ABA programs for children with autism utilized only DTT, and the curriculum focused on teaching basic skills as noted above. However, ABA programs, such as the program implemented at the Center for Autism and Related Disorders (CARD), headquartered in California, continue to evolve, placing greater emphasis on the generalization and spontaneity of skills learned. As patients progress and develop more complex social skills, the strict DTT approach gives way to treatments including other components.

Specifically, there are a number of weaknesses with DTT including the fact that it is primarily teacher initiated, that typically the reinforcers used to increase appropriate behavior are unrelated to the target response, and that rote responding can often occur. Moreover, deficits in areas such as "emotional understanding," "perspective taking," and other Executive Functions such as problem-solving skills must also be addressed. The DTT approach is not the most efficient means to do so.

NATURAL ENVIRONMENT TEACHING

Although the DTT methodology is an integral part of ABA-based programs, other teaching strategies based on the principles of behavior analysis such as Natural Environment Training (NET) may be used to address these more complex skills. NET specifically addresses the above-mentioned weaknesses of DTT in that all skills are taught in a more natural environment in a more "playful manner." Moreover, the reinforcers that are used to increase appropriate responding are always directly related to the task (e.g., a child is taught to say the word for a preferred item such as a "car" and, as a reinforcer, is given access to the car contingent on making the correct response). NET is just one example of the different teaching strategies used in a comprehensive ABA-based program. Other approaches that are not typically included in strict DTT include errorless teaching procedures and Fluency-Based Instruction.

RELIABLE MEASUREMENT

Reliable measurement requires that behaviors be defined objectively. Vague terms such as anger, depression, aggression, or tantrums are redefined in observable and quantifiable terms, so their frequency, duration, or other measurable properties can be directly recorded (Sulzer-Azaroff & Mayer, 1991). For example, a goal to reduce a child's aggressive behavior might define "aggression" as: "attempts, episodes, or occurrences (each separated by 10 seconds) of biting, scratching, pinching, or pulling hair." "Initiating social interaction with peers" might be redefined as: "looking at classmate and verbalizing an appropriate greeting."

ABA interventions require a demonstration of the events that are responsible for the occurrence, or nonoccurrence, of behavior. ABA uses methods of analysis that yield convincing, reproducible, and conceptually sensible demonstrations of how to accomplish specific behavior changes (Baer & Risley, 1987). Moreover, these behaviors are evaluated within relevant settings such as schools, homes, and the community. The use of single case experimental design to evaluate the effectiveness of individualized interventions is an essential component of programs based upon ABA methodologies.

This process includes the following components:

- Selection of interfering behavior or behavioral skill deficit
- Identification of goals and objectives
- Establishment of a method of measuring target behaviors
- Evaluation of the current levels of performance (baseline)
- Design and implementation of the interventions that teach new skills and/or reduce interfering behaviors
- Continuous measurement of target behaviors to determine the effectiveness of the intervention
- Ongoing evaluation of the effectiveness of the intervention, with modifications made as necessary to maintain and/or increase both the effectiveness and the efficiency of the intervention. (MADSEC, 2000, pp. 21–23)

As the MADSEC Report describes above, treatment approaches grounded in ABA are now considered to be at the forefront of therapeutic and educational interventions for children with autism. The large amount of scientific evidence supporting ABA treatments for children with autism has led a number of other independent bodies to endorse the effectiveness of ABA, including the U.S. Surgeon General, the New York State Department of Health, the National Academy of Sciences, and the American Academy of Pediatrics (see reference list below for sources).

SOCIALLY SIGNIFICANT BEHAVIORS

"Socially significant behaviors" include reading, academics, social skills, communication, and adaptive living skills. Adaptive living skills include gross and fine motor skills, eating and food preparation, toileting, dressing, personal self-care, domestic skills, time and punctuality, money and value, home and community orientation, and work skills.

ABA methods are used to support persons with autism in at least six ways:

- To increase behaviors (e.g., reinforcement procedures increase on-task behavior, or social interactions)
- To teach new skills (e.g., systematic instruction and reinforcement procedures teach functional life skills, communication skills, or social skills)
- To maintain behaviors (e.g., teaching self-control and self-monitoring procedures to maintain and generalize job-related social skills)
- To generalize or to transfer behavior from one situation or response to another (e.g., from completing assignments in the resource room to performing as well in the mainstream classroom)
- To restrict or narrow conditions under which interfering behaviors occur (e.g., modifying the learning environment)
- To reduce interfering behaviors (e.g., self-injury or stereotypy)

ABA is an objective discipline. ABA focuses on the reliable measurement and objective evaluation of observable behavior.

References

Baer, D., Wolf, M., & Risley, R. (1968). Some current dimensions of applied behavior analysis. *Journal of Applied Behavior Analysis*, 1, 91–97.

Baer, D., Wolf, M., & Risley, R. (1987). Some still-current dimensions of applied behavior analysis. *Journal of Applied Behavior Analysis*, 20, 313–327.

Maine Administrators of Services for Children with Disabilities (MADSEC) (2000). *Report of the MADSEC Autism Task Force.* Myers, S. M., & Plauché Johnson, C. (2007). Management of children with autism spectrum disorders. *Pediatrics,* 120, 1162–1182.

National Academy of Sciences (2001). *Educating Children with Autism.* Commission on Behavioral and Social Sciences and Education.

New York State Department of Health, Early Intervention Program (1999). *Clinical Practice Guideline: Report of the Recommendations: Autism / Pervasive Developmental Disorders: Assessment and Intervention for Young Children (Age 0–3 years).*

Sulzer-Azaroff, B. & Mayer, R. (1991). Behavior analysis for lasting change. Fort Worth, TX : Holt, Reinhart & Winston, Inc.

US Department of Health and Human Services (1999). Mental Health: *A Report of the Surgeon General.* Rockville, MD: U.S. Department of Health and Human Services, Substance Abuse and Mental Health Services Administration, Center for Mental Health Services, National Institutes of Health, National Institute of Mental Health.

Doreen Granpeesheh, PhD, BCBA-D, has devoted over 30 years to the study and treatment of autism spectrum disorder and is recognized as a leading expert in the field. Dr. Granpeesheh earned her PhD in psychology from the University of California, Los Angeles (UCLA). She is a licensed psychologist in California, Texas, and Arizona, as well as a Board Certified Behavior Analyst—Doctoral. Dr. Granpeesheh is a pioneer in the field of autism treatment and recovery and also a very active member of the autism community. With endless endurance and a resilient spirit, Dr. Granpeesheh leads educational efforts for parents, teachers, and healthcare providers; takes part in conferences; and joins in walks and other efforts to promote awareness of autism spectrum disorder and the resources available to treat it. In 1990, Dr. Granpeesheh founded the Center for Autism and Related Disorders, which currently provides ABA treatment through its 108 sites across the US.

PACIFIC AUTISM CENTER: APPLIED BEHAVIORAL ANALYSIS

R esearch has shown that the use of applied behavior analysis (ABA) is effective for reducing maladaptive behaviors and increasing communication, learning, and social behavior.

A well-known study of ABA was done at UCLA by Dr. Ivar Lovaas (1987). In the study, there were three groups of autistic children. The first group received 40 hours of 1:1 behavioral intervention. The second group received 10 hours of the same interventions. The third group received 10 hours of interventions, but at off-site locations with independent providers. The study showed that 47 percent of the group that received 40 hours of 1:1 behavioral interventions reached normal intellectual functioning and were able to be mainstreamed into classrooms with their peers without any assistance.

Our treatment philosophy is to follow what the research has shown. Although there is no guarantee of recovery, we can assure parents that children will improve significantly using ABA depending upon the age when a child starts services. Our behavioral treatment model addresses developmental milestones and each child's strengths. Our model utilizes an interdisciplinary team approach focusing on the acquisition, generalization, and maintenance of newly acquired skills.

The effectiveness of our services is dependent in part on the early identification of autism. We believe that with early intervention a child will need less intensive and restrictive services in the future. This is the reason for our focus on preschool-age children. With early interventions, there is an increased chance that a child will reach the potential of becoming indistinguishable.

Parents should know that recovery from this very debilitating disorder is possible for some children with the appropriate ABA program. An appropriate program has three main components:

- Duration (commitment to several years of implementing the treatment)
- Intensity (30–40 hours a week of ABA services)
- Quality (provided by well-trained, well-supervised, and well-managed staff who are sharp enough to understand the ABA principles and who care enough to follow through with them)

The Pacific Autism Center (PAC), based in Honolulu, Hawaii, has taken steps to ensure the highest-quality programs their preschool and elementary learning center. They have partnered with the Center for Autism and Related Disorders (CARD), one of the world's leading organizations effectively treating children diagnosed with Autism Disorders. PAC has contracted with CARD to provide program consultation and ongoing staff training. PAC selected CARD because of its strong history in the field of ASD, its experienced and educated staff, and its reputable curriculum that, when implemented effectively, leads to long-term successes and in some cases recovery.

You can contact the Pacific Autism Center at pacificautismcenter@hawaii.rr.com

Contributing Author Laura Cook, President, Pacific Autism Center—The President of Pacific Autism Center, Laura Cook, is dedicated to providing only the highest-quality ABA services. Mrs. Cook is a parent of an autistic child who is fully mainstreamed in a regular education classroom with no additional support. After five years of intensive treatment, her child is considered to be on the cusp of full recovery. Mrs. Cook's leadership in the autism community and personal insight into understanding the road to recovery through quality programming and provider skill development makes her a valuable asset to this organization.

MAXIMIND LEARNING PROGRAM

Alan was deemed unschoolable. He was an affectionate and sensitive child who enjoyed conversation, but his autism and ADHD had crippled his academic and social skills. He was extremely restless, impulsive, and distractible; had minimal social awareness, restricted interests, repetitive behaviors, and poor voice modulation; and suffered from motor and vocaltics.

By the age of nine, Alan had gone through eight different public and private schools because he could not be sufficiently accommodated. Among them were two highly reputed schools exclusively dedicated to serving children like Alan, but even there, he posed too great a challenge. His parents then tried home schooling but this proved equally unsuccessful. Numerous interventions and tutors were tried but to no avail, although dietary changes and supplements did provide some amelioration of symptoms. He was completely unable to read, write, or do math, even at Grade 1 level. How can we help children like Alan? Over the past 50 years, thousands of experts including scientists, doctors, psychologists, educators, and occupational therapists have developed a variety of useful intervention that could be roughly divided into two types: work-arounds and fixes. Work-arounds include things like medication, tutoring, and counseling. They may provide some benefit, but the underlying causes are not addressed, so doses often need to be increased over time and tutoring can seem never-ending. ABA is more of a fix—new behaviors are learned and academic and social skills grow. Real learning and change have occurred.

To be clear, there can be a place for medication for some children, especially in early stages of kick-starting some initial early attention to learning. However, medication does not of course replace or fix the underlying need for "hard-wire" neurological learning of new behaviors and cognitive skills.

The MaxiMind Learning approach is in this second category of neurological (neural pathway) learning. It is a multimodal, activity-based treatment methodology specifically designed for children with ADHD, autism, and learning disabilities. Its techniques are clinically effective, scientifically developed, medically endorsed, and (possibly most important) fun for kids to do. Treatment protocols are customized through intake assessments, which are then repeated postcourse to analyze efficacy of treatment.

To understand how MaxiMind Learning works, we need a bit of neuroscience. There are approximately 100 billion nerve cells with 1,000 trillion connections in the human brain. Mankind will probably never fully model even one of those nerve cells, yet with modern-day imaging we are learning a lot about autistic brains.

Succinctly put, the key difference is in connectivity. Studies have shown that for some people diagnosed with autism, connections are weaker from the front of the brain to the back, from the left side to the right, and from the outer regions to the inner. Because of these differences, complex activities like reading and writing, making decisions, driving a car, controlling emotions, and managing relationships—all activities that rely on good connectivity between various parts of the brain—are performed poorly and in some cases can't be executed at all. Therefore, logical theory suggests that if brain-regions-connectivity is increased, coordination processes and performance is also boosted. This is why MaxiMind Learning's neurodevelopmental therapies 113 can deliver such a wide range of improvements for children like Alan.

Children work one-on-one with a MaxiMind Brain Training Coach, a specially trained and certified teacher, who guides each child through customized courses consisting of 24, 40, or 60 sessions, depending on the need. For most children, one 40-session course is sufficient, but children on the autism spectrum typically require a 60-session course to get lasting, significant improvements, and some will return after a year or so for a second course.

Due to limited resources, Alan's parents signed him up for a 40-session MaxiMind Brain Training Course rather than the recommended 60 sessions. His training regimen consisted of hundreds of sensory integration exercises while listening to engineered classical music delivered through bone-conduction headphones, followed by neurofeedback focus training, and some fine motor, cognitive, and reading exercises. An integral component of the therapeutic value is in the coaching. Children like Alan need to engage in order to perform, and MaxiMind coaches create that engagement by providing lots of interest and positive reinforcement together with the guidance.

We gave Alan a medical-grade, computerized cognitive test that he did both before and after the course. All areas tested improved. Executive Functions, Attention, Information Processing Speed, and Motor Skills improved most dramatically.

Alan's parents also filled detailed rating forms before, during, and after his MaxiMind Brain Training Course. These forms assessed 58 behaviors on a 1-4 scale. The overall improvement was dramatic with no behaviors getting worse, and the great majority getting better. Here is a selected short list of some common areas of challenge that most parents are interested in:

Sensory & Sensory Motor

Bothered by background noise, loud, unexpected sounds	**MUCH BETTER**
Bothered by textures on body, face, or hands, having nails cut, hair combed	**BETTER**
Constantly on the move, seeks intense crashing or rough play	**BETTER**
Has poor balance and falls easily, avoids balance-related activities (bike riding)	**BETTER**
Has difficulty sitting still, wiggles a lot, esp. if trying to pay attention	**MUCH BETTER**
Struggles with fine motor skills, like handwriting	**BETTER**
Makes disruptive noises or sounds	**MUCH BETTER**

Auditory / Language

Needs to be given directions repeatedly before responding	**MUCH BETTER**
Difficulty with spelling	**BETTER**
Poor grammar, doesn't speak in complete sentences	**BETTER**
Does not transition smoothly from one activity to another	**MUCH BETTER**

Social / Emotional

Irritable, short-tempered	**BETTER**
Easily overwhelmed, frustrated by daily life activities	**BETTER**
Does not sleep well, can't get enough rest	**BETTER**
Has frequent mood fluctuations	**BETTER**

Organizational / Attention / Cognitive

Is distracted easily, not able to stay on task	**MUCH BETTER**
Has poor short-term memory	**BETTER**
Disorganized with school assignments, belongings, schedule	**BETTER**
Has difficulty getting/finding clothes, getting dressed in the morning	**MUCH BETTER**
Can't remember sequential tasks—e.g., do A, then B, then C	**MUCH BETTER**

Alan's mother reported that after just seven sessions, he was noticeably more self-aware, communicative, accountable for his behavior, and actively involved in clean-up times, all of which was a refreshing change. These improvements continued throughout the program.

Even before completing the MaxiMind Course, Alan's functioning was so much improved that he was able to enroll in a mainstream private school where he attended three hours a day and made great strides daily in reading, writing, and comprehension with the help of a dedicated teacher's assistant. By the time the course was over, his social life had "launched," and for the first time, he started enjoying school, saw success in his studies, and developed a can-do attitude to his class work and assignments. Now four years later, improvements are maintained. Alan still requires accommodation and educational assistance, but he is now thriving and has fully integrated into school life.

In the fall of 2016, a new imaging study was published analyzing similarities and differences in "white matter" connectivity between the brains of children diagnosed with either ASD, ADHD, or OCD versus neurotypical children. There were similar connectivity deficits noted in all three diagnoses. The authors, representing a large collective of neurodevelopmental doctors and scientists, suggest that there is strong reason to believe that interventions that boost "white matter" connectivity will also remedy the symptoms of these three conditions.

What we propose here is that MaxiMind's Brain Training methodology is one such connectivity-boosting intervention and merits consideration for a follow-up study with these same children or others like them to observe both the anticipated behavioral improvements that are witnessed by hundreds of parents and teachers as well as the connectivity enhancements that we claim underlie them.

When Arnie Gotfryd, a scientist and educator, finally realized that no tutoring, counseling, or medicine could help his son succeed in school, he began exploring alternatives. Eight years later, in 2010, having seen considerable success not only with his own child, but with many others as well, he templated his system and launched a multimodal intervention he called Maxi Mind. Six years and 400 clients later, his Maxi Mind Learning methodology has enjoyed tremendous success delivering lasting improvements in focusing, learning, and self-regulation for a wide diversity of children with special needs. His vision is to make this therapy accessible to every child in need and seeks energetic, like-minded partners who can help make this dream a reality.

THE HANDLE® PROGRAM

Getting Beyond the Labels with HANDLE®

Many of us live with, work with, and interact with children and adults who are experiencing sensory, cognitive, motor, learning, social, and behavioral difficulties. We often recognize that these individuals may be struggling with an underlying condition, and we may simply explain their behavior as part of the label we, as a society, have placed on them. However, what we sometimes fail to recognize is that these individuals are focusing an extraordinary amount of energy attending to their inner needs. They simply have to expend more energy focusing on their inner needs than communicating in the traditional sense with those around them. Consequently, they have less mental energy available to develop and learn in our traditional sensorial world.

What is HANDLE®?

Just as no two fingerprints are alike, no two people have the same arrangement of pathways that carry messages to, within, and from their brain. Each of us acquires slightly different neurodevelopmental patterns. Many children and adults who experience difficulties in learning, task performance, or social interaction have neurodevelopmental differences that interfere with neural processing. For example, when systems that support vision or the sense of body in space are weak, then reading, math, general efficiency, and even social skills may suffer. Trauma may further complicate matters. HANDLE®, the Holistic Approach to NeuroDevelopment and Learning Efficiency, is a holistic and developmental approach to neurological systems. It incorporates research and techniques from the fields of medicine, rehabilitation, reflexology, psychology, education, and nutrition, emphasizing non-drug methods to address root causes of disordered behavior. HANDLE® Practitioners and Screeners use a nonjudgmental multisystems approach to assess irregularities in neurodevelopment. They use this approach to provide insight into which parts of the person's brain are immature, damaged, or disorganized. Through facilitation of neuroplasticity and synaptogenesis, within the paradigm of Gentle Enhancement®, Providers guide the gentle reorganization of the systems through neural rehabilitation.

Behavior as Information Output

Our behavior is communicating what we are not able to express with words. In many cases, we are not consciously aware of what our behavior is communicating, nor where the behavior originated. We can relate this to an information input/output model. If we are to accept that behaviors are the output of our thoughts, feelings, emotions, ideas, and needs, then what is our input? What needs to be expressed? Independency and Interaction Model–The Substrata for Mental Processing.

Information Input

Our senses are the windows into our brain. Our senses allow us to take in information about our world. Judith Bluestone, originator of HANDLE®, created a hierarchical schematic to illustrate how the development of the basic senses and neurological processing regulates behaviors and learning for most neurotypical people. It is entitled the Sensory-Motor Independency and Interaction Model–The Substrata for Mental Processing.

Needs

Sometimes our underlying needs are difficult to define, and even more difficult to recognize in others. Those who have studied Maslow's Hierarchy of Needs are already aware that safety and security are foundational needs. Safety and security require our constant attention and energy. For most neurotypical individuals, this is done subconsciously without us even being aware of the energy expenditure or, in fact, that we are expending any energy in this regard. For those with challenges or inefficiencies, the expenditure can be profound and can indeed consume most of our energy and attention. This leaves us very little energy to develop and learn.

Attentional Priorities

Self-protection is a Primary Attentional Priority. We all protect ourselves in the areas of our greatest vulnerability. Whenever possible, we consciously or subconsciously find ways to protect ourselves. In the current context, we find ways to protect our vulnerable sense(s).

The world around us is a sensorial place. We must find ways to manage sights, sounds, physical sensations, and other stimuli taken in by our senses. We are constantly adjusting to the world around us. Frequently, environmental offenders may be competing for our attention. Some of our attention may be directed toward the tag in our shirt, the seam in our socks, the tuna sandwich next to us, the lighting, the background conversation, or the open area behind one's back, to list a few. Some of us are able to attend to this information input with ease and can relax, concentrate, learn, and develop.

There are individuals who are highly sensitive to environmental factors such as sights, sounds, or tactile sensations, or who may have a poor sense of gravity. Others may feel insecure in shared space. Their foundational systems are not able to efficiently absorb and process the stimuli from their world. Disorganized neurological systems may allow varied stimuli to enter the consciousness at the same priority level, causing sensory overload, and a consequential shutdown of systems. These individuals may be paying extra attention to sounds, lights, or other information in their environment. This utilizes energy and attention for self-regulating and self-monitoring what should be automatic, as these individuals subconsciously make it a priority to attend to their own sense of safety and security.

As an analogy, assume that we all wake up each morning with 100 units of energy. There are individuals amongst us who utilize the majority of the available 100 units of energy attending to, self-monitoring, and self-regulating foundational neurodevelopmental systems that the neurotypical person rarely acknowledges on a daily basis. When the systems are not integrated (automatic), there is significantly less energy available for higher cognitive functions, such as learning, to occur with ease and efficiency. These individuals are utilizing valuable resources, physically, mentally, and emotionally attending to foundational systems, which take precedence over academic achievement, social development, and growth. A lack of focus, concentration, or attention is often seen as a lack of motivation or as laziness. Labels such as ADD and ADHD may not accurately reflect the experiences, as everyone is always attending to something. The question is, to what are they attending?

Disorganized or underdeveloped foundational neurodevelopmental systems utilize attention and mental energy to self-monitor and self-regulate what should be automatic, leaving less energy and attention for higher cognitive functions.

Processing Information–The Balancing of Stimuli versus Needs

When the neuropathways are underdeveloped, or become disorganized, messages may be transmitted at a sluggish pace, may be discarded, or may be confused when new messages come along. When neuroprocessing is not efficient, individuals may be hypersensitive or hyposensitive to sights, sounds, tactile sensations, or other stimuli being received. This needs to be balanced with their attentional priorities, and their inherent need for safety and security. Such stimuli may be entering the consciousness at the same intensity and priority level, causing sensory overload, and a consequential "shutdown".

Shutdown/Overload

When there is a sensory overload, the brain is susceptible to becoming overwhelmed by normal sensory input, resulting in a shutdown of one or more of the neural systems. This can then lead to disorganization in the neurological systems that provide information to the brain via the senses. An individual may seem to be hypervigilant and paying attention to certain lights, sounds, or other information, or seem disconnected. These shutdown strategies, usually generated subconsciously, are necessary for that individual to achieve feelings of safety and security, the basic requirement of all of us. behavior is communication. Perplexing behaviors are often a direct response to sensory overload, the result of neurological dysfunction. The brain is then susceptible to becoming overwhelmed by normal sensory input, resulting in a shutdown of parts of the neural systems. This may result in emotional meltdowns, or what may be more properly termed flare-ups. Individuals may act out in anger and frustration over not being able to concentrate on, comprehend, or respond appropriately to the tasks at hand.

I have a flare-up . . . please help me! behavior may be a direct response to sensory overload, the result of neurological dysfunction or immaturity.

Sympathetic Division of the Autonomic Nervous System

Neurologically, a shutdown/overload is the engagement of the Sympathetic Division of the Autonomic Nervous System—a flight, fright, or freeze response. This is a physiological response to stress, or perceived distress, by the body to ensure survival. When the body has invoked the Sympathetic Division, the individual is not available to learn and organize systems. Many individuals activate this stress response too frequently, and for long durations.

It is the important recognition of the shift, the state change, from the Parasympathetic to the Sympathetic Divisions of the ANS, on which the foundational HANDLE® paradigm of Gentle Enhancement® is founded. Stressed systems do not continue to organize, they shut down.

Promoting Neuroplasticity and Synaptogenesis

Neuroplasticity and synaptogenesis are lifelong processes through which the brain continues to develop and change in response to the world around us. HANDLE® promotes the development of neuropathways by providing organized, predictable, reliable, repeatable movement-based information to the brain, supported by an optimal internal environment. Across the lifespan, the brain continues to adapt in relation to input, through neuroplasticity and synaptogenesis. The brain and the nervous system are in a constant stage of change, except when in the presence of stress. Imposed demands on the developing systems, when conflicting with an individual's internal need, inhibit typical neurodevelopment and can even cause developmental disorders. Toxicity and nutrition are two environmental factors that greatly affect neurodevelopment. HANDLE® recognizes that organized movement, supported by an optimal internal environment, organizes mental processing, influences the body's biochemistry, helps mold the actual structure of the brain, and leads to effective myelination of neural pathways.

Neurodevelopmental Readiness

Neurodevelopmental Readiness is a frequently overlooked component in therapeutic and educational models. Readiness is neurodevelopmental in nature and thus requires organized, predictable, reliable, repeatable, and non-stressful movement supported by proper nutrition. Demanding achievement before there is readiness leads to problems. Neurodevelopmental Readiness can be visualized as the rungs on a ladder, with neurodevelopment as the bottom rung, followed by attention, behavior, organization, academics, and memory as the top rung.

Gentle Enhancement® is the key

Learning

Differences in sensory processing (in any of the systems) influence one's preferred learning modalities. Serious disorders in one system and/or significant disorders in a number of systems create learning challenges that will remain until the foundational systems are organized and integrated. Ideally, all senses must be organized and integrated in order for the individual to effectively take in and process sensory information from the world around them. Individuals often spontaneously compensate, yet these strategies trade immediate action or effectiveness for efficiency.

Sit Still & Listen: The Dilemma—Which one shall I choose? For example, jumping, spinning, any rapid & vigorous movement may be self-protective, shutting down an overloaded vestibular system.

HANDLE® Assessments and Programs

HANDLE® is provided to clients of all ages by Practitioners and Screeners through an Evaluation process. The Evaluation process shows a provider which neurodevelopmental systems are under stress and helps to provide information about the root cause of presenting concerns. The Practitioner draws inferences about the nervous system by observing how the client is completing tasks, in addition to examining their developmental history through interviews with parents and other caregivers, as appropriate. The Evaluation process is largely observational, with a certain amount of interactive tasking and challenges, appropriate to the developmental level of the individual. It is very much focused on the client. Judith Bluestone observed that clients think we want to see what we've asked them to do. When in fact we want to see how they're doing it. The body tells you so much when you know how to read it—the things it avoids doing, the things it seeks, the ways it moves. It gives you a mirror to what's going on in the brain. Following the Evaluation, the HANDLE® provider develops a program focused directly on the needs of the client. The HANDLE® Gentle Enhancement intervention is based on modern neuroscience, and the activities are anchored in anatomy and physiology. The individualized program of activities takes 20 to 40 minutes and is done daily, at home or at school.

HANDLE® has helped

Individuals diagnosed with: Learning Disabilities; Autism Spectrum Disorders; ADD/ADHD; Dyslexia; Tourette's Syndrome; Brain Injury; Stroke; Cerebral Palsy; Bipolar Disorder; Obsessive Compulsive Disorder; Dyspraxia; Dysgraphia; Dyscalculia; CHARGE & other Rare Syndromes Families concerned about: Perplexing Behaviors; Language Delays; Organizational Issues; Memory Problems; Disorders Deemed Psychological in Nature; Sleep Disorders; Work Efficiency; Social Interactions; Mental Health; Maximizing Learning Potential.

The Founder

Judith Bluestone did her graduate work in neurological impairment, behavioral disabilities, and special education. She had over 15 years of advanced study including: education, counseling, human development, neuropsychology, visual processing, sensory-motor integration, nutrition, reflexology, and more. Her doctoral studies were in neurodevelopment. Judith spent 11 years in Israel, where she designed therapeutic activities for at-risk young children, teaching preschool and kindergarten teachers how to integrate the activities into the curriculum. She succeeded, where everyone else had failed, in mainstreaming the children. It was there that she developed many of the insights that were to become the HANDLE® approach.

Judith was the recipient of many prestigious awards, including the 1989 National (Israel) Annual Early Childhood Education Award for the program of screening and early intervention that she designed and supervised for its implementation in Givat Olga. The program reduced the need for special education in young people from nearly 50 percent to approximately 4 percent of the targeted age group. She also received the 2002 Case Western Reserve University Distinguished Alumni Award for her outstanding contribution (through HANDLE®) to the fields of education and neurorehabilitation and to those served through those fields, and the 2004 Jacqueline Kennedy Onassis Award in addition to a National (USA) Jefferson Award for Outstanding Public Service for creating and sharing HANDLE® to enhance the quality of life of individuals and families in her community, country, and the world.

Valerie MacLean, a Neurodevelopmental Educational Therapist, is a HANDLE® Supervisory Practitioner and Instructor and Director of the Phoenix Centre for Neurodevelopment and Osteopathy, located in Peterborough, Ontario, Canada. Additionally, she has graduated from The Canadian College of Osteopathy in Toronto, and has over 30 years of healthcare experience. With a solid background within the medical and educational fields, Valerie has developed a specialty in autism, and in mental health. She is a frequent speaker at national and international conferences and celebrates the opportunity to present the neuroscience anchoring the HANDLE® approach.

LISTENING, SPEAKING, MOVING, AND AUTISM

Note: The following article is adapted from: Billie M. Thompson, Ph.D, and Susan R. Andrews, Ph.D, *Tomatis, Mozart and Neuropsychology : An Historical Commentary on the Physiological Effects of Music.* Integrative Physiological and Behavioral Science, Official Journal of the Pavlovian Society. July-September 2000, Vol. 35, No. 3, 174–188.

D r. Alfred Tomatis was an ear/nose/throat physician in France who discovered that a sound listening training program he developed for singers to retrain their voices was beneficial to autistic children and adults, too. Dr. Tomatis was the first to recognize the role of the ear in the production of the voice. He made his discoveries and developed what ultimately became known as the Tomatis Method through his early work with two diverse groups of people simultaneously: professional singers who had difficulty producing sounds they once had easily produced, and ammunition factory workers who had suffered hearing loss (Tomatis, 1977, 1991). By comparing the audiograms and spectrographs of the two groups, Tomatis discovered the first law, that "A person can only reproduce vocally what he is capable of hearing."

The reasons the program could work for both groups is that the ear has a big job of analyzing movement two different ways: 1) Movement of sound waves, and 2) Movement of muscles to keep us balanced upright and able to move in three dimensions: up-down, left-right, and forward-backward. We listen to sounds of voice, music, nature, technology, and our own movements. To help an autistic child or adult function better, we have to start with improving listening, our most basic and intrinsic sense.

Listening in the Womb

Tomatis was among the first to postulate that the fetus hears (Tomatis, 1963). Listening actually begins in the womb. The ear and the neuron tracks between the ears and the brain are already fully developed and operational in the fifth month of pregnancy (Tomatis, 1987). Before birth, the fetus begins to listen to the mother's voice at 4.5 months in utero. It can attend to the voice, distinguish sounds it makes, and begin to remember sounds such that we recognize the sounds in words at birth. For decades preceding other researchers, Tomatis contended that the voice of the mother speaking and singing plays a key role in the child's language acquisition and development and in social communication skill development (Tomatis, 1963). If human auditory development is similar to that of animals, then research (Abrams et al., 1987) supports Tomatis's contention that it is the ear that plays a vital role in developing human potential. Abrams found that, at least for fetal sheep, normal growth and maturation of the brain depends on an intact auditory system.

The Ear-Voice Connection

Tomatis showed that the two anatomically separate organs, the ear and the larynx, are in fact part of the same neurological loop. Therefore, changes in the ear immediately affect the voice, and vice versa. Both the quality of voice and speech fluency are largely affected by the quality of the ear's ability to listen. The French Academies of Medicine and Science documented the validity of this theory at the Sorbonne in 1957 (Le Gall, 1961). Tomatis hypothesized that if the defective ear can be "retuned" or reeducated to hear missing or faulty frequencies, then these same frequencies are instantly restored in vocal emission. Consequently, he developed a method to specifically stimulate the rich interconnections between the ear and the nervous system.

The Tomatis Method

Though Tomatis retired in 1995, his Method continues to evolve and to offer solutions in many human arenas: educational, developmental, personal growth, language, musical, and rehabilitative conditions. The Tomatis Method involves delivering sound stimulation through special earphones that provide both bone and air conduction. Specially formulated audiotapes that are not available commercially to the general public are used for the music input. The sound is provided over an intense but relatively short time span. In general, a subject listens from one to two hours daily during intensive "sessions" that are separated by breaks to allow for integration of neurological stimulation. For some types of training, 30 to 60 hours of session are sufficient. For others with developmental and/or rehabilitative needs, the training might continue until goals have been achieved. An Initial Assessment and reassessments determine program design and progress. There are four main ways that the music and sound programs can be modified in order to customize and maximize the therapeutic benefits. First, a set of filters modify the sound so that it is regulated to focus evenly on the specific frequency band range of a good functioning ear. The filters can be set to improve reception for a particular language and to develop a "musical ear," which Tomatis considered to be an ideal listening ear. Second, stimulation of the middle ear is achieved by alternating sound from one channel, set to relax the muscles, to another channel, set to tense or focus the muscles.

Repetition of this alternation action over time conditions the ear to operate more efficiently to perceive and analyze sound properly. Third, the balance of sound from right and left is alternated and varied. For example, in the case of a child diagnosed with autism and with delayed speech, the most direct route to the speech center in the left side of the brain is through a dominant right ear. Sound intensity fed via earphones to the left ear is progressively reduced so as to prepare the right ear to become the lead ear for listening and audio-vocal self-monitoring. Fourth, the timing delay of sound reception between the bone and air conduction can be changed to slow down the processing of information internally and to awaken the individual to attend to incoming information. The delay is gradually changed to support a more rapid response to incoming information.

Autism and the Field of Sound Listening Training (SLT)

By definition and diagnosis, persons with ASD have communication delay and challenges. The speech and language difficulties can range from mutism to speaking just a few single words to full sentences and conversation in higher functioning individuals. What is still unknown is what causes the language delays so central to autism. Genetics and brain development likely play a role. Some suggest allergies and toxicity may cloud the brain or directly attack the nervous system. Regardless of cause, Sound Listening Training can stimulate the listening-vocal system such that neural development occurs, laying the foundation for learning to communicate, for success in school, social interaction, and family relationships.

Beyond Tomatis's research, one of the first research studies documenting the presence of auditory processing problems in autistic children was by Dr. Stanley Greenspan and Dr. Serena Wieder, founders of the DIR "Floortime" model. They identified that 100 percent of the 200 cases of children with Autism that they researched in their practice in 1993 had an auditory processing problem. Learning begins with listening to sounds, our most basic skill in language development. It is the foundation for developing social communication skills and for acquiring language.

EnListen

In 1986, Dr. Billie Thompson began study and work in the field of sound listening training. Following initial training with Dr. Tim Gilmor and Paul Madaule at the Toronto Listening Centre, she trained directly with Dr. Tomatis. She was the Founding President of the International Association of Registered Certified Tomatis Consultants. Through her work with over 7,000 children and adults (of which 3,000 are autistic), she developed what is widely considered the most advanced sound listening training system called EnListen®.

The EnListen® software program was introduced in 2005. Since then, it has provided individualized programs to hundreds of autistic children, teens, and adults. An Assessment and Program Decision Model was developed for Certified Practitioners to use to provide an individualized program sequence with appropriate frequencies, filters, timing delays, content, delivery times, and delivery lengths for each listener. EnListen can be delivered by the parent at home using a Windows-compatible computer. Bone and air conduction headphones are used to deliver the program daily for the length of listening intensive (typically 2 hrs/day for 15 days or 90 minutes/day for 20 days). The voice may be used with an external microphone to modify what the subject hears so that missing frequencies are restored to the ear and voice.

EnListen programs can be started with autistic children as early as 18 months of age. Despite parents' understandable concerns, young children learn to keep the headphones on usually on the first day. Parents are taught how to provide activities and structure for the child so that he or she keeps the headphones on and can benefit from the sound listening training.

A number of sound listening training brands provide varied methods and programs for parents to choose from. But it is important to keep in mind that other programs including "Auditory Integration Training" (AIT) do not provide the level of customization that can be achieved through EnListen. To help families make an informed decision, the EnListen office can provide a list of considerations of the ways different programs can vary.

You can also go online to order books by Dorinne Davis. *The Tree of Sound Enhancement Therapy* and *Cycle of Sound* (www.thedaviscenter.com), as well as other books, provide details about 21 varied types of sound stimulation training programs for which she is certified to provide. She has a DETP (Diagnostic Evaluation Therapy Protocol) that assists in determining the best order of these programs and understands the breadth of the SLT field better than anyone.

Sound Listening Training can lead children and their parents to educational and personal breakthroughs. Programs are a comprehensive approach to developing communication, language, and learning abilities that are based on listening. When used with young children, it can enhance auditory processing and speech so that socialization, attention span, and behavior improve. This field includes many independent companies and providers that use a range of equipment to deliver filtered sounds of music and voice that retrain the ear to attend, discriminate, and process auditory information. It also includes parent consultation and coaching to learn effective interaction strategies, raised expectations for communication, and consistent structure to guide the child to learn what appropriate behavior is and what it is not. With some programs, both parents and child participate in Sound Listening Training.

Listening is the most important and most basic of human communication and learning skills. And since good listening can be lost through accident, illness, trauma, or stress at any age, no one is immune to poor listening. The training offers an exciting new avenue to better listening, learning, and communication.

DR BILLIE M. THOMPSON has worked in the Sound Listening Training field since 1986. Dr. Thompson is widely considered to be one of the world's foremost experts and an international leader in the field. Her training with Dr Alfred Tomatis in France and subsequent practice with 7,000 children and adults has made her among the most experienced professionals and researchers in the industry. She was first trained at the Toronto Listening Centre by Dr. Tim Gilmor and Paul Madaule. She founded and directed five Sound Listening & Learning Centers and provided outreach programs in 30 cities, making Listening Programs available to over 6,000 families (1986–2003).

She edited the English translations of two of Tomatis's books, *The Conscious Ear* and *The Ear and Language*. She was the Founding President of the International Association of Registered Certified Tomatis Consultants (2001–2004) and Editor of the May 2004 Ricochet Journal of Tomatis Method International Research. In 2004, she left the Tomatis group and in 2005 introduced the EnListen® proprietary software designed and developed by her husband, Dr. Kirk Thompson. EnListen works on Microsoft computers and uses all of the controls Tomatis used with the Electronic Ear (she could use them because all his patents had expired). EnListen software expanded the choices for filters, delays, and intensity. Dr. Thompson has provided programs to 3,000 autistic children and some adults since 1986 and developed an Assessment and Program Decision Model for determining individualized EnListen programs for each client.

THE MILLER METHOD®: A COGNITIVE-DEVELOPMENTAL SYSTEMS APPROACH FOR CHILDREN ON THE AUTISM SPECTRUM

We maintain that each child, no matter how withdrawn or disorganized, is trying to find a way to cope with the world. Our task is to help that child use every capacity or fragment of capacity to achieve this. Because the ability to assess and respond to the outside world is essential for survival, we have developed specialized training systems and instructional equipment to help make this possible. Because the ability to understand others and to express oneself is fundamental, we have developed methods for teaching communication through signed and spoken language. And because a disordered child affects all around him, we work closely with parents and families to create a supportive but sufficiently demanding home life so that new capacities to cope that have begun to flourish at the Center may generalize to home and elsewhere.

The Miller Method addresses children's body organization, social interaction, communication, and representation issues in both clinical and classroom settings. Cognitive-developmental systems theory assumes that typical development depends on the abilities of the children to form systems—organized "chunks" of behavior—that are initially repetitive and circular but that become expanded and complicated as the children develop. As the children become aware of the distinction between themselves and their immediate surroundings, their systems, previously triggered only by salient properties of the environment, gradually come under their control.

Children then combine their systems in new ways that permit problem solving, social exchanges, and communication with themselves and others about the world. In contrast, developmentally challenged children become stalled at early stages of development and progress to more advanced stages in an incomplete or distorted fashion. Many on the autism spectrum present an impairment in the ability to react to and influence the world. Lacking a sense of the body in relation to the world, salient stimuli drive them into scattered or stereotypic behavior from which, unassisted, they cannot extricate themselves. This results in aberrant systems involving people and/or objects as well as a hardening of transitory formations found in normal development, e.g., hand inspection and twiddling, or intense object preoccupation.

The Miller Method uses two major strategies to restore typical developmental progressions: (1) The transformation of children's aberrant systems (lining up blocks, driven reactions to stimuli, etc.) into functional behaviors; (2) The systematic and repetitive introduction of developmentally relevant activities involving objects and people. Activities are chosen to fill developmental gaps. This process is facilitated by narrating the children's actions while they are elevated 2.5 feet above the ground on an Elevated Square and similar challenging structures. Elevating the children enhances sign-word guidance of behavior and bodyother awareness as well as motor-planning and social-emotional contact. It also helps children make the transition from one engaging object or event to another or from object involvement to representational play. Parents play an integral role in the program by generalizing the children's achievements at the Center to the home and elsewhere.

How do you assess the children?

We assess the children in two ways. First, with the Miller Diagnostic Survey (MDS), which is completed by parents and transmitted to us. This provides a broad overview of how the parents see their child in their everyday life. Second, with our Umwelt Assessment, which carries the assessment a step further by determining not only what the child does but how close the child is to achieving the next stage in development. The Umwelt Assessment examines the unique way in which each disordered child experiences reality. We observe the manner in which the child reacts or fails to react to different parts of a situation.

Figure 1 below indicates what we mean. (Child's variable engagement with suspended ball)

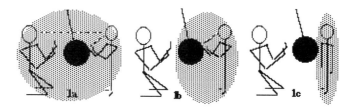

1a. Represents a child enjoying a repetitive pushing-ball game in which adult and child push a swinging ball back and forth. The dotted lines to both ball and adult indicate that the child's reality system includes awareness of both the ball and the adult.

1b. The dotted line indicates the child has a more limited reality system that includes the ball, demonstrated by pushing it whenever it arrives, but not including the adult.

1c. Shows an even more circumscribed reality system, since here the child fails to react even when the ball bumps into him or her. The child is neither focused on the ball nor the adult.

What do you do about more limited reality systems once you discover them?

We expand and transform limited reality systems, and we enrich the child's repertoire by introducing new ones through spheric activity. When, through their work at the Center, the children learn to tolerate "stretching" their reality systems or to accept new ones via repetitive spheres of activity, and can make transitions from one event to another without distress, their abilities to cope with different life situations improve dramatically.

For example, for the child in Figure 1b. whose reality includes the ball but not the adult, we find ways to include the adult within the child's object system or change it from a child-object system to a child-adult-object system. For the child in 1c., we try to find out what gets in the way of the child's failure to react to the ball even when it hits the child. We determine if there are circumstances where the child can become aware of the ball. Some disordered children, for example, become more aware of an object when it approaches very slowly, others when they have repeated opportunity to push the ball.

For children whose reality does not include simple systems such as climbing up stairs to go down a slide, we introduce a repetitive sphere of activity that guides the child up the steps, to sit and to slide down and repeat the sequence. To help the child succeed, we may pace the activity quite rapidly so that the child can connect one part of it with another and, eventually, own the system.

How do you help children generalize what they learn at the Center to the home?

We build in the ability to generalize learning by the way we teach particular functions. For example, suppose a child is being taught to put cups on cup hooks. First, the worker helps the child put the cup on the hook by working hand-over-hand until the child can do this without support. Then, the worker moves about a foot or two away from the child so that the child must turn toward the adult to get the cup and then turn toward the cup hooks.

Ultimately, the child learns to perform the cup-on-hook task while accepting cups of varied shapes and colors from different locations, presented in different positions, and presented by different people. This learning—occurring with the help of at least one parent—makes it possible for the child to perform such tasks at school, at home, and elsewhere.

How do you deal with tantrums and other asocial behavior?

We view tantrums as a failure in the child's ability to cope with people or things in his or her surroundings. We try to understand the meaning of the tantrum—since this varies from child to child. For one child, it may come about because he or she cannot cope with the shift from one situation to another and needs help with this. For another, it may stem from a feeling of loss triggered by a teacher turning to another child. Whatever the source of the tantrum, we do not deal with it by "time out" (placing the child in a space removed from teacher or other children). Instead, we try to meet the need being expressed, to signal transitions from one activity to another more clearly, and to use repetitive (and often reassuring) rituals to help the child reorganize. If all else fails, we hold the child while talking to him or her calmly about what is happening in the classroom, what will happen next, etc.

What is different about how you teach language?

We find, in accord with other developmental theorists, that language begins with directed body action toward or with objects and events. We also find that when children with ASD are placed on elevated boards two to four feet above the ground, they become more aware of their bodies, better focused, and far more able to cope with obstacles or demands directly confronting them. Our research has shown that many children who cannot follow directions on the ground can do so in these elevated board situations. When we place obstacles in their paths and "narrate" what the children do as they climb over, in, through, and across these obstacles, the children develop a repertoire of meanings that can readily be transferred to the ground. Since these "narratives" are accompanied by manual signs and words related to their actions, the children soon become sign and word guided activities.

Goals of the Miller Method®

The goals of the Miller Method are to:

- Assess the adaptive significance of the children's disordered behavior.
- Transform disordered behavior into functional activity.
- Expand and guide the children from closed ways of being into social and communicative exchanges.
- Teach professionals and parents how to guide the children toward reading, writing, number concepts, symbolic play, and meaningful inclusion within a typical classroom.

Biography

Contributing Author Arnold Miller, Ph.D., is with the Language & Cognitive Development Center in Newton, MA.

For more information, visit www.millermethod.org, write to Dr. Miller at Arn-Mill@aol.com, call 1-800-218-5232, or write to the Language & Cognitive Development Center, Inc., Suite 5, 154 Wells Avenue, Newton, MA 02459.

THE BERARD METHOD OF AUDITORY INTEGRATION TRAINING (AIT)

Individuals with auditory and sensory processing problems have difficulty interpreting daily experiences. Their capacities to hear and communicate are compromised. Behavioral issues and social skills are often affected as a result. The Berard method of Auditory Integration Training (AIT) helps reorganize the brain to improve auditory and sensory processing capabilities. Participants use headphones to comfortably listen to AIT auditory stimulation. This reorganizes the dysfunctional sensory center so that the brain no longer gets overloaded with disorganized information.

Language, learning, and social abilities develop more normally and participants are better able to excel as a result. Participants often benefit from just ten days of AIT training, with two 30-minute sessions a day. This method of auditory training was originally developed by Dr. Guy Berard, a French ear, nose, and throat physician, who successfully used this technique with thousands of people in Europe. The Berard system of AIT has since become regarded as the most effective approach available for enhanced listening skills, language, learning, and sound tolerance.

Indications an individual could benefit from AIT

The following difficulties may present the opportunity to benefit from AIT:

- Poor attention
- Slower thinking and processing
- Difficulty listening, understanding and remembering incorrectly, understanding and following directions
- Brain "traffic jams" when processing sensory information
- Hindered ability to put ideas in sequence
- Sound hypersensitivity and hyposensitivity
- Low tolerance for distractions

Why is it important to retrain the system?

Dr. Guy Berard developed AIT as a procedure to retrain a disorganized auditory system that prohibits the efficient processing of information. AIT is relatively quick to administer, readily accepted by the individual, and requires minimum follow-up by other professionals. Berard AIT has important relevance for parents and educators of young children because the focus of this intervention is on retraining the system to improve its performance rather than teaching compensating strategies to help children cope with an inefficient system. By improving the performance of the auditory processing system, individuals benefit more from other education support services, and their rate of progress is increased.

Dr. Berard believes that auditory hypersensitivity and auditory distortions, sequencing problems, and delays in auditory contribute to inefficient learning. He states that AIT is a method of retraining the ear to listen and to process sounds in a more normal manner, without distortions and delays. How we listen to and process sounds affects our alertness, attention span, concentration, information processing, and the way we express ourselves verbally and in writing. When the listening process is not working properly, it can interfere with our entire system and its ability to function. All of these auditory problems contribute to the cognitive fatigue and variable performance that are so common among individuals with learning disabilities and ADHD. These individuals expend much energy trying to decode or translate the scrambled and distorted messages they receive. Their performance will depend upon the amount of energy, interest, and motivation they have at any given time. Other variables such as voice quality, pitch and rate of speech delivery of the speaker, background noises, and visual cues also impact the performance of these individuals.

Are there data to document results?

The Attention Deficit Disorders Evaluation Scale was used to monitor progress with 48 children who participated in AIT. Rapid improvement was seen in the first three months, with the median percentile reaching the 50th percentile, a gain of 24 percentile points. A pilot study was conducted at IDEA

Training Center, in North Haven, Connecticut, with a group of 14 children with varied diagnoses, but all with identified sensory integration difficulties, to see if the anecdotal reports of sensory improvements could be quantified.

The children participated in a standard program of AIT. Parents completed a sensory checklist prior to AIT, and then at one month, three months, and six months post-AIT.

The checklist contained items typically seen on sensory integration checklists and included areas such as vestibular hypersensitivity, vestibular hyposensitivity, tactile discrimination, self-regulation, play interactions, etc. At the end of six months post-AIT, the median percent of improvement was a 79 percent decrease in sensory problems. This means that half of the children achieved even better than 79 percent improvement and half of them did not achieve that much.

How can I find a Berard AIT Practitioner?

To learn more about whether AIT may be a useful intervention for someone you care for, visit www. IdeaTrainingCenter.com or contact Ms. Brockett to discuss your situation. To locate a Berard AIT practitioner, visit www.Dr. GuyBerard.com. This site provides a list of International Instructors of AIT.

Contributing Author Sally Brockett, M.S., Southern Connecticut State University—Ms. Brockett is the Director of the IDEA Training and Consultation Center in North Haven, Connecticut. She founded the Center in 1992 to focus on interventions for developmental disabilities after 12 years as a special education teacher with all categories of disabilities. After she trained in France with Dr. Guy Berard, the Berard method of auditory integration training (AIT) and consultation became a special focus of her work. Ms. Brockett is a founding member of the Society for Auditory Intervention Techniques (SAIT) and has served on the Board of Directors since its beginning. She is the current president of the society. Ms. Brockett is a frequent presenter at state and national conferences. She is on the Professional Advisory Board for the Developmental Delay Resources and president of the Autism Society of Connecticut South Central Region.

MUSIC THERAPY AND ASD

He stares at his hands as they twirl his favorite toy. His mom looks at him with love in her eyes and begins to move closer to him as the music builds in rhythm and verbal cuing. Repetitive words are sung, such as "Joshua is moving, his mom is moving, their hands are touching and they start dancing." The mom reaches for her son's left hand as he continues to manipulate his toy in his right hand. Her hand begins to move to the improvised song that continues to mimic the couple's every move, including the emotion that is so evident. Suddenly her son drops his toy, clasps both of his mom's hands, and begins to jump up and down around the entire living room. Fleeting moments of eye contact ensue between the two. Later, the mom comments that this would be one of the few close interactions they would experience that day. A neighbor looking through the window would see an energetic child and a smiling mother.

Research has shown that music can be an engaging and attractive stimulus for children with autism. Several studies have documented music therapy as a successful treatment modality to engage the child in social, emotional, cognitive, communication, and motor learning activities. People with diagnoses on the autism spectrum often demonstrate a natural affinity to music, making it an excellent therapeutic tool to develop all areas of self.

The above music therapy session is but one example of a family being affected by the relational qualities of music. Music therapists around the world are facilitating sessions in a variety of styles with the same primary aim: for individuals with autism to experience a heightened opportunity for learning, community contribution, and personal growth. Some therapists, like in the scenario described above, strongly support the entire family unit by encouraging family members to participate in weekly sessions. Other music therapy opportunities include peer group therapy and individual sessions. Music therapy, once a "fringe" form of care for persons with autism, is becoming ever more viable and popular with this special population.

Although music therapists around the world use different methods, there are some universal themes in their approach when working with individuals with autism. They consistently emphasize two main areas of importance in their work: (1) the use of improvised music, and (2) the relationship between the therapist and the client through a shared musical experience. Within these broad goals, music therapists work in a variety of ways, often influenced by theoretical models of music therapy and related professions.

The music therapist uses improvised music to reflect back and build on sounds and movements made by the child, much the same way a parent communicates with their infant child. Therapists also initiate and direct through improvised and precomposed music interventions that support speech development, including vowels, speech blends, and phrasing. Call and response is also a popular technique, as music naturally supports inflection to indicate questions posed and answers.

Some music therapists highlight active music making as the main therapeutic agent leading to changes in the child's emotional state: "The emotional life of a child is reached directly by music . . . if he stands at a drum, he is given sticks and asked to beat to the music, then immediately, as he becomes active, he becomes directly, personally involved in rhythmic activity and in musical experience. . . . As the child becomes actively engaged in such music he experiences its emotional content closely." (Nordoff, P. and Robbins, C. (1971). *Therapy in Music for Handicapped Children*. Page 50.)

Other music therapists believe that the therapy is "in the music," and that the relationship between client and therapist is solely a musical one. While others still see music not as the therapy itself, but as a means to a therapeutic end: "The act of playing is not the focus . . . . The focus is the relating and its meaning. The relating goes on whether there is playing or not, and the clue to the meaning is not hidden somewhere in the music, but in the shared experience of the therapist and patient." (John, D., 1995.) The therapeutic relationship in music therapy is a tool in the treatment of psychosis. (In: Wigram, T., Saperston, B. and West, R., eds. The Art and Science of Music Therapy: A Handbook. Page 160.)

No one model of working can be applied to every child, as each child responds in his own way. Work with one child may require sessions that focus on the child's emotional state, while work with another child may require a more structured, activity-based approach.

For 30 minutes a week, six young boys come together for music therapy. Starting in child-sized chairs and sitting next to their aides, the boys begin their familiar musical greeting to welcome one another by name, signaling the beginning of the session. They soon move into speech vocalizations and phrasings, concentrating on extending the breath. The aides encourage each child independently in a style that best suits the child, such as the use of PECS, face-to-face imitation, or quiet gestures. The music therapist continues to facilitate several interventions, including instrument improvisation and vocal and verbal practice through inflection, melody, and rhythm.

The boys each have different responses. For some, success is that they have stayed within a group context for five minutes. For others, it is that they have answered a closed question with no prompting or that they have selected an instrument and shaken it three times before passing it back to an aide. And for others, it is that they have selected an instrument, traded it with another child, then sat back in their chair indicating that they love music and their friend by their positive, smiling affect. The fact that many individuals with autism can participate successfully and often with others, in music activities, contributes to music therapy's value as an effective therapeutic tool for the child.

The following examples of music therapy interventions address key goals.

Speech/language development

Singing and speech share many similarities, yet are accessed differently by the brain. Language skills such as asking and answering questions, maintaining a conversation, and using new vocabulary are embedded in song lyrics that are repeated session to session.

Practicing oral-motor imitation exercises, to strengthen functional use of the lips, tongue, jaws, and teeth, are repeated through vocalization exercises (singing single or combinations of vowels and consonants, with proper inflection and breath support). Lining out a song (leaving out the last word or few words in a song sentence) supports memory development, comprehension, and sentence completion.

Social and emotional development

Every instrument possesses a personality and, depending on how it is played, can reflect or demonstrate many emotions. A percussion instrument may also provide a point of mutual contact between the therapist and the child when other attempts at social interaction are rejected or unnoticed.

Cognitive development

Songs aid in memory of new or challenging academic concepts by organizing information into smaller pieces, making them easier to translate and retain.

Music engages children in an optimal learning environment, especially those who may be easily distracted. Educational research supports the idea that our ability to learn and later use new concepts and information is strongest when we are motivated by meaningful material presented to us. Melodies and rhythm are useful in teaching language concepts, body image, and self-help skills.

Motor development

Research is highly conclusive in supporting rhythm as an external time-keeper for movement. Music therapy is often recommended as a direct intervention for students with severe physical impairment or basic goals such as imitating movement. In these cases, musical instruments are used with song cueing to target various grasps, improve coordination, and increase duration of participation.

They are swaying again. Not to a greeting this time, but to the closing melody. A personalized song that says, "You are wonderful, amazing, beautiful, and I am so lucky to be with you." The music therapist adds a special line today: "and together we find happiness, we are happy together, and Mommy loves you so much."

The training of a music therapist involves a full-degree curriculum of music classes, along with selected courses in psychology, special education, and anatomy, with specific core courses and field experiences in music therapy. Following coursework, students complete a clinical internship and a written accreditation file or board exam. Registered music therapy professionals must then maintain continuing education credits to remain current in their practice. For more information in Canada, visit www.musictherapy.ca. For more information in the U.S., visit www.musictherapy.org.

Contributing Author Jennifer Buchanan is an Accredited Music Therapist (MTA) from Calgary, Alberta, and past president of the Canadian Association for Music Therapy. She is a frequent guest lecturer at national conferences, universities, and association meetings as well as an author. Ms. Buchanan has inspired and developed many music therapy programs in schools, universities, health care facilities, and private and government centers, through her long-established company, JB Music Therapy. To learn more about JB Music Therapy, visit www.jbmusic.ca.

REACHING THE CHILD WITH AUTISM THROUGH ART

I wrote the book *Reaching the Child with Autism through Art* to help general education art teachers include students on the autism spectrum in their classes. Too often children on the autism spectrum are "left out" of art class because they are difficult to reach. The lessons in this book have been "autism tested" and given the "lick, sniff, twiddle" seal of approval by children with autism everywhere.

From the introduction

Art is a feeling, an aura, a pleasant memory.

Art is an expression of self. A state of mind. An act not always recorded.

There should be no failure in art—only the release of creativity.

All children benefit from art, but children on the autism spectrum in particular, who may experience difficulties with communication, social interaction, and sensory perceptions, can benefit from the creativity and good feelings art produces.

Art leads the child in a positive direction.

Art helps in the development of a positive self-image. Art also helps to develop:

- Figure–ground discrimination
- Concept development
- Spatial relationships
- Form discrimination
- Sequencing
- Fine motor skills
- Directionality
- Cause and effect
- Body in space

- Perceptual motor skills
- Tactile/kinesthetic awareness
- Attention span
- Pride in accomplishment
- An appreciation of beauty in the environment

Art, as I perceive it, does not always have to result in "something to take home." When there is a finished product, it is for the pride of both the adult and the child. The act of doing is for the enjoyment and development of the child alone. While in college, I was fortunate enough to have an art instructor who did something all the students thought radical. He took away the brushes and canvas and made us use everyday objects in the creation of our art projects. There was resistance from the students at first. Then we started having fun. There was competition to see who could create the ugliest piece, and I won. I concocted a collage of cooked and uncooked popcorn, paint, and plastic bubbles on a background of fungus-ridden wood.

My mother, however, thought this was a beautiful piece of art. She displayed it proudly in her living room for years, until her house burned down. When the "work of art" was destroyed, you would have thought that she had lost a masterpiece. (When there is a finished product, it is for the pride of the parent.) Although the class set out to outdo each other in grossness, something strange happened. This approach to art released such a creative surge that I went on to make some hauntingly beautiful pieces using pictures of my grandmother's birthplace combined with string, sandpaper, and paint.

I got an A in the course, but I'll never forget my professor's comments as he surveyed my work. He said, "I don't know if this is the biggest collection of trash that I have ever witnessed, or if it is the birth of an artistic genius." I don't think this teacher ever knew the full impact of his course on me. Trash or artistic genius did not matter. The enjoyment and growth I experienced in that course changed the way I looked at the world around me. I began questioning, and I began trusting my abilities and instincts, instead of reaching for comfortable truths.

Through my long and varied positions within education, I have found art to be a valuable component of many a child's education because they are all children first and foremost, not this disability or that. Always teach to the child's ability, not their disability.

Experiencing art should lead to an unfolding awareness of self and the environment.

To grow, To expand,
To begin building trust within yourself, and to have fun doing it,
To me, that is ART!

Reaching the Child with Autism through Art is divided into collage, painting, play, and sculpture experiences.

Each experience is in an easy-to-read format with Objectives, Choices, Suggested Directions, and Notes. Many optional suggestions are included to take into account a child's individual needs. For example, if a child is tactile, defensive, and doesn't want to engage in messy activities, he or she can wear rubber gloves while finger painting.

Contributing Author Toni Flowers is an award-winning educator whose work with autistic children won her the Autism Society of America's coveted Teacher of the Year award in 1989. *You can write to Ms. Flowers at tflowers@jcs.k12.in.is.*

THE MOST OVERLOOKED SOLUTION TO A CHILD'S READING PROBLEMS

If your child has been diagnosed with an autism spectrum disorder, will you take just a moment and reply to the questions below?

Is your child disruptive or does he or she try to avoid near-point (close up) tasks? Does he or she have illegible handwriting, or write uphill or downhill on paper?

Does your child seem to have no depth perception or frequently bump into things? Does your child avoid all eye contact, choose not to look at the blackboard, have a stiff-legged walk, appear to overuse peripheral vision, or poke at the sides of the eyes? Does your child seem unable to catch even a large ball or appear to have other eye-hand coordination problems? If your child is reading, has he or she child complained that words on a page jump around, or skip lines when reading aloud? Does your child skip over the punctuation at the end of a sentence? Does your child seem to know a word on one page and not recognize the same word on the very next page?

If you answered yes to several of these questions, then your child may have an undetected visual/perceptual problem that may have been mistaken for normal "autistic" behaviors. If this is the case, as you read on, you will learn how these problems may be easily corrected with the proper diagnosis and visual activities treatment.

If you have ever taken your child for a regular eye exam, you may have been told that he/she has 20/20 vision and naturally assume that they have the ability to read easily or can participate in sport activities with no problems. In addition, you may think that all of the other behaviors listed above are simply "autistic" in nature and must require behavior modification or can be taught with numerous repetitions. This may not be the case at all.

Why 20/20 eyesight is not good enough for your child

You may be surprised to learn that your child's 20/20 eyesight diagnosis (even with corrective lenses) is completely unrelated to reading or eye-hand coordination activities at near point. When your child covers one eye during an exam and reads a chart with letters at 20 feet away, he or she is using an outdated chart from the 1800s, known as the Snellen Chart, which simply says that your child can see a certain size letter from 20 feet away! This chart only measures clearness and sharpness of eyesight using a stationary target.

How many children read books from 20 feet away, and isn't there more to reading and sensory motor activities than distance at 20 feet away?

Eyesight and vision myth

It is important to know that your child needs both eyesight and strong vision to be able to read and perform everyday activities. Yes, few parents or teachers realize that eyesight and vision are very different skills. Eye doctors who specialize in learning-related vision disorders tell us why and how a treatment known as "vision therapy" can make a world of difference for your autistic child.

Eyesight, or the ability to see, is present at birth. Vision has to be learned as your child grows. Eye doctors who specialize in learning-related vision screenings tell us that vision is so complicated it involves about 20 visual abilities and more than 75 percent–90 percent of all pathways to the brain. Visual skills allow your child to comprehend and make meaning from what he or she sees.

When a child does a variety of activities, such as coloring, jigsaw puzzles, building blocks, playing with jacks, running, jumping, playing baseball or basketball, riding a bike, building forts, skating, and many more, he or she is learning skills that will make him or her a great reader later on.

Today, however, millions of children are doing very different things from those you did when you were a child. You are correct if you think they are indoors more of the time. They are sitting in front of a computer screen at a very young age (sometimes as early as age one), watching thousands of hours of television (studies show that children watch anywhere from three to seven hours of television per day), and playing video games for hours on end. Your autistic child may be hyperfocused on small things for untold hours.

While these indoor activities may have some value, when too excessive they actually limit your child's visual development and will cause reading problems in the future. The human visual system is not designed for constant near-point activities. Your child may develop so much visual stress, he or she will have to work twice as hard to get the same results as other kids. In addition, your child won't learn how to develop eye movement skills like tracking (so they can read smoothly and not skip a line), eye-focusing skills, eye-aiming skills, visual perception, peripheral vision, eye-hand coordination (involved in playing sports, copying from the book to the paper or from the board to the paper), right-left directionality (know the difference between a, b, and d and p and q), and much more.

When your child enters school or is reading at home, his or her visual problems may actually worsen. Children are required to read far more material than you ever had to as a child. The demand on their visual systems is much heavier than it was for you. Since visual skill testing is limited or absent, and your child may not be able to verbalize what he or she is feeling, you also have no way of knowing whether there is further stress on the visual system like eye turns or lazy eye, both of which make reading and other activities very painful and difficult.

Thus, if you have an autistic child, "normal" autistic behaviors such as looking through or beyond objects, aversion to light, lack of reciprocal play, fear of heights, poor reading skills, or inability to participate in sports activities may all be related to a weak visual system. This system is so critical to behavior and reading that it can impact nearly every activity your child does.

The following chart shows the relationship between vision skills and everyday tasks your child performs.

Why your child must have a comprehensive learning-related vision exam and follow-up vision therapy activities, if prescribed.

Since eyesight and vision are at the very core of your child's ability to read and learn many activities, it is critical that you provide your child with a compre-

VISIONS SKILLS NEEDED FOR TYPICAL READING, CLASSROOM, AND OTHER TASKS

Classroom Tasks	Tracking	Visual Memory	Figure Ground	Eye Movement Control/Fixation	Simultaneous Focusing At Near	Simultaneous Focusing At Far	Sustaining Focusing At Near	Sustaining Focusing At Far	Eye Teaming/Sustaining Alignment At Near	Eye Teaming/Sustaining Alignment At Far	Central Vision	Peripheral Vision	Depth Awareness	Color Retention and/or Contrast	Gross Visual Motor	Fine Visual Motor	Visual Perception/Directionality/Closure	Eye Hand Coordination	Simultaneous Alignment At Near	Simultaneous Alignment At Far
Reading	X	X	X	X	X		X		X		X	X	?			X	X		X	
Copying (CB to Desk)	X	X	X	X	X	X					X	X			X	X	X	X	X	X
Copying (At Desk)	X	X	X	X	X		X		X		X	X			X	X	X	X	X	
Writing	X	X	X	X	X		X		X		X	X		X		X	X	X	X	
Discussion	X	X	X				X				X	X					X			X
Demonstration	X	X	X	X		X					X	X	X	?	X		X			X
Movies, TV	X	X	X	X		X		X		X	X	X	?				X			X
P.E., Dancing	X	X	X	X	X	X		X	X	X	X	X	X		X		X	X		X
Arts, Crafts	X	X	X	X	X		X	X	X		X	X	X	X		X	X	X	X	
Play	X	X	X	X	X	X	X	X	X	X	X	X	X	X	X	X	X	X	X	X
Computers	X	X	X	X	X		X	X	X		X	X				X	X	X	X	
Taking Notes	X	X	X	X	X		X				X	X				X	X	X	X	

hensive, learning-related vision exam before embarking on other therapies. A number of "autistic" symptoms may be a vision problem in disguise.

Specially trained optometrists, known as developmental or behavioral optometrists, can properly diagnose and treat your child. Once your child has this exam, he or she may be prescribed a very specific series of exercises and visual activities, and you may be very surprised to discover that many of the behaviors you thought were "autistic" in nature improve or disappear altogether.

For more information on vision therapy, download the Eye-Q Reading Inventory at www.howtolearn.com/ireadisucceed.html, administer it to your child, and visit the website listed on the Inventory to find a doctor in your area who can give your child the comprehensive, learning-related vision exam he or she deserves. If you choose to do some of the vision activities at home, you can find out more by taking a look at the I Read I Succeed Program, already proven to help thousands of autistic children improve their reading and behavioral abilities.

Contributing Author Pat Wyman, M.A.—Pat Wyman is known as America's Most Trusted Learning Expert. She is a university instructor of Education, Reading Specialist, and author of several books, including the *Instant Learning™* series, *Learning vs Testing, What's Food Got To Do With It? 101 Natural Remedies for Learning Disabilities*, and a noted expert who testifies on vision screen legislation. She has developed the Eye-Q Reading Inventory and the I Read I Succeed Program and is the founder of a nonprofit organization dedicated to helping all children read at or above grade level at www.ireadisucceed.org. Ms. Wyman is an expert on the www.autismtoday.com website, a frequent guest on radio and television, and has been interviewed on reading improvement, learning, and learning styles in magazines such as *Nickelodon's Nick Jr. Family Magazine* and *Family Circle Magazine*. Ms. Wyman is the founder and CEO of the award-winning website www.howtolearn.com, where you can give your child her Personal Learning Styles Inventory and find out more about her mission to help children succeed in reading, learning, and life.

SCOTOPIC SENSITIVITY SYNDROME AND THE IRLEN LENS SYSTEM

There is growing evidence, based on both research and personal reports, that many autistic individuals see their world in a maladaptive, dysfunctional manner. Researchers at UCLA and the University of Utah have found evidence of abnormal retinal activity in autistic individuals. Additionally, there are many visual problems that are often associated with autism, such as reliance on peripheral vision, tunnel vision, hypersensitivity to light, and stereotypic (repetitive) behavior near the eyes, such as hand flapping and finger flicking. Donna Williams, an autistic adult, has written several books about her life and has often commented on her vision. She once wrote: "Nothing was whole except the colours and sparkles in the air . . ." and "I had always known that the world was fragmented. My mother was a smell and a texture, my father a tone, and my older brother was something which moved about."

Scotopic Sensitivity/Irlen Syndrome is a visual-perceptual problem that occurs in some people with learning/reading disorders, autism, and other developmental disorders. People with Scotopic Sensitivity/Irlen Syndrome experience "perceptual stress" that can lead to a variety of perceptual distortions when reading and/or viewing their environment. Scotopic Sensitivity is triggered by one or more components of light, such as the source of the light (e.g., fluorescent lighting, sun), luminance (e.g., reflection, glare), intensity (i.e., brightness), wavelength (i.e., color), and/or color contrast. As a result, the person may experience:

- Light sensitivity: bothered by brightness, glare, types of lighting
- Inefficient reading: letters on page move, dance, vibrate, jiggle
- Inadequate background accommodation: difficulty with high contrast
- Restricted span of recognition: tunnel vision or difficulty reading groups of letters
- Lack of sustained attention: difficulty maintaining attention

The Irlen Lens System, developed by Helen Irlen, was designed to treat Scotopic Sensitivity/Irlen Syndrome. Helen Irlen has developed two methods to treat Scotopic Sensitivity: (1) the use of colored transparencies or overlays to improve reading, and (2) tinted glasses to improve visual perception of his/her environment.

Transparencies

Transparencies or overlays are used to reduce perceptual stress while reading. For some people, letters/words on a page are not perceived clearly and/or not perceived in a stable manner (i.e., letters and words appear to move). White backgrounds, the most common, may overtake and dominate the perceptual system, and the black print of the text may fade into the background. Other symptoms may include having difficulty reading for relatively long periods of time, developing headaches, and feeling dizzy. It is possible that, for some, the high contrast between black print on a white background provides excessive stimulation to the visual system and thus interferes with the reading process.

In the Irlen Lens System, colored transparencies are placed over printed text with the result that these problems may be reduced or eliminated. A colored overlay, such as a light blue transparency placed over the text, will reduce the contrast between black and white as well as reduce the dominance of the white background. The optimal color of the transparency required depends upon each person's unique visual-perceptual system.

Glasses

In addition to reading problems, people with Scotopic Sensitivity/Irlen Syndrome may have difficulty perceiving their surroundings. Many autistic individuals wear tinted glasses, which were prescribed by Helen Irlen or at one of her 76 worldwide diagnostic clinics. They have reported rather remarkable benefits. After wearing her glasses, Donna Williams wrote: "These [Irlen] glasses would have changed all that. Faces and body parts and voices would have been whole and understood within a context of equally conjoined surroundings." Other autistic individuals report seeing better, feeling more relaxed, being less bothered by sunlight and/or indoor lighting, and have fewer perceptual distortions that can affect small and gross motor coordination.

Helen Irlen has developed effective methods for determining if a person suffers from Scotopic Sensitivity/Irlen Syndrome. She has also designed a standardized set of procedures that can be used to determine the correct color prescription for the transparency and the tinted lenses.

For more information, write to Irlen Institute/PLD, 5380 Village Road, Long Beach, California 90808, U.S.A. or Irlen_Institute@compuserve.com

---

Contributing Author Stephen M. Edelson, Ph.D., Experimental Psychology— Dr. Edelson has worked in the field of autism for 25 years. He is the director of the Center for the Study of Autism in Salem, Oregon, which is affiliated with the Autism Research Institute in San Diego, CA. He is also on the Board of Directors of the Oregon chapter of the Autism Society of America and is on the Society's Professional Advisory Board. His main autism website is www .autism.org.

Helen Irlen has trained people throughout the world in the use of her methods.

VARIOUS EDUCATIONAL APPROACHES TO CONSIDER

The autism bomb hits the mark, and life is never the same again for the person on the autism spectrum or for the family members, educators, doctors and others who provide support. The first questions that bubble up are: "What should I do?" and "What is the best intervention for my child with autism?" During the mid-1960s there were very few choices for a child who became non-verbal, had tantrums, and very little body-to-environmental awareness. At that time an autism diagnosis was considered as a sentence to a life of dependency with either family members or in an institution. Perhaps, with luck and a lot of hard work, employment in a sheltered workshop was a possibility.

Interventions

There are now myriad interventions, approaches and techniques for working with children on the autism spectrum. Many parents and others who support people with autism wonder which one is the best? Is it Applied Behavioral Analysis (ABA) as originally developed by Ivar Lovaas? What about the Treatment and Education of Autistic and related Communication handicapped Children (TEACCH)? Is Developmental Individual-Difference Relation-Based intervention (DIR), often referred to as "Floortime," better than Relational Developmental Intervention (RDI)? And then there is Daily Life Therapy (DLT), developed in Japan and available in the Boston area for the past two decades. There's also the Miller Method (MM), which has been developed over the past 40 years.

I haven't even gotten to techniques such as Powercards, Sensory Integration, Picture Exchange System. What about all those biomedical interventions, such as gluten/casein Free diets, chelation and other heavy metal detoxifications? Re-framing the quest for the best methodology to "Which methodology is best for this person at this time?" will be much more helpful.

Although all well-designed approaches and techniques should be considered when supporting a person with autism, for purposes of space I shall concentrate on the educational/behavioral methods and save the others for future exploration.

Six educational approaches

We shall look at six promising methodologies for working with children on the autism spectrum as mentioned above: ABA, TEACCH, Daily Life Therapy, DIR, the Miller Method, and RDI. When implemented by competent professionals well versed in both the method and the characteristics of the child they are working with, all of these approaches can offer great benefit. The challenge is to match the method to the child's needs as close as possible. This decision has to be made by the parents and/or other significant caretaker along with others who are familiar with both the child's needs and the methods available.

Given that autism initially was thought to be behavioral in nature (Rutter, 1999), the behavioral method is the oldest of approaches. The ease of measuring and assessing physical behavior also contributes to the popularity of this method. Although commonly thought of as a method even though it is not, the Treatment and Education of Autistic and Communication Handicapped Children (TEACCH) places its main thrust on preparing the person with autism to function in the typical community and work environment. A third approach, Daily Life Therapy, as developed by Dr. Kiyo Kitahara (1984), of Tokyo, takes a more Platonic (1968) view by stressing an order of the physical, emotional and intellectual parts of the child. Further, the pharmacological approach sees autism as stemming from chemical imbalances that can be corrected via medication. An offshoot of this approach is the use of medicine to address secondary psychological issues such as excess anxiety and depression that can arise from being on the autism spectrum. The developmental models more closely address the developmental delay aspects of the autism spectrum. Believing that those with autism get stuck at a particular developmental level, progress is encouraged by techniques to spur development on.

Developmental Individual-Difference Relation-Based intervention (DIR), of which Floortime is a part, as developed by Stanley Greenspan, stresses building an emotional bond (Greenspan & Wieder, 1998) with the child, whereas the Miller Method, while sharing a developmental component with DIR, takes a more cognitive-systems approach with the implementation of elevated structures (Miller & Eller-Miller, 1989; 2000). RDI takes many concepts of the Miller Method for developing fluency in experience sharing activities and relationships with others.

The behavioral approach

The behavioral approach, Applied Behavioral Analysis (ABA), is based on operant conditioning that is originally derived largely from the work of Pavlov and Skinner (A. Miller, personal communication, July, 1999). Heavily influenced by the work of these behaviorally oriented psychologists, Dr. Ivar Lovaas began work in the 1960s (Sallows & Tamlynn, 1999) and developed a variant of this behavioral method that is sometimes referred to as the Lovaas Method.

The behavioral methods are concerned with examining and shaping the visible actions of the person being worked with. In the strictest sense, the brain is viewed as a black box with inputs (antecedents) that result in behaviors that are either reinforced or extinguished by ignoring unwanted behaviors or providing negative consequences. The work of the behavioral-cognitivists such as Edward Tolman (1960) expands the behavioral model to include more cognitive developmental and environmental aspects of a person's existence. A very useful concept developed and used extensively by practitioners of the behavioral methods is the concept of Antecedent, Behavior, and Consequence when conducting a Functional Behavioral Analysis.

Treatment & education of autistic and communication handicapped children

A program known as the Treatment and Education of Autistic and Communication Handicapped Children (TEACCH) is often erroneously thought of as a method. However, it is a public health program of services that is available in North Carolina for autistic people. It makes use of several techniques and methods in various combinations depending upon the individual person's needs and emerging capabilities (Trehin, 1999). Like other reputable approaches to working with people on the autism spectrum, TEACCH does not claim to cure autism but strives to allow them as much independence as possible in the world around them. Concentrating on the strengths of a person with autism, as opposed to the person's weaknesses, the major thrust of TEACCH reaches toward the improvement of communication skills and autonomy to the maximum of the child potential (Trehin, 1999). Education is used as the medium to achieve that goal. Although the shaping of behavior is an important aspect of the program, behavior is not treated directly as in behavior modification. Rather, TEACCH strives to understand and deal with the underlying causes for any aberrant behavior (Trehin, 1999).

Daily Life Therapy

Daily Life Therapy was developed by Dr. Kiyo Kitahara of Tokyo in the 1960s. Originally a regular kindergarten school teacher, she derived her method from working with a child with autism who was included in her classroom (Kitahara, 1984).

Placing heavy emphasis on group dynamics, the method incorporates physical education, art, music and academics, along with the acquisition and development of communication and daily living skills (Boston Higashi School, 1999). Specifically, Dr. Kitahara's method focuses on social isolation, anxiety, hypersensitivity and hyposensitivity, and the apparent fragility of children with autism.

According to Dr. Kitahara (1984), stability of emotions is gained through the pursuit of independent living and development of self-esteem. Mastery of self-care skills allows for the development of self-confidence and a desire to attempt other adaptive skills. The second focal point, extensive physical exercise, is used to establish a rhythm of life. Many of the exercises are founded upon principles of sensory integration and vestibular stimulation that lead to coordination and co-operative group interaction.

Vigorous exercise releases endorphins, which help reduce anxiety. In addition, exercise has been found to reduce incidences of self-stimulatory behavior and aggression (Allison, Basile, & MacDonald, 1991; Elliot, Dobbin, Rose, & Soper, 1994; Koegel & Koegel, 1989), along with hyperactivity and night wakefulness while increasing time on task. Children also learn how to control their bodies as they master riding a bicycle, rollerblading, the balance disk and other Higashi exercises. Physical education is carried out in different-sized groups, thus serving as a bridge to social development. Stimulation of the intellect with academics, including language arts, math, social studies and science is compatible with typical school curricula to prepare each student for inclusion opportunities. In the Higashi program, medication is not recognized as a therapeutic technique for working with children on the autism spectrum. Finally, art and music provide opportunities to gain mastery and appreciation for aesthetics.

Developmental Individual-difference Relation-based intervention

Developed by Stanley Greenspan, "Floortime"—which is a part of DIR—is an interactive-developmental approach for working with children with autism. As indicated in The Child with Special Needs (Greenspan, 1998), Floortime is based on heavy parental involvement. The method strives to bring the child through the six developmental milestones of self-regulation and interest in the world, intimacy, two-way communication, complex communication, emotional ideas, and emotional thinking through ever-expanding circles of communication.

This intensive one-on-one method involves a three-part therapeutic approach. The parents are employed to help their child master developmental milestones. The entire program revolves around this component. The second leg consists of specialists, such as speech pathologists, occupational and physical therapists, educators and/or psychologists, who use Floortime techniques to deal with specific challenges and to facilitate development. The third part relates back to the parents who work on their own responses and styles for working with the child. Floortime is similar to ordinary play with the child, except that the child's partner plays a very active developmental role. The parent or professional in a Floortime session takes the child's lead but does so in a way that encourages the child to interact. The parent or clinician actively follows the child by building on what the child does. It is structured in such a way that the child needs to communicate with the other person.

The Miller Method

The Miller method, which embodies developmental, cognitive, and systems components, builds on the work of Heinz Werner, Jean Piaget, Lev Vygotsky and Ludwig von Bertalanffy (Miller & Eller-Miller, 1989). The developmental aspect of the approach looks at children with autism spectrum disorder as being completely or partially stuck at earlier stages of development and therefore structures its interventions to spur on development. The cognitive aspect strives to promote cognitive development by structuring the environment so as to be conducive to increased cognitive development. This emphasis on thought processes contrasts with other, more behaviorally oriented approaches, which devote most of their focus to stimuli and response as the explanations of the way child with autism functions in the world. Finally, the systems address the roles systems play in restoring normal development in two ways. The first is to build on the repetitive behaviors (systems) the children have managed to achieve. A system is defined as a coherent organization (functional or non-functional) of behavior involving an object or event (A. Miller, personal communication, July, 1999). Systems range from quite small (mini-systems) such as flicking light switches on and off to quite elaborate such as taking groceries from a bag and putting them where they belong in cupboard or refrigerator (A. Miller, personal communication, July, 1999). The hall-mark of a successfully formed system is a desire in the child to continue the activity after it has been interrupted. The second way is to teach children certain behaviors by introducing repetitive activities. These activities or systems are designed to teach behaviors to a child who has not been able to otherwise develop them spontaneously by him or herself. (Miller & Eller-Miller, 1985)

The use of elevation in working with children on the autism spectrum is a technique unique to the Miller Method. Dr. Miller has created a series of devices designed to make it possible for very disordered children to function in a goal-directed manner unavailable to them on the ground. When obstacles and sign language are introduced with these structures, they make it possible for disordered children to understand and use signs and spoken words for the first time. (Miller & Eller-Miller, 1985)

The idea of using elevated structures was discovered by accident after Dr. Miller observed some children on the autism spectrum playing on a construction site. A child known for rocking and being relatively unaware of his environment was seen moving from rock to rock in a goal-directed manner across a ditch. Upon reaching one side, he would turn around and go back to the other side. Struck by the contrast between the child's encapsulated rocking and his goal-directed manner of crossing the ditch, Dr. Miller and his wife placed a plank across the ditch and guided the child gently across it. (Miller & Eller-Miller, 1989). The two were amazed as this deeply involved child with autism crossed the ditch with the same directed intensity he exhibited while working his way from rock to rock across the ditch a few moments before.

Shortly thereafter, they started working with children as they stood on and walked across planks set up between tables. The Millers noticed an increased "awareness and sudden increase in intention" (p. 23) as the child proceeded across the board. This awareness seemed to be as a result of an edge experience that occurs when people find themselves in a precarious situation.

Another unique feature of the Miller Method is that it works in a way that honors the need for repetitive actions and routines and issues of sensory sensitivities affecting the child with autism. Miller maintains that "each child, no matter how disordered, is still trying to make sense of the environment" (Miller, http://www. millermethod. org, 1999); even the smallest piece of functioning will be exploited to lead the child from a reliance on ritualistic behaviors to developing a set of functional repertoires. In addition, the method appears well suited for working with the diverse range of presentation that exists within the autism spectrum.

Relational Development Intervention

Relational Development Intervention is a six-stage model treatment approach developed by Steven Gutstein designed to teach people with autism to participate in experience-sharing interactions, as opposed to being solely restricted to instrumental social interaction.(Gutstein, 2000) Instrumental social interaction relies on rote scripts and is conducted to obtain a specific endpoint.

In other words, people serve as "instruments" or the means to an end in order to obtain something we want—like information, money, food, or any other commodity. One such example is ordering a hamburger from a McDonald's cashier. The challenge is to lead this population towards experiencing sharing interaction where people are related to as ends unto themselves, in order to create common experiences. Experiences sharing interactions introduce novelty and variety in our lives. An example of such an experience might be two friends deciding to take a walk in the woods for the sheer beauty of seeing the trees.

Conclusion

I have only barely begun to scratch the surface in describing some of the salient aspects of six methodologies for working with children on the autism spectrum. Additionally, there are many other approaches for helping those with autism. It is only with complete and unbiased information that parents, educators and others who support people on the autism spectrum can make informed decisions on the best approach or combination of methods for educating persons on the autism spectrum.

It is also important to realize that no matter how effective these methods are for developing ways for people on the autism spectrum to function in society, there will always be residuals of the autistic condition that make their presence known. Some examples include difficulty with subtle social situations, such as office politics, facial recognition, sensory issues, and using multiple modalities simultaneously when taking in information and dealing with tasks that involve unstructured information such as remembering directions to a location or a shopping list of items.(Grandin, 1995; Williams, 1992)

Our goal should be to help persons with autism understand and use their strengths to work around any presenting challenges so they, just like everyone else, has an equal chance at living a fulfilling and productive life.

For more information, visit Mr. Shore's web site, www.autismasperger.net/.

References

Allison, D.B., Basile, V.C., & MacDonald, R.B. (1991).Brief report: Comparative effects of antecedent exercise and larazapam on the aggressive behavior of an autistic man. *Journal of Autism and Developmental Disorders*, 21, 89–94.

Boston Higashi School. (1999). Daily life therapy. *In Daily life therapy guidelines* (p. 23). Randolph, MA.

Elliot, R.O., Jr., Dobbin, A.R. Rose, G.D., & Soper, H.V. (1994). Vigorous, aerobic exercise versus general motor training activities: Effects on maladaptive and stereotypic behaviors of adults with both autism and mental retardation. *Journal of Autism and Developmental Disorders*, 24, 565–574.

Grandin, T. (1996). *Thinking in pictures: And other reports from my life with autism*. New York: Vintage Press.

Greenspan, S. & Wieder, S. (1998). *The child with special needs: Encouraging intellectual and emotional growth*. Reading, MA: Addison Wesley.

Gutstein, S. (2000). *Autism Aspergers: Solving the relationship puzzle: A new developmental program that opens the door to lifelong social & emotional growth*. Arlington, TX: Future Horizons.

Kitahara, K. (1983). *A method of educating autistic children: Daily life therapy: Record of actual education at Musashino Higashi Gakuen School, Japan*. Brookline, MA: Nimrod Press

Koegel, R. L., & Koegel, L. K. (1989). Community-referenced research on self-stimulation. In E. Cipani (Ed.), *The treatment of severe behavior disorders. Behavior analysis approaches* (pp. 129–150). Washington, DC: American Association on Mental Retardation (Monograph No. 12).

Lovaas, I. O., & Simmons, J. Q. (1969). Manipulation of self-destruction in three retarded children. *Journal of Applied Behavior Analysis, 2*, 143–157.

Miller, A. & Eller-Miller, E. (1989). *From ritual to repertoire: A cognitive-developmental systems approach with behavior-disordered children*. New York: Wiley-Interscience.

Miller, A. and Eller-Miller, E. (November, 2000). "The Miller Method: A Cognitive-Developmental Systems Approach for Children with Body Organization, Social and Communication Issues". Chapter 19.(pp 489–516) in (Eds.) Greenspan, S & Weider, S. *ICDL Clinical Practices Guidelines: Revising the standards of practice for infants, toddlers and children with developmental challenges*.

Plato. (1968). *The republic of Plato*, (2nd ed). Translated by Allan Bloom.

Reading, MA: Basic Books.

Rutter M. (1999). "The Emanuel Miller Memorial Lecture 1998. Autism: Two-way interplay between research and clinical work." *Journal of Child Psychology and Psychiatry and Allied Disciplines*, 40, 169–188.

Sallows, G., & Tamlynn, D. (1999). Replicating Lovaas' treatment and findings: Preliminary results. In Autism 99 Conference. Available: www .autism99.org/html/pmpapers/Frames/fr_nav_mainpage_to.cfn.

Tolman, E. (1960). *Purposive behavior in animals and men.* In Century Psychology Series. New York: Irvington Publishers.

Trehin, P. (1999) *Some Basic Information about TEACCH.* Available: web.syr .edu/~jmwobus/autism/papers/TEACCHN.htm#Section_0.1.

Williams, D. (1994). *Nobody nowhere: The remarkable autobiography of an autistic girl.* London: Jessica Kingsley Publisher

Contributing Author Stephen Shore, Ed.D., Boston University—Diagnosed with "Atypical Development with strong autistic tendencies," Mr. Shore was viewed as "too sick" to be treated on an outpatient basis and recommended for institutionalization. Nonverbal until four, and with much help from his parents, teachers and others, he is now completing his doctoral degree in special education at Boston University with a focus on helping people on the autism spectrum develop their capacities to the fullest extent possible. In addition to working with children and talking about life on the autism spectrum, Mr. Shore presents and consults internationally on adult issues pertinent to education, relationships, employment, advocacy and disclosure, as discussed in his book *Beyond the Wall: Personal Experiences with Autism and Asperger's Syndrome,* and *Ask and Tell: Self-advocacy and Disclosure for People on the Autism Spectrum*, and numerous other writings. A board member of the Autism Society of America, he serves as board president of the Asperger's Association of New England as well as for the Board of Directors for Unlocking Autism, the Autism Services Association of Massachusetts, MAAP, and the College Internship Program.

THE MULTI-TREATMENT APPROACH TO AUTISM

"The whole is greater than the sum of its parts"

Note: This article is based on an earlier one that I wrote and published in *The Autism File USA* magazine, Issue 30, 2009. And while I have modified and updated it, and added a few new ideas, the main challenges that parents faced in 2009 in navigating the field of autism treatments, frustratingly, remain the same many years later. I have hope, though, that the field will soon recognize the enhanced value that an integrated multi-treatment approach can have.

A young couple sits in a doctor's office. Both of them feel anxiety brewing in their stomachs. They have waited two months for this appointment. The doctor, from behind his desk, confirms their worst fears: with a certain neutrality of emotion, he explains a diagnosis of autism spectrum disorder for their three-year-old. After he negotiates their tears and shock, he hands them several brochures introducing them to local autism support centers along with a list of resources to contact and public services waiting lists they should sign up for. They have dozens of questions flooding into mind. At home, without even taking off their shoes or coats, they Google "Autism" . . . over 82 million links . . . where do they begin?

82 Million Choices

Sensory Integration Therapies and special "autism diets," socialization peergroups, Auditory Integration Therapy, Lovaas and Applied Behavior Analysis (ABA), early intervention, home-based, school-based, residential care, TEACCH, Boston's Higashi School, Irlen lenses, promises of a cure, vitamin B12, swimming with dolphins, acupuncture, play therapies, The Son-Rise Program, Relationship Development Intervention, Floortime, physical therapy, music therapy, equestrian therapy, and Integrated Multi-Treatment Intervention (IMTI) could all possibly play a role.

To add to the overwhelming number of choices parents have to make, the field of autism is, more than other professional fields, I would argue, particularly proprietary: "Our method works best. We understand your child best. Be careful about what others tell you." So, there are hundreds of choices, and . . . they are all the best! Each one promotes its success stories. They all have genuine endorsements from parents, including my program. So how should parents choose? Which is best for their son? Six months after the diagnosis, the couple is still spending its most valuable resource, time, on researching treatments, reading recommended books, making phone calls to check on waiting-list status, and feeling as confused and directionless as they had the first moment they heard the doctor say "autism."

Despite the rhetoric, most parents figure out at some point, one year or two or even three years after committing to a single approach, that their child's needs cannot be met by just one method. Parents learn quickly stereotyped repetitious behaviors all impact a wide range of developmental steps. The symptoms manifest across a spectrum. Each child is uniquely complex. The young couple observes their own son's range of ability and disability. In their search for answers, they recognize parts of their child in other families' anecdotes and testimonials, but never exactly the same. Ultimately, each family must design a unique "treatment map" for their child's uniquely complex disorder.

Parent as Director, Negotiator, Diplomat

And so this young couple begins to design a multi-disciplinary program for their child, and, like thousands of other parents, they find themselves in the role of negotiator and diplomat communicator between competing professionals. The physical therapist strongly recommends that the child get outside on the playground several times per day, but the intensive behavior therapist strongly recommends the child work indoors in 1-to-1 training for as many as 40 hours per week. Meanwhile, the local school principal and school psychologist are threatening that the child will suffer from lack of socialization if they are kept at home and not in school.

Parents are left to negotiate these different views and to fit the puzzle together. In what order do they fit best? All at once? And how much of each different treatment should a child receive; full-time, part-time, once per month, and how should a family distribute their limited financial resources among the myriad choices? If they can only afford two, which should they prioritize that will make the biggest difference?

A family I recently guided through this decision process explained, "We heard about some great success stories about kids on special diets and supplements; we'll put all of our money in that direction if you think it will work . . . but our doctor is pushing us to go ahead with the IBI training full-time if we can afford it. We're already stretched with finances and we're hoping you can help us figure out what we should do . . . we just want to do what is best for our son." This summarizes perfectly how every parent I've ever worked with feels.

During my twenty-five years working in autism treatment, this predicament that parents face hasn't changed. How is it possible that as a field of professionals we haven't collaborated enough to provide parents with a set of guidelines for how to choose amongst all of the therapies for their unique child? Yes, some organizations have drafted guidelines, mostly ABA associations that implore parents to only consider scientifically proven methods of which they continue to claim falsely that ABA is the only one. It's time the field moved toward more comprehensive and cooperative systems of treatment.

Parents of children with autism are already stretched well above maximum capacity; committed to loving and providing the best for their special child, they shouldn't also be put in the position of special education program designer, coordinator, and manager all while navigate through a field of such polarized professionals.

An Integrated Approach

Children with ASD and their families would benefit greatly from a next-generation treatment protocol: Integrated Multi-Treatment Interventions.

As diverse as the explanations and theories are of the causes of autism, we can agree that autism has a biological/physiological (body) component, a cognitive (mind) component, and a social/emotional (psychological) component, among others. I encourage parents to place various treatments they research into one of these three categories and to aim toward trying at least one from each. Some of course fit into more than one.

> *Current research supports the idea that the factors contributing to the behavior, communication, and learning challenges of people on the autism spectrum are multifaceted; therefore, I believe, treatment should be multifaceted, too.*

Some research on what is called "eclectic" treatment approaches doesn't support combining methods. However, in my opinion, these studies have not yet explored a truly integrated model such as IMTI. "Integrated" is the key word. There is still much to be learned about how to sew together complementary and sometimes seemingly diametrically opposed approaches into education and treatment. But concluding that it can't work just keeps us stuck in the same uncoordinated field. We have to figure this out.

Treatments such as ABA-based Behavioral Intervention (called IBI in Canada), play therapies such as Floortime, and The Son-Rise Program and biomedical treatments each specialize in a narrow yet important range of strategies. Each is based on a particular theory and etiology of autism and its treatment. More important, most of the highly specialized programs either do not interface with other possible complementary treatments or flat- out reject and criticize treatments that are different from their own. Some proponents of ABA, for example, have been fairly vocal in rejecting play therapies, biomedical treatments, and any other "not scientifically proven" approach. In the same way, ardent play therapists denounce behavioral methodologies as somehow less humane. Ironically, Dr. Ivar Lovaas himself, considered the pioneer of ABA, wrote in his seminal instruction manual, *The ME Book,* that ". . . no one approach will solve all the problems of developmentally disabled persons. Rather, the persons who try to help these individuals need to draw upon a variety of concepts and teaching techniques." Furthermore, "The 'teacher-therapist-parent' has to be flexible, innovative, and able to draw upon a variety of techniques and procedures"(p. 3, 1981).

With a nod to Dr Lovaas's prescient remarks, I believe that the extreme "we're right, you're wrong" positions simply aren't inclusive enough and that a diplomatic meeting in the middle would lead to a multifaceted approach that would be even more appropriate and more effective than any single approach alone.

There is top-tier research underlining the fact that children with autism require a range of supports. A group of America's leading psychologists and specialists surveyed and studied the field of autism treatment for more than a year and concluded, "No single intervention has been shown to deal effectively with problem behaviors for all children with autism." (Educating Children with Autism, National Research Council Report, 2001.) For many readers, this idea is neither new nor controversial. Yet, in my practice, I continue to hear on a weekly basis of parents who have been directed by their doctor or local autism information center to only consider ABA/IBI and to dismiss any other treatments as false hope and potentially harmful. I meet therapists and school officials often who sincerely believe that IBI is the only scientifically "proven" treatment; that special diets are all baseless fads; and that parents who find that massage calms their child down are most likely being taken advantage of by a quack therapist. Just last year, I participated in a funding meeting with an Ontario IBI service provider who has the authority to determine the direction of hundreds of children's programs. He leaned over in my direction, nudged me in confidence, and claimed that "Sensory Integration Therapy was known and proven to be not helpful, at best, and potentially harmful, at worst." He explained that he would definitely not approve (i.e., provide funding for) any home-based program that included Sensory Integration activities.

It is important to note that in the past five years or so, many service providers and professionals have begun to promote what is most often called a multidisciplinary approach to treatment. Teams of professionals from various disciplines usually include an ABA therapist, a physical or occupational therapist, a speech and language therapist, and a school psychologist, among others.

An individualized education/service plan is designed and implemented. While this is a huge step in the right direction, the various different therapies are typically provided separately from one another, often in separate locations by different therapists who are often not in daily communication. The design of the education plan is multidisciplinary, but the implementation and the actual educational experience of the student is anything but cohesive.

The Integrated Multi-Treatment Approach

After working in the field of autism for many years as a therapist, I was frustrated with having to choose to work in either one or another specific methodology. When I returned to Canada following twelve years of work and studies in the USA, for example, I was offered work with a provincial IBI service provider, but it was made clear to me that I would not be allowed to practice anything but strict IBI methods with the children. Years before, during a year of work abroad consulting for a US-based treatment center to about seventy-five families in the United Kingdom, I was reprimanded for spending too much of the allotted time talking about biomedical treatments rather than sticking exclusively to the center's proprietary treatment. In one particular case, it was painfully evident that the young boy of four years old whom I was hired to help needed medical attention. His bloated stomach, chronic constipation, and repetitive self-gagging, pushing his fingers down his throat, were all distracting him from gaining any benefit from the play therapy we were providing. Yet the restrictions of the play-therapy center limited my ability to best help this child and family.

With this as background, I finally created a new approach that draws from a "menu" of evidence-based strategies, methods, and programs called Integrated Multi-Treatment Intervention (IMTI), which from its inception has remained committed to being flexible and evolving as new research adds to our knowledge. For example, for some children I design a program that is heavily focused on play-therapy and socialization, while for others the emphasis is on a more structured curriculum-based IBI approach. Many have elements of both. The strength of the "IMTI effect," as I call it, is derived from the interaction between the diverse elements. Order and timing of the mix is critical.

Each program is unique, yet there are some principles that underlie the foundation of any successful multi-treatment design. The following is a description of some of these principles, further illustrated with anecdotes:

Learning is a biological process, so physical health must be the priority before behavioral training and cognitive education. Joshua had already been attending playschool. He was diagnosed with Pervasive Developmental Disorder (PDD) and was verbal, but he often struggled to pay attention. He was hyperactive and sometimes mixed up his words and thoughts. He didn't interact typically with his peers, and his parents agreed he was not ready for school. After reviewing his physical health history, including nutritional and diet details, I recommended that the amount of processed sugar be reduced in his diet. Along with replacing sugared snacks with fruits, vegetables, and natural foods (not without protests from Joshua and animated coaxing from us), Joshua's mother was careful to maintain his calorie intake and worked closely with their family doctor to monitor vital health indicators.

Four weeks later, at their monthly in-home training day, everyone agreed that Joshua's overall demeanor had changed positively. Throughout forty minutes of the therapy session, Joshua sat focused and still at the table as he cooperatively took turns with the Jenga building block game. He then followed his father's directions to try some sit-ups and push-ups for fun, and later he sat sweetly at his mother's side as they read a story together. Joshua was, without question, calmer with improved attention span. I also noted his language was less chaotic. Joshua still had many learning challenges to work through. The dietary changes were not a magic cure and did not resolve most of the issues he faced with his PDD, but by addressing Joshua's physical health first, he was able to attend more readily to the many hours of focused learning he needed to do to catch up to his peers. Using data collected from a medical lab, their family doctor will now take the next steps to design and implement a specific protocol to ensure that Joshua will continue to improve his physical health and, consequently, his studentship in the IMTI program.

Start by considering the physiological health of the child and possible underlying links to the autistic behavior. Under the supervision and direction of a medical doctor, biological treatment can kick-start a child's development and add momentum to the multi-treatment effect.

Learning happens more easily in cooperation with a teacher that a child trusts, feels respected by, and enjoys. As obvious as this principle is, surprisingly few models of therapy prioritize *maintaining* a positive and dynamic therapist-student relationship, after the initial get-to-know-you (pairing) phase. With socialization as a "core deficit" for people with ASD, it is especially crucial that caregivers and therapists engage people with autism in extremely thoughtful and respectful ways. Far too often, I have witnessed a therapy goal imposed upon a child against their will, in the face of protest, through struggle and conditional manipulation. The therapist prioritizes completing the treatment protocol over maintaining the integrity of the relationship. In that moment they believe that the target objective is somehow more important for the child to learn than their actual learning experience itself. Sadly, the experience of struggle and lack of trust push the child further from willing participation and further from wanting to learn.

I was once asked to review and provide feedback on a videoed sensory integration therapy session. A state-of-the-art day school for students with autism uploaded a video focused on one particular student as he was led through a multistation activity rotation in his school gymnasium. About ten minutes into the video, the child was led to an oral-motor station that, frankly, was painful to watch. The therapist asked the child to lie down on a gym mat, which he did. But within seconds of seeing the therapist pull the electric toothbrush from his bag, the child jumped up and ran across the large gymnasium. Two other therapists entered the scene to help corral the young student and return him to the mat. However, this time he was held down and literally rolled up in the gym mat with his arms at his sides so that he was swaddled and not able to avoid the imminent oral-desensitization treatment. The main therapist then straddled the student-wrap, held the child's head in place, and proceeded to push the electric toothbrush in and around the child's mouth. While the oral-motor objective was indeed completed, the damage to the student-therapist relationship far outweighed any sensory integration gains. The school staff had not established trust, rapport, or cooperation with this young student. They were stuck in a vicious cycle of having to use restraint strategies that just led to more avoidance and resistance and the consequent need for more restraint.

Today, there are many excellent strategies and programs that can be effectively used to build rapport and cooperation with students. Play therapies, models of socialization, and communication strategies, when put in place first, help to establish more willing studentship; this way, more structured curriculum-based models such as IBI can be more useful to the child, who is no longer struggling against learning but is enjoying trying. This example begins to dissolve the debate between choosing either play therapy or IBI toward using them in a complementary way. Invest a good amount of time to build the student-therapist relationship first and then use structured learning second.

Multi-treatment should not mean "all at once." Understandably, with the pressure of early intervention, educators and parents rush to provide as many treatment services as early after the diagnosis as possible. While no one argues time is of the essence, timing is equally important. I have spent the past ten years studying, experimenting with, and specializing in the order and timing of programming within the multi-treatment model. Some treatments are more effective if followed by or preceded by other treatments. For example, my students typically make greater gains and benefit more readily from peer group play after a successful phase of intensive one-to-one adult-directed structured programming (of between three months up to or over one year). If this order is reversed or done concurrently, the children don't seem to benefit as much from the peer play. I am currently writing a paper discussing the developmental basis for this.

The effects and benefits of each individual treatment are maximized by carefully considering the order and timing of the total treatment plan. In contrast, when a multidisciplinary team implements a variety of treatment protocols all at the same time, the child may be subjected to too many different behavioral expectations and different therapist styles at once. For example, I was once asked by a family to find a solution to their son's toilet training. He had learned the routine and had been almost entirely independent but was wetting his pants since starting at a new school. In the child's morning behavioral center program, students were expected to ask permission to use the bathroom to practice social communication, while in the afternoon at the child's school he was encouraged to simply go on his own will to develop independence. He became confused by the two opposing expectations, felt anxious, and held until he wet his pants. Both of the goals, independence and social communication, were good in their own right, but combined they were opposing. The stresses on the child of "all at once" programming can be compounded when a child is enrolled in diametrically opposed treatments such as half-day ABA/IBI and half-day socialization play therapy. While a child will make some gains in each type of program, the benefits that each type can provide simply won't be maximized.

There are many complex and interdependent variables to consider when designing multi-treatment programs. The success of the IMTI program has been exciting and promising. It is my hope that many parents and professionals will benefit from adopting these strategies that ultimately could begin to form bridges between treatments. Working together, I believe we can create more positive effects combined than they we ever can manage apart.

Jonathan Alderson, Ed.M., is an autism treatment specialist and founder of the innovative Intensive Multi-Treatment Intervention Program (www.IMTI. ca). A graduate of Harvard University, with experience as a Curriculum Specialist Coordinator with Teach for America, he trained at the Autism Treatment Center of America in Massachusetts and worked as Administrator and senior family trainer in their Son-Rise Program. He has worked with over 3,000 children and families. Now based in Toronto, he is a contributor for the Huffington Post, a member of the Seneca College behavioral Sciences Advisory Committee, and cochair of the Young Professionals for Autism Speaks Canada Advisory Board. He has lectured on his multidisciplinary approach to autism treatment throughout Canada, the USA, England, Ireland, Holland, Spain, Australia, Israel, and Mexico. He is the author of *Challenging the Myths of Autism,* which has inspired educators and parents to consider a radical reframing of how we think about and treat people diagnosed with autism. His book has been honored with a 2018 Teachers' Choice Award, the 2017 Readers' Favorite Gold Medal Award, the Mom's Choice Gold Award, the American Non-Fiction Authors' Association Silver award, and the 2012 International Book Award for Best Parent-Resource.

6

HELPING CHILDREN WITH ASD GAIN SOCIAL SKILLS

CREATING A CULTURE OF INCLUSION THROUGH AUTISM DEMYSTIFICATION®

Note: About Friend 2 Friend Social Learning Society

Founded in 2002, Friend 2 Friend Social Learning Society is a non-government-funded charitable organization with one mission: to foster mutual friendships between children with autism and their peers.

Beyond building friendships, the Society's programs focus on the development of group identities and a better understanding of inclusion and diversity (Wolfberg, McCracken, & Tuchel, 2014). To accomplish this goal, the Society delivers a variety of unique and innovative peer play and friendship programs including their signature Autism Demystification® Programs and the Integrated Play Groups® Programs. To date, Friend 2 Friend has provided its signature Autism Demystification® Programs to more than 200,000 children. For more information about Friend 2 Friend Social Learning Society programs and services, see www.friend2friendsociety.org

"I want friends."

If you ask anyone what they remember most about school, the answer is almost always "My friends." Friendships are what motivate us to get up in the morning and to go to school or work. Imagine what it must be like for a child on the autism spectrum to attend school every day knowing that no one will ask them to sit beside them at lunch, or to play after school or invite them to a birthday party.

My son, like so many other individuals I know on the autism continuum, wants the one thing that we all want: to have friends and be accepted for who he is.

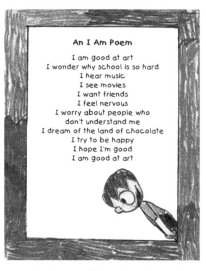

An I Am Poem

I am good at art
I wonder why school is so hard
I hear music
I see movies
I want friends
I feel nervous
I worry about people who
don't understand me
I dream of the land of chocolate
I try to be happy
I hope I'm good
I am good at art

"I wonder why school is hard."
But it is clear to me that my child as well as other children with autism are at risk of social isolation and probable peer bullying that may affect their psychological well-being (Wolfberg, Bottema, & DeWitt, 2012).

Poem by Iain Robbins (age 8, son of Heather McCracken)

Watching my son suffer from social isolation in the school environment, I felt compelled to do what I could to change this situation, not only for my son, but for others who experience these same social difficulties. In 1997, I began reading everything I could get my hands on about friendships between typically developing children and those with special needs. Within a year, I found the book that would set me on the course I had been searching for. Dr. Pamela Wolfberg's book *Play and Imagination in Children with Autism* describes her Integrated Play Groups® model that brings children on the autism spectrum ("novice players") together with their peers ("expert players") to play and interact together in such a way that true friendships begin to emerge. Wolfberg's book inspired me to learn more about how the Integrated Play Groups® model might help my son foster friendships through peer play.

"I worry about people that don't understand me."
With the knowledge that an evidence-based socialization program like IPG exists, I became ever more aware of the void in our community including

schools, preschools, and daycares of specialized educational programs to address social inclusion of children with autism.

I began designing the model and programs in a way that went beyond simply "awareness" of what autism is, but rather to create real understanding. As a parent of three, it was important to me that all my children (and others) would find the program fun and engaging, but more important, they would feel safe; how the program is presented and the language is used is critical to create a space in which both children with and without autism can interact without inhibition and without feeling stigmatized. I felt strongly that I didn't want to create just another "awareness" program that simply informs people about autism. Instead, I envisioned *demystification* programs: to provide authentic learning experiences that dissolve preconceived judgments and foster genuine understanding and empathy. Opening the door to real human connection and friendship.

What Is Autism Demystification®?

For years I read about people doing "awareness training" that was neither a model for action nor evidence-based, and that often singled out and identified the child with autism by removing them from the classroom and talking about them without them. I was determined to create a model that resolved these issues and that went beyond "awareness." I had done some reading on the term *demystify* and felt this was a much better way to describe our goals. Autism Demystification® brings about a better understanding of autism in general in a nonjudgmental way that builds healthy levels of acceptance toward all individuals on the autism spectrum, while at the same time building prosocial communication competences in both the peer group and child with autism.

Some of the guiding principles of the Friend 2 Friend Autism Demystification® are:

- The Programs are play-based, tapping into children's intrinsic ability to learn through play.
- The Programs *NEVER single out or identify* any one individual as being on the spectrum.

- The Programs use and encourage affirmative language and a shared vocabulary that avoids "us and them" language.
- The Programs use real terminology to describe characteristics of autism.

Friend 2 Friend Autism Demystification® Model

Our research-based model uses a systematic approach to educate both individuals with autism and their peer groups in an inclusive, fun, age-appropriate, and sensitive manner. We promote understanding of neurodiversity by using language that helps participants view "different" as normal. For example, "different kinds of minds" and "we are all different in our own way." "Everyone has affinities and everyone has challenges" and that "being a good friend means accepting differences," rather than viewing differences as deficiencies. We promote empathy toward individuals on the autism spectrum using age-appropriate tools (e.g., puppets and Simon Says game) and by modeling, labeling, explaining, and normalizing the characteristics of autism, while never singling out any one individual with autism or individuals who may be participating in the program. Empathy is the key to friendships and is one of the ultimate goals of the programs and the teaching model.

While the Friend 2 Friend Autism Demystification® model aims to shift perspectives and build empathy toward individuals with autism, just changing attitudes is not enough. The model provides participants with concrete tools. "The Seven Friendship Tips" teach participants prosocial communication strategies that enhance social interactions with individuals on the autism spectrum. We have found that when peers know *how* to communicate and interact with an individual on the spectrum, they are more than willing and confident to do so. A few example Friendship Tips are:

1. Get your friend's attention. Move closer to your friend and say his or her name to get your friend's attention before you start talking.

2. Wait. Give your friend extra time to think about what you are saying and then answer you.

3. Give your friend choices. When you want to play, instead of choosing a game for them, offer your friend choices of things they like to do.

"I dream of the land of chocolate"

After several years of extensive research, development, and field-testing, the Friend 2 Friend Autism Demystification® model and programs were launched. In 2002, with the support of my family, we founded the Friend 2 Friend Social Learning Society, a non-government-funded, nonprofit charity based in Vancouver, BC, Canada. Our signature Autism Demystification® programs (Puppet Program for children ages 3–11 and Simulation Game Program for children ages 12–18) was well received in my son's school and many others since.

The model is evidence-based and has now been tested for more than 15 years. The programs have had a profound impact on the way thousands of children and adults think about and interact with individuals with autism.

When I dream of the land of chocolate, it is a place where individuals with autism have friends and feel accepted for who they are within their communities. I'm proud that the Friend 2 Friend Autism Demystification® model and programs have moved us a little closer to making this dream a reality.

References

McCracken, H. (2006). *That's What's Different About Me Puppet Program Manual*. Shawnee, KS: Autism Asperger's Publishing Company.

McCracken, H. (2009). *Demystifying Autism: The Friend 2 Friend Simulation Game Program*. Vancouver BC: Friend 2 Friend Social Learning Society Publisher.

McCracken, H. (2010). *Can I Play Too?: The Friend 2 Friend Puppet Program Manual*. Vancouver BC: Friend 2 Friend Social Learning Society Publisher.

McCracken, H. (2017). *You Don't Know, Jack: The Friend 2 Friend Autism Demystification®Puppet Program* Vancouver BC: Friend 2 Friend Social Learning Society Publisher.

Wolfberg, P.J. (2003). *Peer play and the autism spectrum: The art of guiding children's socialization and imagination.* Shawnee, KS: Autism Asperger's Publishing Company.

Wolfberg, P., McCracken, H. & Tuchel, T. (2008). *Fostering peer play and friendship: Creating a culture of inclusion.* In K. Dunn Buron & P.J. Wolfberg (eds.), Learners on the autism spectrum: preparing highly qualified educators. Shawnee Mission, KS: Autism Asperger's Publishing Company.

Wolfberg, P.J. (2009) *Play and imagination in children with autism* (2nd ed.). New York: Teachers College Press, Columbia University.

Wolfberg, P., DeWitt, M., Young, G.S., & Nguyen, T. (2015). *Integrated Play Groups: Promoting symbolic play and social engagement with typical peers in children with ASD across settings. Journal of Autism and Developmental Disorders* 45 (3), 830–845. (DOI) 10.1007/s10803-014-2245-0.

Heather McCracken is the founder, program and executive director of Friend 2 Friend Social Learning Society. Heather is a parent of three; one of her sons is on the autism spectrum. As creator of the Friend 2 Friend Autism Demystification® Model and Programs, Heather leads an interdisciplinary team providing the Friend 2 Friend Autism Demystification® Programs and the Friend 2 Friend – Integrated Play Groups Programs® throughout BC, Canada, the US, and abroad. She also provides training and outreach efforts to establish inclusive peer play and friendships programs worldwide. Heather is widely published with numerous journals, books, and related video productions including: *That's What's Different About Me, Demystifying Autism: The Friend 2 Friend Simulation Game Program*; *Can I Play Too? The Friend 2 Friend Puppet Program;* and *You Don't Know, Jack: Friend 2 Friend Autism Demystification® Puppet Program.* She is also coauthor of a chapter in the award-winning *Learners on the Autism Spectrum: Preparing Highly Qualified Educators.*

SOCIAL SKILLS TRAINING FOR CHILDREN WITH AUTISM

John is three years old, with very limited language skills. When his parents try to sit and play with him, he focuses on lining up play letters on the floor, virtually ignoring his parents. They call his name and he does not respond. They show him other toys and he ignores them. His older sister tries to engage him in a game of peek-a-boo and he shows no interest.

Karen is a 12-year-old with Asperger's Syndrome. Her intellectual and language skills are excellent. She is very articulate and understands most anything someone says to her. Often, when she has a project in school, she either refuses to do it or refuses to compromise with peers or teachers on how to do the project. Her teachers and parents explain that she needs to compromise if she wants to develop friendships with peers and needs to do the work if she wants to get a job later in life. She explains that she has no interest in making friends or ever having a job, and thus there is no need to do the work or compromise with others.

Although very different in their levels of functioning, neither John nor Karen is motivated to learn social skills. Efforts to teach them how to relate to others will be frustrating for all until the issue of motivation is addressed. Table 1 describes several methods of motivating students to learn social skills and many other skills.

The table categorizes methods of motivating students in terms of the language ability of the students (preverbal *versus* verbal reasoner) and the locus of motivation (external/contrived *versus* internal/naturalistic). Preverbal reasoners are students who may have some language but are not yet able to understand "if—then" statements, such as "If you play this with me, then you can have a snack." Verbal reasoners can understand "if—then" statements, so that one can try to motivate them through verbal reasoning. An example: "If you do your math with me, then we can play afterward."

	Extrinsic/ Contrived Rewards	Intrinsic/Naturalistic Rewards
Preverbal Reasoner (Pre-symbolic language)	The reward may have no natural connection to the skill in that the reward may not be available in naturally occurring settings. Use of material rewards such as food, toys, privileges, or social praise provided after skill enactment. Controlled studies have demonstrated effectiveness. This characterized the earlier **Lovaas discrete trial approach**; the more contemporary Lovaas approach utilizes intrinsic approaches as well.	Reward is logically related to student's response. Controlled studies have demonstrated effectiveness. **Pivotal Response Training** often embeds the child's interests into the skill lesson, and intersperses challenging tasks in between easier ones to maintain intrinsic motivation. **Verbal Behavior Training** starts with "mand" training in which the child learns to request favored items or activities, so that the reward is intrinsic to the learning situation. **DIR®/Floortime™** follows the lead of the child to gain motivation. **RDI** attempts to make social referencing fun and engaging in and of itself
Verbal Reasoner	Extrinsic rewards are provided as above, often through the accumulation of symbolic rewards such as tokens or points on a behavior chart. Controlled studies have demonstrated effectiveness. Make socializing fun. Have students teach others the social skills.	Explain rationale for working on challenging skills; that it will help the student reach their own future goals. For students who seem not to care about their future, increase self-awareness of strengths and talents to establish future goals prior to focusing on their challenges. Have students teach necessary skills to others to help them feel competent themselves. Make socializing fun through high interest activitiesLink skill-goals to student's personal goals. Promising but not true controlled outcome studies yet.

Table 1

External/contrived motivation refers to providing students with a reward that may be unrelated to the activity or response they are making. For example, if a student is able to greet others when prompted, an external reward might be a special snack or access to a toy. The reward here is not logically related to the response (i.e., greeting) and is not naturally built into the situation (i.e., the instructor must provide the reinforcement).

Internal motivation refers to situations in which the student's behaviors naturally provide them with rewards because the activity itself is rewarding or because the student's responses bring its own rewards. For example, if a child enjoys playing follow the leader, then playing the game is itself rewarding and there is no need to provide another reward. Similarly, if a student learns to request a toy from others and receives the toy, then the request naturally leads to its own reward, receiving the toy, and there is no need for other rewards.

Motivational strategies for nonverbal reasoners

The motivational methods listed for nonverbal reasoners include strategies often associated with "early intervention." The goals are often to build crucial skills that are prerequisites for later learning in school and social settings. These skills include joint attention (attending to others and attending to what others point out), the ability to label objects, request objects, follow simple directions, and answer simple questions. The interventions associated with applied behavior analysis (ABA) have been subjected to the most rigorous controlled evaluations of outcome and demonstrate excellent results in about 50 percent of autistic students in terms of intellectual, language, adaptive, and early social skills.

ABA approaches include Discrete Trial Intervention (DTI) (Lovaas, 2003), Natural Language Paradigm (and its more recent cousin Pivotal Response Training) (Koegel and Koegel, 2005), and Verbal Behavior Training (Sundberg and Partington, 1998). Although these approaches share a basic structure of teaching behavior through cueing, prompting, and rewarding students, they differ in their emphasis on teaching in natural environments and utilizing internal/naturalistic *versus* external/contrived motivational systems.

A discrete trial has five components: a cue, a prompt, the student's response, a reward, and data collection. Early DTI interventions often emphasized compliance and labeling of objects. For example, if a child was learning colors, the child might get a cue, "Point to the blue car." Then the instructor might prompt the student to touch the blue car. If the child responded correctly he might then get a favored reward, such as a piece of candy. Here the reward is not naturally related to the response. Earlier DTI approaches have been shown effective in improving students' abilities to respond to adult cues, but they are not always as successful in increasing students' spontaneous language or generalizing skills in natural settings.

In contrast, Verbal Behavior Training and Pivotal Response Training occur in more natural settings and capitalize more on the students' own interests. In the first phase of verbal behavior training, the emphasis is on teaching children to spontaneously request, utilizing the students' own interest in activities, food, objects, wanting a break, or wanting attention while in a more natural play environment. As such, the students are typically highly motivated, since their responses lead to naturally rewarding consequences (i.e., getting what they requested). Similarly, Pivotal Response Training begins with assessing what the students are interested in and then beginning a discrete trial centered on that interest. For example, if a youngster shows an interest in playing with a car, the adult might hold the car out and cue, "What color is the car?" If the youngster says "car," the adult might cue and prompt, "What color is the car? Is it blue?" And when the child says, "blue car," the child would get to play with the car.

Greenspan's "Floortime" DIR (Developmental Individual-Difference, Relationship-Based) model also capitalizes on the student's own interests, emphasizing following the lead of the youngster as the adult plays with the student in an effort to target various developmental skills (the interested reader should see Greenspan & Wieder, 1998). Although there are some semi-structured play activities in this model, cues, prompts, and rewards are not used in the same systematic way as in ABA methods.

Another promising approach is Relational Development Intervention (RDI) (Gutstein & Sheely, 2002). RDI outlines a systematic set of activities that encourage students to want to engage in social interaction because of the joy in the social activity and not because of a contrived/external reward for interacting. Early activities to build joint attention might include imitation games like follow the leader or "follow my eyes to the prize," where students have to look at an adult's eyes to find where the adult hid a prize in the room (the adult is looking in the direction of where the prize is hidden). Although these activities have not yet been empirically tested, the concept is reasonable: engage students in activities that limit overstimulation and require attending to others.

Motivational strategies for verbal reasoners

Verbal reasoners understand "if—then" statements. For example, if you learn how to interview for a job, you might get that job. External motivational strategies focus on finding incentives (rewards, privileges) for practicing new skills. Often tokens or points are earned on a behavior chart and exchanged for short- and long-term rewards.

For many students, external rewards are not necessary. Internal motivational strategies start with linking social skills training to students' goals. If students want friends, a job, good grades, or to be able to engage in an activity (sports, clubs, or a birthday party), then teaching crucial skills can be linked to these goals. For example, if a youngster wants to go to a birthday party, one can motivate him to learn how to play the games that they will play at the party and other crucial skills to maintain himself at the party. Similarly, many adolescents who never wanted to learn social skills suddenly develop motivation to learn certain skills in an effort to help them find a date.

Strategies cannot be so straightforward for the student who seems to have no goals, has become depressed, and is withdrawing from the social world entirely. Such students may need to deny a need for skills training. It takes a modicum of self-esteem to tolerate thinking about one's difficulties. One way around such resistance is through counseling that allows them to expand their senses of their talents and strengths before targeting areas that need improvement. For most students, it is helpful to have someone else point out two to three strengths for every diffculty that is highlighted. The student can be asked directly what talents and strengths they have, and then the counselor can add or refine that list of strengths before suggesting areas in need of improvement. For example, during group sessions, I will ask each member what his or her special talents are and corroborate these positive descriptions. Then I might say, "There are some minor issues I want to address with you guys so that you can continue to do as well as you are doing." Then comes the lesson on a skill topic.

There are several more ways to motivate engagement for skill lessons including: using entertaining role-plays and social games; linking skill lessons to fun group activities or projects; and creating skill lessons to teach others (see Baker 2003 in press.) This last method involves students creating picture books (see later discussion of making social skill picture books), videos, or live skits, so that they can demonstrate the skills to other students. As such, they can learn a skill in order to "help others" without having to acknowledge that they themselves needed to learn it.

With some motivation to socialize, skills can be more easily taught and generalized. What follows is a description of the components of social skills training, including teaching skills, generalizing skills, and targeting typical peers.

The components of social skills training

All social interaction and social problems involve at least two people. A social difficulty can be defined as both a skill deficit for the student with a social disability and a problem of acceptance of that student by peers or the community. Thus intervention must focus on teaching skills for both the student with a disability and typical peers. All too often we strive to "fix" the child with the disability and virtually overlook the "typical" peers who may be ignoring, teasing, or rejecting the student. Moreover, including typical peers as a focus for intervention may yield results much sooner, as typical peers may learn to be understanding of the student with a disability more quickly than the child with a disability can learn to interact more appropriately with peers. We might begin to target peers at the age that many students enter school environments and typically begin to interact with peers, by about three to four years of age.

Consistent with this view, I believe effective social skills training for individuals with ASD and their peers consists of at least four components. The student with ASD requires: skills training lessons to teach explicitly the social skills that do not come naturally for ASD students; and activities to promote generalization of skills in the situations where they are needed. Typical peers and the student's community require: sensitivity training lessons, so that they are more accepting of, and engaging with, students with ASD; and activities to promote generalization of sensitivity to ASD students.

Skill lessons

Skill lessons include a variety of strategies geared to the students' cognitive/language functioning. For verbal reasoners (i.e., students who can understand verbal explanations), we might break down a skill into its component steps, *explain it, model it,* and *role-play it* until the youngster can demonstrate the skill and understands why it is important. Let's say a student with good verbal skills always wants to do things his way and that conduct gets in the way of developing peer relations. We decide to teach him how and why to compromise. We teach him how to ask what others want, say what he wants, and to offer to do a little of both. We explain that when you do a little of both (i.e., compromise), the other person will be happy and may want to play with you again or be your friend.

Using this straightforward approach, we have broken down into simple steps over 70 such social skills related to play, conversation, emotion management, and empathy in a manual on social skills training for children with social communication problems (see Baker, 2003).

For very young students (three and under) with very little language or ability to attend to others, we might begin with the early intervention strategies described earlier (Discrete Trail Intervention, Verbal Behavior Training, Pivotal Response Training, Floortime—DIR, and RDI). For students who have developed some language but still have difficulty understanding verbal explanations, I have translated a subset of the skills that appear in the manual (Baker, 2003) into picture form (see the *Social Skills Picture Book*, Baker, 2001). Instead of explaining skill steps with words, we show a picture sequence. Thus, for a skill-like compromise, the pictures demonstrate a student asking to play a game with another youngster who says he wants to play another game. We show them pictures of the students compromising and playing a little of both games with both looking happy. Then we show them pictures of the same people not compromising, not playing with each other, with both looking upset. Of particular benefit is making your own picture books, so that students have pictures of themselves engaged in the right (or wrong) ways to demonstrate a skill. After the pictures are shown, students should still role-play the skill so that they can actually go through the motions of the skill steps.

Another strategy called cognitive picture rehearsal utilizes cartoon-like drawings on index cards combined with positive reinforcement principles (Groden & Lavasseur, 1995). Cognitive picture rehearsal always includes drawings or pictures of three components: the antecedents to a problem situation, the targeted desired behavior, and a positive reinforcer. The pictures are displayed on index cards. On the top of each card (or on the back of the card) is a script describing the desired sequence of events. Children are shown the sequence of cards until they can repeat what is happening in each picture. The sequence is reviewed just before the child enters the potentially problematic situation.

For example, a cognitive picture rehearsal was created for Matt, a seven-year-old who would throw tantrums when his teacher told him to get off the computer. Cards 1 and 2 illustrated the antecedent to the problem situation: Matt is playing at the computer, and then the teacher tells him it is time to get off the computer. Cards 3 and 4 showed Matt engaged in the desired target behavior: thinking that the teacher will be happy if he gets off the computer and give him a chance to use the computer later, and then saying, "Okay, I'll get off the computer." Cards 5 and 6 show the positive rewards of engaging in the desired behavior: Matt receiving a point on a reward chart and the teacher letting Matt use the computer again later because he had cooperated earlier.

Social Stories™, developed by Carol Gray and colleagues (Gray et al., 1993), uses stories written in the first person to increase students' understanding of problematic situations. Beginning with the child's understanding of a situation, a story is developed describing what is happening and why, and how people feel and think in the situation. While the story contains some directive statements (i.e., what to do in the situation), the focus is on understanding what is happening in the situation.

The following situation provides an example in which Social Stories™ may help an individual with autism deal with a social problem.

Peter was a 13-year-old who frequently got into fights at lunchtime because he believed that other students in the cafeteria were teasing him. He said that several other boys who sat on the other side of the cafeteria always laughed at him. He would give them "the finger," and then they would start a fight with him. When Peter was observed at lunch, it was apparent that the other boys were laughing, but not at him. They were at least 50 feet from Peter, not looking at him, and laughing with one another, presumably about some joke or discussion they were having.

We developed the following social story for Peter, starting with his perspective that others might be laughing at him:

"When I am in the cafeteria I often see other boys laughing and I think they are laughing at me. Lots of students laugh during lunchtime because they are talking about funny things they did during the day, or funny stories they heard or saw on TV, movies or books they read. Sometimes students laugh at other students to make fun of them.

"If they are making fun of other students, they usually use the student's name or look and point at that student. If the other students are laughing, but they do not look or point at me, then they are probably not laughing at me. Most students do not get mad when others are laughing, as long as they are not laughing at them. If they do laugh at me, I can go tell a teacher rather than give them the finger."

Like cognitive picture rehearsal, Social Stories™ are read repeatedly to children until they have overlearned them and are then read again just prior to the problematic situation.

Generalization

Generalization refers to the ability of an individual to use a new skill in situations beyond the training session, and hopefully to use the new skill spontaneously without prompting from others. To achieve this level of fluidity with a new skill, individuals must practice and repeat the skill steps a great deal. As a result, it is unrealistic to think one can generalize many new skills at once. In my experience, true generalization occurs when individuals are reminded about or rehearse no more than one to three new skills every day for several months. Although individuals can learn the concept of many more skills during skill lessons, they may only be able to generalize one to three new skills at a given time. Generalization of a skill involves three steps: priming before the situation in which the skill is needed; frequent facilitated opportunities to practice the skill; and review of the skill after it is used.

Priming involves some reminder to the individual of what the skill steps are just prior to needing the skill. For example, just before going on a job interview, an individual might go over how to answer anticipated questions. Or just prior to starting a frustrating task at school or at work, the individual might review options for dealing with frustrating work. Priming can be verbal and/or supplemented by a visual aide. Verbal priming involves someone verbally explaining the skill steps prior to the situation in which they will be needed. Cue cards, behavior charts, copies of skill lessons (see Baker, 2003), Social Stories™, cognitive picture rehearsals, and social skill picture books can serve as visual aides that depict the skill steps.

If students want to change their behavior but can't remember the skill steps, then cue cards or copies of the skill lessons may be ideal. We might write one to three skills on an index card and laminate it. Then we might ask a parent, teacher, or employer (or the students themselves) to review the skill steps prior to the situation in which it will be needed. Although it is ideal for the student to see the skill steps immediately prior to the situation in which they need to use the skill, this may not always be practical. Instead the parent, teacher, employer, or student might review the skill once in the morning prior to school or work, once at lunch, and then again at the end of the day so that the student at least has to think about the skill three times per day.

If a student has not fully agreed to try a new skill and thus is lacking in "internal" motivation to perform the skill, then a behavior chart can be used in which external rewards are contingent on demonstrating certain targeted skills.

In order to practice the new skills, students need opportunities. Facilitated opportunities involve creating daily situations in which the skills can be practiced and coached. Sometimes those opportunities are naturally built into the day. For example, a student learning to deal with frustrating work may always have his or her share of challenging work to do during the day. Other times, the practice opportunities need to be carefully planned or created. For example, a student who never initiates conversation with anyone may be asked to call someone on the phone once a day or join others for lunch and initiate conversation once during that period.

After situations have occurred in which skills were needed, the student's performance can be reviewed to increase awareness of the skill. If a youngster is on a reward chart, the reason why the student received the reward (or not) should be reviewed with him or her to enhance learning.

Peer sensitivity

Sometimes youngsters with ASD are ignored, yet often they are actively teased or bullied. Students with ASD may do nothing to deserve such teasing, and other times they may provoke such reactions with unintentional "irritating" behaviors like perseverating on a topic, making loud noises, or having angry meltdowns. When students are harassed, teased, or rejected because they look or behave differently, it is crucial to explain to others the unintentional nature of their behaviors and how others can help. We often talk with peers not only about the unintentional nature of their difficult behaviors, but the strengths and talents of the individuals with ASD and about examples of successful, famous figures who may also have had an ASD.

Generalization of Peer Kindness

We ask peers to do three things to help their ASD classmates and one another: (1) include others who are left out; (2) stand up for those who are teased; and (3) offer help to those who are upset. To help these kind behaviors generalize into the daily routines of the students, we might create a lunch buddy program, where peers volunteer to eat and hang out with the ASD student on a rotating schedule. We might also introduce a reward program to recognize and reward"kind" behaviors toward fellow students. We may also train peers in how to engage ASD students in play, including how to get their attention and what kinds of games to initiate (i.e., games the ASD student can play). Our experience and a growing body of research suggest that including typical peers as targets for training can have profound effects on the development of social skills and overall happiness of ASD students in school environments (Baker 2003; Wagner, 1998).

For more information about Dr. Baker and the Social Skills Training Project, visit www.socialskillstrainingproject.com.

References

Baker, J. E. (2001). *Social skill picture books.* Arlington, TX: Future Horizons, Inc.

Baker, J. E. (2003). *Social skills training for students with Aspergers syndrome and related social communication disorders.* Shawnee Mission, Kansas: Autism Aspergers Publishing Company.

Baker, J.E. (in press). *Social skills training for the transition from high school to adult life.* Arlington, TX: Future Horizons, Inc.

Baker, J.E. (in press). *Social skill picture book for teens and adults.* Arlington, TX: Future Horizons, Inc.

Gray, C., Dutkiewicz, M., Fleck, C., Moore, L., Cain, S.L., Lindrup, A., Broek, E., Gray, J. & Gray, B. (eds.), (1993). *The social story book.* Jenison, MI: Jenison Public Schools.

Greenspan, S. I., and Wieder, S. (1998). *The child with special needs: Encouraging intellectual and emotional growth.* Reading, MA: Addison-Wesley.

Grodon, J., and LeVasseur, P. (1995). *Cognitive picture rehearsal: A system to teach self-control.* In K. A. Quill (ed.), *Teaching children with autism* (pp. 287–306). Albany, NY: Delmar Publishing.

Gutstein, S. E., and Sheely, R. K. (2002). *Relationship development intervention with children, adolescents and adults: Social and emotional development activities for asperger's syndrome, autism, PDD, and NLD.* London: Jessica Kingsley Publishers Ltd.

Koegel, R. L., and Koegel, L.K. (eds.) (2005). *Pivotal response treatments for autism: Communication, social, and academic development.* Baltimore, MD: Brookes Publishing Co., Inc.

Lovaas, O.I. (2003). *Teaching Individuals with Developmental Delays: Basic Intervention Techniques.* Austin, TX: PRO ED, Inc.

Sundberg, M.L., and Partington, J. W. (1998). *Teaching language to children with autism or other developmental disabilities.* Behavioral Analysts, Inc.

Wagner, S. (1998). *Inclusive programming for elementary students with autism.* Arlington, TX: Future Horizons, Inc.

Contributing Author Jed Baker, Ph.D.—Dr. Baker is the Director of the Social Skills Training Project in Maplewood, N.J. He is on the professional advisory board of ASPEN (an information network for parents of children with Asperger's Syndrome). He is a behavioral consultant for several New Jersey school systems, where he provides social skills training for students with pervasive developmental disorders and learning disabilities. He directs and supervises social skills training for students at Millburn Public Schools. In addition, he writes lectures and provides training across the country on the topic of social skills training for individuals with Asperger's Syndrome and related PDDs. He has recently published both a manual on social skills training for children with Asperger's Syndrome and a social skill picture book to aid in social skills training.

LEARNING STYLES AND AUTISM

Learning styles refers to the ways people gain information about their environments. People can learn through seeing (visually), hearing (audi-torily), and/or through touching or manipulating an object (kinesthetically or "hands-on" learning). For example, looking at a picture book or reading a textbook involves learning through vision; listening to a lecture live or on tape involves learning through hearing; and pressing buttons to determine how to operate an iPad involves learning kinesthetically.

Generally, most people learn using two to three learning styles. Interest-ingly, people can assess their own interests and lifestyle to determine the ways in which they obtain much of their information about their environment. In my case, when I read a book I can easily understand the text. In contrast, it is difficult for me to listen to an audiotape recording of that book—I just cannot follow the story line. Thus, I am a strong visual learner, and a moderate, pos-sibly poor, auditory learner. As far as kinesthetic learning, I am very good at taking apart objects to learn how an object works, such as a vacuum cleaner or a computer.

One's learning style may affect how well a person performs in an educa-tional setting, especially from junior high on through college. Schools usually require both auditory learning (i.e., listening to a teacher) and visual learning (i.e., reading a textbook). If a person is poor at one of these ways of learning, he/she will likely depend mostly on his/her strength (e.g., a visual learner may study the textbook rather than rely on the lecture content). Using this logic, if one is poor at both visual and auditory learning, he/she may have difficulty in school. Furthermore, one's learning style may be associated with one's occu-pation. For example, those individuals who are kinesthetic learners may tend to have occupations involving their hands, such as shelf stockers, mechanics, surgeons, or sculptors.

Visual learners may tend to have occupations that involve processing visual information, such as data processors, artists, architects, or manufacturing part sorters. Moreover, auditory learners may tend to have jobs that involve processing auditory information, such as salespeople, judges, musicians, 911 operators, and waiters/waitresses.

Based on my experiences and those of my colleagues, it appears that autistic individuals are more likely to rely on only one style of learning. By observing the person, one may be able to determine his/her primary style of learning. For example, if an autistic child enjoys looking at books (e.g., picture books), watching television (with or without sound), and tends to look carefully at people and objects, then he/she may be a visual learner. If an autistic child talks excessively, enjoys people talking to him/her, and prefers listening to the radio or music, then he/she may be an auditory learner. And if an autistic child is constantly taking things apart, opening and closing drawers, and pushing buttons, this may indicate that the child is a kinesthetic or "hands-on" learner.

Once a person's learning style is discovered, relying on this style to teach can greatly increase the likelihood that the person will learn. If one is not sure which learning style a child has or is teaching to a group with different learning styles, then the best way to teach could be to use all three styles together. For example, when teaching the concept "jello," one can display a package and bowl of jello (visual), describe its features such as its color, texture, and use (auditory), and let the person touch and taste it (kinesthetic).

A common problem of autistic children is that they run around the classroom and do not listen to the teacher. Such a child may not be an auditory learner—and so is not attending to the teacher's words. If the child is a kinesthetic learner, the teacher may choose to place his/her hands on the child's shoulders and then guide the student back to his/her chair, or go to the chair and move it toward the student. If the child learns visually, the teacher may need to show the child his/her chair or hand them a picture of the chair and gesture for the child to sit down.

Teaching to the learning style of the student may affect whether or not the child can attend to and process information presented. This, in turn, can affect the child's performance in school as well as his/her behavior. Therefore, it is important that educators assess for learning style as soon as an autistic child enters the school system and that they adapt their teaching styles to the strengths of the student. This will ensure that the autistic child has the greatest chance for success in school.

Contributing Author Stephen M. Edelson, Ph.D., Experimental Psychology—Dr. Edelson has worked in the field of autism for 25 years. He is the director of the Center for the Study of Autism in Salem, Oregon, which is affiliated with the Autism Research Institute in San Diego, CA. He is also on the Board of Directors of the Oregon chapter of the Autism Society of America and is on the Society's Professional Advisory Board. *Dr. Edelson's main autism website is www.autism.org.*

AUTISM AND SPEECH

Note: This article originally appeared and is published on Eustacia Cutler and Temple Grandin's website on the page "Writings by Eustacia Cutler" at http://www.templegrandineustaciacutlerautismfund.com/eustacia-cutler/writings-by-eustacia-cutler/.

> I think Temple is going to talk, but let's speed up the process. Here's the address of Mrs. Reynolds. She teaches speech.
> — Dr. Bronson Caruthers, Children's Hospital, Boston, 1947

It took Temple three years with Mrs. Reynolds to learn to talk, and, as we all know, she hasn't stopped talking ever since.

*   *   *   *

For thousands of years, speech has played a major role in the way humans connect to one another. Yet it remains puzzlingly elusive for many on the autism spectrum. Is it the process that's difficult or its intention? Sounding out the words or what the words stand for?

The Process

We humans, along with other warm-blooded animals, are social creatures. All of us weave a reciprocal social story that serves our particular tribe, herd, pack, or pride. We react, imitate, love, scheme, bond, remember, raise and teach our young, use vocals and eye contact to connect.

But here's the difference between us humans and animals:

As far as we know, most animal scenarios involve only the risks and joys of the physical world surrounding them. Long ago we humans achieved another more imaginative scenario: one that reached beyond what was actually happening to what we might make happen.

Anthropologist Loren Eiseley puts it this way:

> *He [man] was becoming something the world had never seen before.*
> *A dream animal—living at least partially within a secret universe*
> *of his own creation and sharing that secret universe in his head with*
> *other, similar heads. Symbolic communication had begun.*
>
> —*The Immense Journey*, Vintage, pp. 120, 1957

We don't think of speech as "symbolic communication"; we think of it as natural. But when you break down the steps those long-ago-dream-animals had to go through in order to share their secret thoughts with one another, it turns out that words are highly motivated, cooperative, and, yes, symbolic.

I looked up *word* in Webster's dictionary, and old Noah defines it as "*. . . an articulate sound or series of sounds which symbolizes and articulates an idea.*"

To do this, first we had to develop a mutual idea (concept) of what each animal or action was for. Then we had to turn our old animal sounds (growling, barking, snarling) into unique individual vocals that would stand for (symbolize) that animal (bear, wolf, cat) or action (chase, fight, flee).

Achieving these two steps gave us a huge advantage over other animals, but it only worked if the group understood it both collectively and individually. Each human had to get the gist of the steps on his own.

Despite the odds, we accomplished it:

> *. . . long before previously thought, in some cases more than 40,000*
> *years . . . We have sufficient evidence to the effect that Neanderthals*
> *possessed a symbolic culture.*
>
> —Dr. Joao Zilao, prehistorian at the University of Barcelona,
> *New York Times*, 2012

Miraculously, somewhere in the lost eons of prehistory, speech got programmed into our genetic makeup . . . Except for those on the autism spectrum. With autism, the knack for this interreciprocal act appears to be missing or skewed (or maybe both). As a result, those on the spectrum don't get what we're up to, and here's what's interesting: we with a full deck of neurological cards don't always get what they're up to.

What's Not Working?

The best way to illustrate this logjam is to lay out how it does work for most of us. And for that I turn to the story of Nicholas, my youngest grandson, twenty years ago when he was a baby, just about to start talking.

The first word his grandmother heard him say wasn't "Mama" or "Dada," but "Oreo." He looked at us, pointed at the cookie jar, and said, "Oreo." We all laughed. But I knew that the steps of his bioneurology were complete.

Step 1 He understood the idea of what a cookie was for. This, in professional linguistic terms, is called conceptual thinking.

Step 2 He understood location: he was sitting in his high chair, the place where he got things to eat. If he wanted a cookie, he sensed he better ask for it quick before someone took him out of that place. Understanding location and its relevance to the action is called context.

Step 3 He looked at us and pointed to the cookie jar. He understood he had a different mind from us and he'd have to get the cookie idea from his head into our heads (i.e., shared information).

Step 4 He could put all this together and act on it. This is called executive function.

The neurology for these steps had to develop in Nicholas before he could talk. And most crucially, he had to understand the idea of what "words" themselves are for. When many people with ASD learn to talk, their voices are often loud and robotic, as if they learned the act of talking, but not the idea behind it. And they tend to use words solely as a device to gain physical wants (e.g., food, comfort, escape).

If that's how it shapes up in their heads, it raises the same old question: is the knack for symbolic thinking missing or skewed? Despite the enormous variety of ability in ASDs, this skill is so frequently and recognizably missing that we can call the lack of it "autism."

How Do You Compensate for What's Not There?

Arthur, a little boy with autism, cannot get the idea of what a shovel is for. If you ask him to point to his sand shovel, he can point to it, and he knows its name. But if you ask him to point to the thing he digs with, he's lost. Though in time he may understand what his own sand box shovel is for, he cannot understand that his father's winter snow shovel serves the same purpose, and that the motorized excavating shovel digging out a hole in the garden for a summer swimming pool also serves the same purpose.

How can he compensate for this gap?

For a possible solution I look to my daughter Temple, who, early on, dismissed conceptual thinking with the remark *"I don't go for this flighty idea stuff. I work from the ground up."*

She compensates for her gap by memorizing visually every situation that happens to her. She refers to them as *"My videos . . . whenever I meet a new situation, I take out my videos and use the one that fits it best."*

She calls her system "categories," and it works amazingly well for her—primarily because she has a phenomenal memory, instant recall, and a top-notch brain to put it together. But it goes no further than the physical world around her, as does the animal scenario. If that's the nature of her compensation, it could explain why she's so deeply committed to understanding and teaching animal behavior.

Also, despite its value, her "categories" can only compensate for what has already happened. They don't resolve Arthur's problem with the shovels.

If Arthur can't understand how three different shovels resemble one another, he can't *generalize*. Nor can he understand when others generalize. This leaves him unable to understand *relevance* (how things relate to one another).

Look at how we, the general public, turn the word "shovel" from a noun into a verb and in the process broaden our interpretation of the word.

In WWII, when train engines ran by coal, the words to the pop song "Chattanooga Choo Choo" went: *"Shovel all the coal in, gotta keep her rollin' . . ."* And in all eras, parents say to their children, *"Eat nicely. Don't shovel food into your mouth."*

The visual images conjured up by these two quotes are so different that it's hard for Arthur (who is a visual thinker like Temple) to see that it's not the images that relate, but the nature of what the word "shovel" conjures up in each image.

We neurotypicals don't have to figure relevance out. Our neurology does it for us. It also allows us to communicate intention (i.e., sharing what we intend to do with another human who might have the same intention). And we can reinforce our intention by combining animal communication with symbolic communication.

For example:
We use battle shouts as a *physical* threat to intimidate the enemy in a fight for ownership of territory. (Think Rebel Yell.) If we win, we use a spoken agreement that *stands for* our new ownership of the territory. Though both acts are intentional, the shout is *physical*, the spoken agreement is *symbolic*.

And the mix of the two is doubly confounding for Arthur. Compensation is not an easy task. Temple and Arthur, though different in their capabilities, both have to work very hard.

The Written Word

> Polonius: *What do you read, my lord?*
> Hamlet: *Words, words, words*
>
> —*Hamlet*, Shakespeare, 1601

Oral traditions are old. Songs and stories have always traveled orally down the decades, giving families and tribes a shared identity. Nevertheless, early on, we humans craved a permanent record of our stories and when trading with one another found we needed something more binding than spoken agreements. Note: Ancient clay tablets mostly record agreed-upon business deals.

So out of spoken language we devised a series of written symbols, each standing for a particular sound. Write the sound symbols together and they turn into words. Write the words together and they become sentences. Abracadabra. You, the reader of the sentences, are now holding in your hand a *physical* object that can be seen, and stored with other objects of value.

This trick is also stored in our genetic makeup—that is, for most of us.

Most of us understand that concepts are generalized ideas. Though people with ASD are tops at visual thinking, there's no way for them to "see" their way to either an idea or a generalization. Speech, too, cannot be seen. It's also fraught with nuance that can defy the best of us.

But here's where Abracadabra is a boon. Words when typed are no longer symbolic. They've turned into physical objects that people with ASD can see and understand as an animal understands his physical environment.

Might that explain why those who can't talk can often type?

*   *   *   *

I remember an autism conference where two middle-aged ASD men were on the platform with the professional speakers. Both of them, almost totally mute, had become friends by typing to each other.

One of them typed for us, letter by letter, in the slow time-eating way a prisoner in solitary taps out a message to another prisoner through the wall. At the same time, he managed to speak the words he was typing. Yes, his voice was loud and robotic. And though he may never understand that words are symbolic communication—or even what symbolism is—the longing in his words was achingly human:

"I-want-you-to-know-that-I-am-intelligent."

Eustacia Cutler, Temple Grandin's mother, earned a B.A. from Harvard; was a band singer at the Pierre Hotel, New York City; performed and composed for NYC cabaret; and wrote school lessons for major TV networks. Her research on autism and other disabilities created the scripts for two WGBH television documentaries: *The Disquieted* and *The Innocents*, a prize-winning first. Her 2006 book, *A Thorn in My Pocket*, describes raising Temple in the conservative world of the '50s, when autistic children were routinely diagnosed as infant schizophrenics.

Her latest book, *Autism Old As Time*, is a collection of essays written to take the reader on a journey through history, examining the impact of autism on the opinions and solutions of writers, poets, and other prominent individuals from the early 19th century through today. While her first book described raising Temple, this book describes the journey that Ms. Cutler took as she came to terms with autism in her life and saw our ever-evolving capacity, as individuals and as a society, to keep reinventing ourselves. She looks at autism from the point of view of the phoenix: that ancient symbol of culture renewing itself.

Ms. Culter has also hosted a series of *Conversations with Eustacia Cutler*, where she interviews autism experts from around the world. These can be viewed on the Temple Grandin Eustacia Cutler Autism Fund website.

Today, Cutler lectures nationally and internationally on autism and its relation to the rapidly emerging bioneurological study of brain plasticity. She discusses what causes rigid behavior in autism, the toll it takes on the family, and how current research into the neural nature of consciousness is pointing toward insightful possibilities of change.

IDIOMS & METAPHORS & THINGS THAT GO BUMP IN THE NIGHT

Note: This section is expanded from *Idioms and Metaphors and Things That Go Bump in Their Heads*, originally published in the Autism/Asperger's Digest, www.autismdigest.com (January–February 2005).

"If the English language made any sense, a catastrophe would be an apostrophe with fur." Doug Larson's words are steeped in truth, of course. But a woeful truth it is for young children with language deficits. The problems are more thorny than furry.

Vernacular English as we speak it is nuanced to the eyeballs (there's one right there), and if you were to stop yourself throughout your day every time you unthinkingly used an idiom, pun, metaphor, double entendre, or sarcastic remark, you would get very little else done.

For our children with autism, it must seem like an impenetrable swamp. With their concrete, visual thinking, their often brilliant associative abilities, and their limited vocabularies, the imagery generated by some of our most common idioms must be very disturbing. Ants in his pants? Butterflies in her stomach? Open a can of worms? Cat got your tongue?

Actually, that very imagery they conjure up is at the root of some of our everyday expressions. When you tell him it's pouring cats and dogs, what you really mean is that it's raining very hard. One interpretation of the origin of this idiom—and there are many—goes back several hundred years to the English floods of the 17th and 18th centuries. After these torrential downpours, the streets would be littered with the bodies of cats and dogs that had drowned in the storm. It looked as if they had rained from the skies. And I am sure this is what a lot of young ones with autism visualize when you say it's raining cats and dogs. Heaven help you if he hears you telling someone it's a dog-eat-dog world or not to throw the baby out with the bathwater.

You wouldn't dream of knowingly issuing instructions to your child in a foreign language, but English can seem that way, even to the unchallenged neurotypicals. A popular Internet essay notes: "Why do we drive on the parkway and park in the driveway? There is no egg in eggplant, nor ham in hamburger; (there's) neither apple nor pine in pineapple. A guinea pig is neither from Guinea nor is it a pig. If the plural of tooth is teeth, why isn't the plural of booth beeth? One goose, two geese. So one moose, two meese? If teachers taught, why didn't preachers praught? We have noses that run and feet that smell. How can a slim chance and a fat chance be the same, while a wise man and a wise guy are opposites?"

When Bryce was quite young, his ultraliteral, concrete thought processes were constantly tripping me up. One day I went into the boys' bathroom and discovered, in the sink, my older son Connor's Michael Jordan action figure with a tub of Danish Orchards Seedless Raspberry Preserves dumped on top. I was truly mystified. "What is this?" I asked Bryce.

"Space Jam," he replied, having just seen the movie. I watched the crimson stain spreading across the sink and oozing down the drain. I truly did not know what the proper response should be. So I did the sensible thing. I nodded and walked away.

The bathroom was in fact the source of more than one run-in with the English language. One memorable afternoon I was helping Connor pack for a weekend trip, gathering up toothpaste, shampoo, and soap.

"Where is your toiletries bag?" I called across the loft.

"WHAT??!!" gasped Bryce.

"I'm looking for the blue bag where Connor keeps his toiletries," I explained.

"TOILET TREES?! HE'S TAKING TOILET TREES ON HIS TRIP???!!!"

Bryce's jousting with the English language grew more sophisticated as he learned to read. At one point he went through a phase where he would become very agitated by the sight of phone booths: "Oh no! Not another one of those!" I eventually found out why—he had recently mastered the fact that "ph" makes an "f" sound, and he found it frankly annoying. (Or did he phind that phact phrankly annoying?) Seeing "phone" all around ticked him off. Speaking of which—why isn't "phonics" spelled the way it sounds?

The bottom line is, communicating with a child with autism is astonishingly easier when we pause to consider our words. It may take a bit of retraining—yours, not his. Reconsider these popular idioms and clichés.

And even when you become aware of the morass of language obstacles your young one faces, you will fall off the wagon occasionally. (See?) When Bryce was about seven, we experienced what I came to call "The Terrible Weary Battle of the Hangnail." It was one of those infamous incidents that escalate inexorably from nothing to warfare before you realize what's happening. And you are left with an episode for which you can be forever unproud.

He came to me with a tiny hangnail on the index finger. The offending finger was being held immobile by the opposite hand. "No big deal," I said, "I'll just nip it off with the nail clippers."

"Nooooooooooo!" He shrieked, gale force. "It will HURT!"

This child had spent his whole life being impervious to true pain and extreme cold. But for reasons I simply could not imagine, this hangnail was an antagonist of Goliath proportions.

First, the usual rebuttals. It won't hurt. I promise. I'll be very quick. Look the other way. No? Then, OK, you can do it yourself. No clippers? Just bite it off. No. We'll numb it with an ice pack first. No. We'll soften it up with a warm bath. No.

Out came plans B, C, D, E, F, and G, like some horrid Cat in the Hat variation. All rejected. Exasperation on both sides escalated sharply.

The evening wore on. Was that me, almost shouting? I knew I was losing it, being sucked in, sucked down, seemingly unable to break the fall. Now two people were miserable instead of one.

"Look," I said. "Here are the choices: I nip it off. You nip it off. Or you just live with it."

"Nooooooooooo!" Scarlet face, tears flying, hair matted with sweat.

Bedtime finally came, and with it, a mom with the determination of Houdini. As I bent to tuck him in, so stealthily palming the nail clipper, I grabbed his finger and the hangnail was history. The pure surprise on his face was unforgettable. "There," I said. "Did it hurt?"

"No."

The next morning I took him on my lap and told him two things. First, he had to trust me. If I tell him something will not hurt, I mean it. I would always be honest with him if something was going to hurt, like a shot. I respected his preference for the truth, however unpleasant. So when I told him it wasn't going to hurt, it wasn't going to hurt.

Just as important, I told him I really admired his tenacity. I explained that "tenacity" meant that he really stood by what he believed, didn't back down, resisted pressure. That took strength and determination. "You really stuck to your guns," I said, "and that can be a very good thing." The words hadn't even cleared my lips before I knew I had goofed. A dark cloud instantly eclipsed a troubled face.

"I don't want to stick to a gun!" he cried, truly alarmed.

And then: "Are you sure you didn't mean . . . *gum?*"

Don't say	Say Instead
It's a piece of cake	It is easy to do
Hold your horses!	Please stop (or slow down)
You are the apple of my eye	I love you very much
You have ants in your pants	It's hard for you to sit quietly
I'm at the end of my rope	I'm about to get angry
Stop beating around the bush	Please answer my question
Bite your tongue!	Please don't speak to me like that
You're like a bull in a china shop!	You are being too rough
I have butterflies in my stomach	I'm nervous/anxious about this
The ball is in your court	It' your turn
Let's call it a day	It's time to stop for now
He can't hold a candle to you at chess	You are better at chess than he
Cat got your tongue?	Is there a reason you can't answer me?
I smell a rat	This doesn't seem right to me

Common Idioms

Our conversation is rife with potentially incomprehensible idioms. How many of these automatically make their way into your speech: catch more flies with honey, bird in the hand, chicken feed, clam up, cold turkey, cook your goose, cry wolf, count your chickens before they hatch, look a gift horse in the mouth, eat crow, fat cat, for the birds, get your goat, high horse, in the doghouse, kill two birds with one stone, let the cat out of the bag, mad as a wet hen, monkey business, pull a rabbit out of a hat, rat race, sick as a dog, get your ducks in a row, snake in the grass, from the horse's mouth, straw that broke the camel's back, wild goose chase, teach an old dog new tricks?

And that's just the animal idioms. How about food idioms? It's cheesy. But that's the way the cookie crumbles. We all know you can't have your cake and eat it, too.

Body idioms? Might cost an arm and a leg! But if you learn it by heart, you'll become an old hand and be able to keep it under your thumb at all times.

Sports idioms, anyone? Hit it out of the park! The ball is in your court now, so if you jockey into position, you'll be able to call all the shots.

It's enough to drive your child up the wall.

Ellen Notbohm suggests visiting her Autism Today website to learn about her other products and services: Visit: http://notbohm.autismtoday.com today! Your comments and requests for reprint permission are welcome at ellen@thirdvaria-tion.com.

Contributing Author Ellen Notbohm—Author, columnist, and mother of sons with autism and ADHD, Ellen Notbohm is coauthor with Veronica Zysk of *1001 Great Ideas for Teaching and Raising Children with Autism Spectrum Disorders*. A columnist for Autism Aperger's Digest, her articles on autism have also appeared in Exceptional Parent, Children's Voice, Language Magazine, numerous parenting magazines, and over 100 websites.

PLANNING THE PERFECT BIRTHDAY PARTY

When it comes right down to it, kids with autism are just like every other kid. Let's help kids with autism through those challenges with the "perfect party for kids with autism" and help others along the way understand autism. Kids grow and learn in different ways—some can read at age 3, others not until third grade. Social graces have to be taught very carefully. For children on the autism spectrum, these challenges are a little bigger.

A LITTLE BACKGROUND INFORMATION: Sometimes it is hard to tell that a child has autism, and at other times it is very clear. A child with autism struggles with these developmental issues on a continuing basis. These five main challenges are:

1. Communication—Most people equate a difficulty in speaking as a sign of autism. That is true in some cases, but not in all. Some children with autism talk just like you and me but can have difficulty communicating their feelings or describing an event.
2. Sensory dysfunction–Many children with autism hear, see, taste, and smell better than most people. "Sensory violation" is a term my good friend Stephen Shore uses a lot when referring to offensive sounds, tastes, odors, or even clothing!
3. Social skill deficits—These challenges overlap, and difficulty in one area can affect others. The one constant is that children with autism have a difficult time making and keeping friends . . . and friends are the primary ingredient of a party!
4. Behavioral issues—Since kids with autism like to do things over and over again, which is called perseveration (per-sev-er-ay-shun), they have a unique ability to develop their area of interest whether it is art, music, dance, acting, or even

computers. It's important to incorporate their talents from the very beginning to help guide your child's life with the goal of helping them thrive and grow beyond their boundaries and into their greatest potential!

5. Physical challenges—Children with autism are very often not real active or may be very clumsy. Social skill deficits often deter those with autism to engage in sports, because sports are competitive. This lack of physical activity often results in clumsiness.

To begin, it's important to try to imagine what it's like to be a child with autism. So, I am going to ask you to take yourself back to when you were around the age of six. What was your favorite toy? Imagine for a moment that you are playing a game with your friends. To win your favorite toy, you have to walk across the room barefoot over ice cubes. When it is your turn, your friend puts duck tape over your mouth. Then, as you are crossing the room, firecrackers start exploding all around you, but you can't see where the noise is coming from. Now let's assess . . .

- How did you get across the ice? Did you walk on your toes to try to avoid contact with the cold, slippery surface? Do you think you might be walking on your toes to avoid contact with the ice cubes?
- How did you feel when the sounds started coming from everywhere? Did you cover your ears?
- How did you feel when your friend put tape on your mouth? Were you frustrated because couldn't say what you're thinking or feeling?
- Were you laughing at the scene, and what other kids would look like? Would they be laughing at you?
- Would any (or all of these) agitate or embarrass you?

All of this sounds very frustrating, doesn't it? You have now walked in the shoes of a kid with autism. Kids with autism love parties, too, and by asking you to think about how the "little" things matter, we hope that you can find activities that are fun for EVERYONE

TIPS FOR PLANNING THE PERFECT PARTY TO INCLUDE KIDS WITH AUTISM

Give your child a voice: It important for your child with autism to participate and see that his opinions and ideas matter. Get them involved in the beginning, whether it is choosing the colors they like, the party favors they want, or the people they'd like to invite. It helps them see the process from start to finish.

Avoid surprises: A party is an "unknown" that can leave kids with autism feeling uneasy and lacking control. Many kids with autism are very visual. Write out a little story, or if your child doesn't read yet, put together a series of pictures or drawings to show what will happen the very day of the party, step by step. This way they will know what to expect and can plan it in their own minds. Surprises are not fun for kids on the autism spectrum.

Inclusion starts with education: While you are inviting your child's friends, be sure to encourage the other children's parents not to be afraid of inviting your child just because he's different. Autism needs to be understood, not feared, and it's our job as parents to help this happen.

Age groups can be key: Keep the guest list appropriate to the child's age. Remember, too many kids may be too much stimulation if your child is sensitive to it.

Educate party guests: (Sometimes parents come, too) prior to and during the party. It is through empathy, not sympathy, that we begin to understand children with autism and their condition. It would be a good idea to print something about autism in the party invitation so kids know what to expect.

Here is an example:

Dear Party Friend,

Your friend, Jonny, has a condition called autism (aw-tis-em). He's a great kid and may be very interested (and good) at art, music, or computers. He sometimes acts different than you but his actions are nothing to be afraid of.

He may not look at you, but that doesn't mean he doesn't see you out of the corner of his eye. It's nothing personal against you. He may seem far away, spin in circles, or may not even talk to you, but that doesn't mean he doesn't care or want to be your friend. Keep trying to find things in common with him, and you will get to know a really great kid.

Sincerely,
Karen, [or, Jonny's Mom, Karen] *Jonny's Mom*

Tone it down: Make sure the party favors are not the loud (in your face) type and that they don't make unexpected sounds. Kids with autism often times are very sensitive to sounds and loud or unexpected noises.

Make a schedule and post it: Select activities that are structured and predictable, not impromptu or spontaneous. Kids with autism like to know what's coming next, and they thrive on structure.

Group play and individual play: Plan activities or games that the children can do by themselves or as a group. Group activities can often be intimidating at the best of times for children with autism, as social interactions may be very challenging for most. If you do plan games, plan quiet ones for those who want to play and maybe some activity tables for those who do not want to play a game. Above all, plan activities that may not escalate into a lot of noise or commotion.

Build the party menu carefully: Food allergies are prevalent in all communities. It is a good idea to ask about allergies before the party or ensure that there are sugar-, wheat-, gluten-, dairy-, and peanut-free choices for everyone. You will have a much calmer party, and everybody will have something to munch on. Besides, who says you can't break the norm by saying good-bye to traditional birthday cake and ice cream?

Redirect and be aware: It can be hard for kids to stay "in the moment" in any given social situation, especially when there's not much feedback from another child. In this case, you can help the regular kids engage with the child with autism by finding a common ground for them to share.

Plan around a successful skill: Find a great strength the child with autism has to focus on and play it up. By doing so, you will help his or her light shine and build their self-esteem. Maybe she likes to draw. Build the party around drawing. Perhaps he loves lining up trains. Expand his common interest and find engaging games for the other kids so they can play with him . . . with his trains. The ideas you can come up with are endless. After we published the *Artism*™ *Art by those with Autism* book, I have witnessed many early artists become phenomenal artists as adults with high self-esteem.

IF YOU ARE GOING TO A PARTY YOU DIDN'T PLAN:

- Talk to the host before you attend. Be sure to explain what to expect.
- Set realistic expectations for your child.
- Talk about the schedule of events for the party.
- Bring alternative food and drinks if needed.
- Explain and review how present time works.
- Talk about manners.
- Be there for your child. It seems obvious, but if you head off an issue before it's a problem, your child will feel more successful.

If you need to leave early, don't assign guilt, but do talk about it later and assess what happened so that your child will have many more successes in the future. Be sure to pass out this information to everyone you meet so they can learn what makes your child with autism "tick." This way we can raise awareness one party person at a time. Most important, have fun with this party plan. By following these tips and guidelines, you will make it an absolutely perfect party for your child with autism for years to come.

I invite YOU to celebrate a "perfect party" with your child with autism!

—Karen L. Simmons, CEO Autism Today

7

POSITIVE TOOLS TO BUILD SELF-ESTEEM

THE STRONGEST URGE OF ALL

Once again, my three-year-old Jonathan refused to walk, and I was forced to drag him across a busy street to keep an appointment with an autism specialist. It was an appointment that I was sure would be a waste of time, as nothing was wrong with my son Jon. As usual, his tantrum was getting unwanted attention from other people, and I was subjected to the stares that implied I couldn't control my child.

I was used to people reacting this way to Jonathan's moods. Heaven knows even some members of my own family didn't understand how special he really was and often gave me well-intentioned but useless advice.

Maternal love can often be a blinding emotion. My continued reluctance to accept the fact that there might be something wrong with Jonathan merely added fuel to my frustration. I was confident that he was an exceptionally bright child, as he had begun reading at the young age of two and his first word wasn't the usual "Mommy" or "Daddy," but "recycle."

For an hour, the doctor asked Jonathan a battery of questions and then said he might have Pervasive Developmental Disorder: a fancy name for what would later be termed "autism." Because he was so young, a definite diagnosis would not be possible. The doctor told us to go home and to come back in a year.

A year! Wait for a year? I knew enough about PDD to know that early diagnosis and treatment during the formative years was crucial. So I immediately sought a second opinion. The next doctor gave Jon tests and also observed his actions. Jon would spin around in circles, couldn't sit still, wouldn't follow simple instructions, and hummed out loud. This doctor also suspected autism and recommended us to another psychiatrist.

So off we went, and thank God we did. The next doctor recommended and found a placement for Jonathan in an Early Intervention Program. But even so, I still needed reassurance of the diagnosis and went to another specialist just to make sure. It was when the last doctor confirmed the fact that I was finally able to accept the reality of Jonathan's disorder.

It was winter 1993 when I placed him into a neighborhood school Early Intervention Program that is designed to help special needs children during the first years of their lives. Therapies, there, focused on enhancing speech, communications interaction, fine and gross motor movement, sensory stimulation, and physical therapy. A bonus of this program was that the ratio of teachers was three for every eight students. Finally, Jonathan was going to get everything he needed, and I could expend some of my energies on other family members.

My husband, Jim, and I had five children, and this made for a busy household and a full life. Kimberly was eight, Matthew seven, Christina six, Jonathan, and baby Stephen who was only 19 months old. And just when you think things have settled down, God gives you another blessing. I became pregnant with our sixth child.

I had never experienced difficulties with any of my previous pregnancies. So I continued on with my hectic schedule. In addition to raising the children, I had started attending conferences on autism, ever hopeful that somewhere would be a cure and maybe this whole thing would go away. Again, this was my maternal urge and a mother's unrealistic hope for a miracle.

Our son Alex, born on April 18, 1994, wasn't even named for three weeks but was just known as "Baby Sicoli." That was because I had not recovered well from the birth and spent three weeks in a coma in intensive care, surviving five major surgical procedures and care from 20 doctors. At times, there was doubt that I would survive, and I had received last rites. But the doctors' skills, combined with the prayers of relatives, friends, and members of prayer groups that I had never met, saved my life.

While it may sound funny, there was another event that gave me that final boost of energy to recover.

Jim came into my hospital room and, through a fog, I heard him say, "Don't worry, honey, I'll take care of the kids." How could he do that and manage the family business, not to mention all the things Jonathan required? This time my maternal urge was a positive emotion that drove me up out of that hospital bed. To this day, many people refer to me as the Miracle Lady.

It was a joyous moment when I was able to hold Alex for the first time. All the children came to visit, and after their initial awkwardness about all the tubes and the breathing machine, they climbed aboard and I gave them wheelchair rides. They were eager for me to come home, and young Stephen even tore the "Sic" off my Sicoli wristband in an effort to show that I was well and ready to leave.

The homecoming was a nervous time for me. I couldn't walk, and stairs were out of the question. Six months were to pass before the tube from my kidney was removed. At the same time as this happened, another milestone event slammed into our lives.

My mother had noticed that baby Alex's eyes "jiggled," and she was also worried that he couldn't support his weight on his little legs. I really didn't think it was a big deal, but I made an appointment with our pediatrician so that it could be checked. Once again, my maternal urges were protecting me against a possible problem.

Our doctor did a thorough examination including a CT scan, and while we were still at the hospital we got the test results. The good news was that it was not a brain tumor; the bad news was Alex had cerebral palsy. I felt like vomiting. No brain tumor? I hadn't even thought of that and had felt sure all the tests were going to be negative. I was in shock about the cerebral palsy, though. Not one, but two children with special needs. Life just wasn't fair.

I went home and cried my eyes out. But after a while I realized that for the sake of everyone, I had to get on with things. Even though I couldn't see it, I kept telling myself there's always a good side to everything. Soon Alex and I began the same journey I had taken with Jonathan: one doctor after another; one test after another. And again, we had more sad news. I had picked up Alex's CT scan from one hospital and carried it with me to a brain specialist the following day. After examining Alex, he said, "I don't know why you're here, there doesn't seem to be anything wrong with this child." "Did you see the scan?" I asked.

He hadn't. He and an intern then viewed it in the examining room with me, and I heard him mumble. "See this groove here, and this one here, you could drive a truck through it." I wondered what on earth he was talking about.

Finally he turned to us and said, "CP is the least of your problems. You will have to watch Alex carefully and you won't be able to be sure till he's five, but he may have major delays. It doesn't look good." I was devastated, and his style didn't give me any kind of reassurance. I still think some doctors should be required to take a "Bedside Manners When Dealing with Patients and Parents" course. It's a course I know many of us would love to help instruct.

Without my really realizing it, my life had now become very full. In addition to raising the children, I was helping with our family business and attending numerous conferences relating to autism, cerebral palsy, and services for children. It was at one of these conferences that a new focus entered my life. What was said by a 12-year-old autistic boy, a speaker at the conference, struck a nerve in both my heart and my soul. "I wish I would've known about my autism earlier. Everyone else knew," he said.

I was filled with resolve that this wasn't going to happen to Jonathan. It was his life, and he deserved to know everything about it. I began to search for a book that would tell him what he needed to know, but I came up empty. No such book existed. So with my usual single-mindedness, I proceeded to write one. To my delight, a publisher accepted the story, and *Little Rainman* was born. It was a surprise announcement for Jim, as I had kept that book a secret. He was still having trouble accepting Jonathan's autism. Every day he would come home and say, "Is Jonathan OK?" He kept hoping Jon would just snap out of it one day.

Little Rainman took off, and, aside from its originally intended audience (children with autism), it is being read by friends, relatives, and teachers of autistic children. The publisher, Future Horizons, says: "*Little Rainman* gives a more simplistic, yet comprehensive explanation of this strange disorder than any other book we have seen." Those kind words mean the world to me. They validated my labor of love for Jonathan.

As I write this, Jonathan is doing fine. Yes, he's still autistic. He goes to a regular school, and we certainly have our moments. His latest "accomplishment" is that he has learned to lie. Most children pick this talent up earlier in life. A recent example was when he told his aide that he had a tummyache and didn't want to go play. Then he went to his teacher and said, "I told my aide I had a tummyache so I wouldn't have to go play." The teacher told the aide what he had said. She said, "Jonathan, a little 'birdie' told me that you didn't want to go play, so you told me you had a stomachache. Is this true?" Jonathan said, "Teacher doesn't have feathers!" With true mother's bias, I view this as an example of wit and humor.

In a couple of months, Alex is going into the same Early Intervention Program that Jonathan attended. At his orientation day, the teacher was so impressed with his progress that she suggested he might be able to start in the advanced class. This made me very happy and made the time I have spent enriching his program over the last two years very worthwhile.

He is just beginning to speak, and we call him our little miracle baby. He walks, runs, and even climbs all over everything. Not that I would ever complain about his high level of activity, I consider it a blessing. He had his first seizure last winter, and it scared the living daylights out of us. I pray that it will not be repeated.

Alex's doctor says his brain scan shows the typical image of someone who is severely crippled and most likely has been confined to a wheelchair. Not that life is always dreadful. I have the good fortune of knowing a local newspaper writer who has cerebral palsy, and his life is very rich. I was thrilled when he took the time to write a delightful article about *Little Rainman*.

I never anticipated the overwhelming response to my book, and I have been told that it is changing the way autistic people are viewed. It demonstrates that they, too, want and need to be loved. They do appear distant and uncaring at times, but this is because autism is a sensory and communication disorder. The very thing they have a hard time with, communication and their lack of social skills, blocks the amount of love they receive. But love, once given, is returned a hundredfold. It would be my hope that these words will be the spark to ignite other mothers to write and share their life experiences as they deal with their children and their own strong maternal urges.

In July of 1996, before the book was printed, I started the Key Enrichment of Exceptional Needs Foundation (KEEN), in Sherwood Park, Alberta. The purpose was to assist people with exceptional needs to become the best that they can be. To this end, we provide funds toward existing programs, equipment, services, and therapies. An important intent of the foundation is to help enrich the lives and minds of parents, siblings, educators of special needs children, and of course . . . special needs children.

In my own case, taking the knowledge I have gained from Jonathan and Alex and applying it to others has certainly enriched my life. I am now thrilled to be distributing all Future Horizon's books on autism across Canada in the hope that this will raise autism awareness and promote diagnosis at the earliest possible age. This, along with many public speaking engagements to different groups about autism and special needs, continues to keep my life full and meaningful.

I thank God daily for my life and for my loving and compassionate husband, parents, and friends. He has given me six wonderful children, including the two who have special needs. My own words are inadequate to describe all they have taught me about love and acceptance. Who would have guessed, a single gemologist jeweller, in ten short but full years, would become a mother of six, almost die, write a book, and start a foundation. My life, although chaotic at times, is really about living with what God has given me.

They say that view of life determines whether your glass is half empty or half full . . . like my maternal urges and love, my cup runneth over! The strongest urge of all.

Karen L. Simmons, CEO and author suggests visiting her Autism Today website to learn about her other products and services: Visit: http:/ simmons.autismtoday. com today!

Contributing Author Karen Simmons Sicoli, CEO, Autism Today, is a mother of six and the author of *Little Rainman*, a story of autism told through the eyes of her son, and coauthor of the *"Chicken Soup for The Soul"* book surrounding exceptional needs. A gemologist by trade, Karen shifted gears to working full-time in the autism community after a near-death experience. She is the founder of AutismToday.com and is active worldwide in promoting a deeper and more personal understanding of autism and Asperger's Syndrome. She makes her home in Sherwood Park, Alberta, Canada.

FACING AUTISM FOR LAW ENFORCEMENT AND FIRST RESPONDERS

Early one morning, nineteen-year-old Reginald Latson sat on the front lawn of the local library in Stafford County, Virginia, waiting for it to open. A nearby-school staff apparently reported a suspicious black male, possibly with a gun, sitting by the library, and soon enough Latson was approached by a police officer. When the officer asked Latson for his name, he didn't respond. The officer searched the young man and didn't find a weapon but reportedly continued to press the boy until a struggle ensued. Latson was ultimately arrested, held in isolation without bail for 11 days, and was convicted and sentenced to two years in jail. Once released during his probation, unfortunately, he got into a physical struggle at a treatment center; police once again were called, and Latson was ultimately sentenced to another 10 years. Three years later, after many pleas and protests from the community, the state governor granted him a pardon conditional on his accepting treatment out of state. During his imprisonment, he was locked in solitary confinement for months, a stun gun was used on him, and correctional officers regularly assaulted him. A lawsuit has been filed against the prison authorities.

Reginald woke up that morning in 2010 to responsibly return a library book. He spent the next three years in prison. News reports suggest it is a potential case of racial profiling, but what is painfully clear is that the judge didn't understand enough to take into account Latson's Asperger's diagnosis. Neither the police involved nor the courts or the correctional authorities appeared to have the knowledge or training to recognize and successfully respond to Latson's symptomatic behaviors. Instead, he was treated as a danger to officers, and apparently society as a whole. Like most people with Asperger's Disorder, Reginald Latson became anxious and shut down his communication when he was confronted by a stranger asking multiple questions very close in his personal space. Not unlike many people, he got uncomfortable when being frisked, and he also didn't fully understand why the officer was going into his pockets or touching him. He panicked. And while the officer also did not know of Latson's diagnosis, it seems unfathomable that the judge lacked any sense of human empathy.

In the past couple of years, persons with autism spectrum disorders have died in interactions with police, some of those interactions captured, in part, on cell phone videos. In the spring of 2016, an autistic adult died after an apprehension struggle with police. His only offense had been to wander away from a group on an outing. In the summer of 2016, an autism support worker was shot by police in the company of an autistic boy. The worker was filmed lying on the ground, with his hands up when he was shot. Some observers say that police intended to shoot the autistic boy beside him but missed.

Clearly stereotypical behaviors, which are generally not dangerous, of some autistic individuals are so greatly misunderstood by first responders that, in some cases, their (over)reactions are fatal. We should acknowledge how far police have come in diversity and special needs sensitivity training. However, if we are to truly serve and protect, *we still need to pursue greater acceptance and, frankly, just learn more about autism and all special populations.*

When officers are empowered with specific knowledge and understanding, then their responses can be more confident and dramatically more successful. For example, the *Toronto Star* newspaper reported the following story: Five years ago Constable Molyneaux, a police officer in Toronto, Canada, who had some knowledge about special needs answered a dispatcher's call to an apartment where a 12-year-old boy was clutching two knives and threatening suicide. The boy had Asperger's Syndrome.

"You model the behavior you want them to display," said Molyneaux. "You bring a deliberate, forced calm. There's an almost exaggerated mellowness to your voice."

Molyneaux noticed paper airplanes suspended in the room and asked the boy about them. In a few minutes, the boy gave up the knives.

It was lucky that Molyneaux was the one who answered the dispatcher's call. He has a child with Asperger's and knows how to handle meltdowns and knew what to expect. Today, Molyneaux provides the only training in autism response that any of the 5,200 Toronto police receive: a one-hour presentation, footnoted below, one time in their career.

Many police and first responders intend to approach people with special needs in a respectful and caring way. No one can respond to every special need effectively; and certainly much less effectively when training and coaching are not provided. It's difficult, though. The range of special needs that police officers may interact with is staggering. And when it comes to autism, the spectrum of behaviors that define the disorder is broad—from "high-functioning" people who have jobs and might be married with children yet who struggle to socialize, all the way to "low-functioning" people unable to communicate, with unusual repetitious behaviors. Both high-functioning and low-functioning individuals with autism are likely to have anxiety and stress levels that can escalate quickly.

There are books and training courses teaching law enforcement officers to "recognize the signs of autism." On one hand, recognition profiles are necessary. On the other hand, they can also unintentionally perpetuate stereotypes. Since autism is a *spectrum* disorder, it's hard for anyone, even specialist doctors who diagnose, to instantly recognize all of the challenges of all people with autism. So should police be expected to do this?

The main idea I share with first responders is to be cautious about stereotyped profiling, very much along the lines of what I discuss in *Challenging the Myths of Autism* (Harper Collins, 2011). For example, if you believe people with autism are aggressive, or can't speak or have mental retardation, then you are likely to misjudge and misinterpret their behavior. You may act in less than effective ways because people with autism aren't all the same.

Recognizing the unique behaviors is the obvious first step: training on how to react, to establish rapport, to gain cooperation, and most important, to avoid potentially fatal reactions should be a mandatory second step. Along with teaching officers to identify the tell-tale signs of autism, here are three immediately useful strategies that can be used regardless of the degree of autism:

1) RECOGNIZE COMMUNICATION DISORDERS/ CHALLENGES:

When approaching a suspect, law enforcement officers use their voice and words to communicate important instructions, yet many people with autism are not able to understand verbal communication or the meaning of voice tone. They may not respond appropriately to simple questions like "What is your name?" and may not comply with simple commands such as "Stop right there." *However, it would be false to conclude that they are ignoring the command or resisting arrest.* Not understanding is different than ignoring.

One communication disorder common in people diagnosed with autism is called "echolalia" in which the person simply repeats almost everything they hear in direct imitation. A police officer may ask, "What is your name," and a person with echolalia would reply with "What is your name?" A common reflex is to think the person repeating your words is mocking you. An officer could easily conclude that the subject is making fun of them.

Even more difficult is that people with autism don't have visible signs or immediately obvious behaviors that let you know they don't understand when you first approach. Communication disorders are a "hidden disability" until you are faced with having to get information or give commands. Note: getting louder isn't the answer, and using a more aggressive tone won't help, either. Your first step should be to not assume that when a person doesn't respond to your verbal communications they are deliberately begin defiant or refusing to comply. Instead, consider that your intended message is simply not getting through.

Signs that an individual may have a communication challenge or be autistic:

- They don't turn their head toward the verbal command.
- They show absolutely no behavioral response to the command.
- They respond to different questions or commands with one single word or phrase repeatedly.

In this situation, it is best to:

√ Stop using verbal language as your main communication style
with them. If they aren't responding to simple questions like
"What's your name," more complex dialogue isn't going to help.

√ Try to position your body to ensure the suspect can see you before
giving further verbal commands.

√ Try smiling and moving in a predictable and nonaggressive
manner. Nonverbal communicators often rely on nonverbal
cues and behavior to understand. They are more likely to pay
attention and try to cooperate with a friendly-looking person
than a serious or angry-looking one.

√ Provide one clear instruction like "Please sit down" and look for
any small behavioral signs, rather than a verbal response, that
they are trying to comply.

√ Use animated/exaggerated physical (but nonaggressive) gestures,
like pointing to where you want them to stand, which they may
understand better than verbal commands.

2) USE APPROACH TECHNIQUES TO GAIN TRUST VS. TRIGGER "STARTLE"

Especially when you suspect a communication challenge, there is a higher
possibility of triggering a startle-and-defense (flight or fight) response: running away, screaming, or aggression, if you:

- Approach too quickly
- Don't establish line-of-sight visual acknowledgment (make sure
they *see* you)
- Sound angry (voice tone)
- Try to establish physical touch/control before they are ready

In this situation, it is best to:

√ Ask yourself who, if anyone, is in danger with things as they are.
If the answer is "no one," or the danger to the subject can be

mitigated without needing to gain immediate compliance by the subject, take a deep breath and proceed slowly.

√ Be patient. If there is no imminent danger, wait longer than usual for the suspect to take the first steps toward you, i.e., for them to begin to cooperate. When they perceive they are in control, they will cooperate much more readily.

√ Lower your body position. Especially for younger children, it will often be better to lower your face and eye level. Drop to one knee, to avoid towering over the child when giving commands. The chances of triggering aggression from this position are greatly reduced.

√ Use your voice tone like a front-line tool to communicate "security" and "friendliness." People with autism will be much more likely to pay attention and not get defensive (i.e., stop listening) when they hear in your tone that you are sincerely trying to help and not hurt. Raising your voice volume will almost always trigger more startle and less cooperation.

√ Provide more reassuring statements than interrogating questions. The statements "You're okay" and "I'm going to help you" will gain trust versus rapid fire questions like "What's your name?" and "What are you doing here?" Your first objective with a person with autism is to establish rapport and to gain their attention before you can assume to begin questioning, probing for more information or seeking their cooperation.

3) RECOGNIZE SUBTLE AND ESCALATING SIGNS OF (DIS)STRESS

For many people with autism, especially nonverbal children, it is common that their level of stress (and consequent presigns of aggression) escalates rapidly. Anxiety is highly comorbid with autism. As most parents of these children will explain, there are some tell-tale signs that identify increased anxiety early on:

- Tension in the extremities (fingers, arms, legs), clenched, or extended

- Increase in hyperactivity (jumping, pacing, vocalizations)
- Increase in stereotypical autistic behaviors (hand flapping, walking on toes, flicking fingers in front of face, screeching, self-talk)

Important Note: While many of these same behaviors if exhibited by a nonautistic suspect might indicate impending aggression or noncompliance toward the first responder, *for people with autism these behaviors may be self-regulating*; They may be the familiar and comforting behaviors the child or adult does to cope with the mounting stress of not understanding the situation, in the same way that some of us pace back and forth when we have a difficult decision to make.

This is usually not an appropriate time to escalate your command and control techniques of shouting commands or physically arresting/controlling the subject.

Instead, if you recognize escalating signs of distress, it is best to:
√ Give the autistic person some room to jump or hand-flap for up to one or two minutes. It is best to not add to their distress with more questions or verbal information. Silence can be a powerful tool to gain rapport and to deescalate the stress.

√ Maintain your position but don't advance, i.e., you don't have to immediately control or stop these behaviors. If they aren't dangerous, the repetitive behaviors may be necessary for the person to calm down. This may be a kind of physical self-soothing by the subject, not aggression directed toward the intervenor.

√ Again, use a calming voice to deescalate tension and communicate statements that "You are safe with me" and "You can relax and listen with me." Model the behavior you would like to see in the subject.

By practicing and using these strategies, you can reduce situations of risk both to the subject and you, the intervenor.

We recommend that you find an opportunity to spend some time with a person with autism outside of an arrest situation. This will begin to demystify autism as a strange "other" disorder.

Police need to identify stereotypical signs of autism, but just as important, to apply this set of skills and restrategize in these fresh ways to gain rapport and cooperation successfully. These strategies have broader benefits, not only with people with autism, but toward good outcomes in addressing, for example, subjects with other mental health challenges and behavioral disorders.

In fact, most of us, however law-abiding and innocent, display increased anxiety and less coherence, in initial interactions with police. A gentler more empathic assessment and approach can produce a safer and more successful interaction with members of the public in the majority of police encounters.

We encourage parents to share this article with local authorities including their local police and fire stations and with their apartment/residence and school security personnel.

Recommended reading:

Challenging the Myths of Autism, Jonathan Alderson (Harper Collins, 2011).
Dennis Debbaudt's First Responder training videos and materials, www
  .autismriskmanagement.com

Jonathan Alderson, Ed.M., is an autism treatment specialist and founder of the innovative Intensive Multi-Treatment Intervention Program (www.IMTI .ca). A graduate of Harvard University, with experience as a curriculum specialist coordinator with Teach for America, he trained at the Autism Treatment Center of America in Massachusetts and worked as administrator and senior family trainer in their Son-Rise Program. He has worked with over 3,000 children and families. Now based in Toronto, he is a contributor for the Huffington Post, a member of the Seneca College behavioral Sciences Advisory Committee, and cochair of the Young Professionals for Autism Speaks Canada Advisory Board. He has lectured on his multidisciplinary approach to autism treatment throughout Canada, the USA, England, Ireland, Holland, Spain, Australia, Israel, and Mexico. He is the author of *Challenging the Myths of Autism,* which has inspired educators and parents to consider a radical reframing of how we think about and treat people diagnosed with autism. His book has been honored with the Mom's Choice Gold Award, the American Non-Fiction Authors' Association Silver award, and the 2012 International Book Award for Best Parent-Resource.

Gordon Mac Scott is a safety and security consultant and trainer based in Toronto, Canada. He is a former policing manager and has served as Board member and chair of arts, youth, immigrant settlement, and community organizations. He is managing partner of the Strategic Improvement Company providing crisis management, training, and safety audit services, as well as policy guidance to government, social agencies, and the private sector. He has lectured at colleges and universities and received numerous awards and recognitions.

I AM . . .: ONE MOTHER'S EXPERIENCE

I am the mother of a child who has special needs. I am the little engine that did. When on my journey in life my tracks led me to a mountain—a diagnosis of autism, or CP, or MR, or a similar disability—I have looked at it with defeat, thinking there was no way. I could climb over it. I then pondered the obstacle before me, and I then said to myself over and over, "I think I can, I think I can . . . ." Then I slowly started climbing the mountain saying to myself over and over, "I know I can, I know I can . . . ." and I made it over that ominous diagnosis and continued my journey. I am the little engine that did.

I am more devoted than Noah's wife. I sometimes feel overwhelmed in my "houseboat," 365 days and 365 nights a year, constantly working with and teaching my child. But when the storms of isolation and monotony become most unbearable, I do not jump ship. Instead, I wait for the rainbow that is promised to come.

I am Xena, real-life warrior goddess of Autism.

With my steel-plated armor I can battle anyone who gets in the way of progress for my child. I can overcome the stares and ignorance of those with no experience of disability in their lives and educate them as to why my child is the way he is and why he does the things he does. With my sword of persistence, I can battle the schools to have them properly educate my child. Yes, I am Xena—and I am prepared for any battle that might come my way.

I am beautiful. I have hairy legs because I get no time alone in the bathroom. I have bags under my eyes from staying up all night with my child. The only exercise I get is the sprint from my house to my car, to take my child to therapy. "Dressed up" to me is, well. . . just that I had a moment to get dressed! They say that beauty is in the eye of the beholder. So even on the days when I don't feel very beautiful, I will know that I am beautiful because God is my beholder.

I am the Bionic Woman. With my bionic vision, I can see through the disability my child has, to see the beauty in his soul, the intelligence in his eyes, when others can't. I have bionic hearing. I can look at my child when he smiles at me and hear his voice say, "I love you, Mommy," even though he can't talk. Yes, I am thankful to be Bionic.

I am Mary. I am a not-so-well-known mother of a special needs child who was brought here to touch the souls of those around him in a way that will forever change them. And it started with me by teaching me things I would never have known, by bringing me friendships I never would have had, and by opening my eyes as to what really matters in life. He has shown me things like the Joy of just living in the moment, the Peace of knowing that God is in control, never losing Hope, and knowing an unconditional Love that words cannot express. Yes, I too am blessed by a special child, just like Mary.

I am Superwoman. I am able to leap over tall loads of laundry in a single bound and run faster than a speeding bullet, to rescue my child from danger. Oh yes, without a doubt, I am Superwoman.

I am Moses. I was chosen to be the mother of a special needs child. I may at times question whether I am the right person for the job, but God will give me the faith I need to lead my child to be the best he can be. And as with Moses, God will give me the small miracles, here and there, needed to accomplish my mission.

I am Stretch Armstrong—the mom who can be stretched beyond belief and still somehow return to normal. I can stretch limited funds to cover every treatment and therapy that insurance won't cover. I can stretch my patience as I bounce from doctor to doctor in a quest to treat my child. I can stretch what time. I have, and share it with my husband, my children, my church—and still have some left over to help my friends. Yes, my name is Stretch. And I have the stretch marks to prove it!

I am Rosa Parks. I refuse to move or waver in what I believe is right for my child in spite of the fact that my views are among those of the minority, not the majority. I refuse to accept the defeatist question, "What can one mother do?" Instead, I will write, call, and rally before the government, if I have to, and do whatever it takes to prevent discrimination against my child and to ensure he gets the services he needs.

I am Hercules, the Greek god known for strength and courage. The heavy loads I must carry would make others crumble to the ground. The weight of sorrow, fear of uncertainty of the future, injustice at having no answers, and the tears of despair would alone possibly be too much, even for Hercules. But then the joy, laughter, smiles, and pride at my child's accomplishments balance the load and make it easy to bear.

I am touched by an Angel, an Angel who lives in a world of his own. And it's a fact. He lives in a world of innocence and purity, a world without hatred or deceit. He lives in a world where everyone is beautiful and where no one is ugly, a world where there is always enough time. He lives in a world where he goes to bed with no worries of tomorrow and wakes up with no regrets of the past. Yes, I most certainly am touched by an Angel, and in some ways his world is better.

I am a true "Survivor." I am the mom of a child who has faced, is facing, and will face some of the most difficult challenges life has to offer. I am ready for the challenge and have God-given endurance to last until the end, along with a sense of humor to cope with all the twists, turns, and surprises along the way. Oh yes, I am a true "Survivor"—and I don't need to win a million dollars to prove it!

I am a mom of a special needs child, all the above, and so much more. Some days I will want to be none of the above and just be a typical mom with a typical child, doing typical things. On those days I will know it's okay to be angry, and to cry and to lean on my family, friends, and church for support, because after all most important I am human.

And on this day, and any other day I feel the need, I will read this as a reminder of just who it is that I am.

Contributing Author Karen Simmons Sicoli, CEO, Autism Today—Karen Simmons is a mother of six and the author of *Little Rainman*, a story of autism told through the eyes of her son, and coauthor of the *"Chicken Soup For The Soul"* book surrounding exceptional needs. A gemologist by trade, Karen shifted gears to working full-time in the autism community after a near-death experience. She is the founder of AutismToday.com and is active worldwide in promoting a deeper and more personal understanding of autism and Asperger's Syndrome. She makes her home in Sherwood Park, Alberta, Canada.

ADDRESSING BEHAVIORAL CHALLENGES FOR THOSE WITH AUTISM

Effective teaching strategies for students with autism require development of a systematic program for addressing problem behaviors. Students with autism often exhibit a wide variety of challenging behaviors, including physical aggression, self-injury, tantrums, and noncompliance. These behaviors are disconcerting to staff and parents and should be resolved. Developing effective behavior intervention programs is often the most important step for the classroom or home. The following are important elements of an effective program:

- Reviewing the elements of a functional assessment
- Developing and writing a behavior intervention plan
- Identifying the principles of active programming
- Teaching replacement skills
- Reviewing environmental controls
- Implementing compliance training
- Planning reactive programming
- Developing a crisis management plan

An effective program for managing problem behaviors focuses on two main strategies: proactive programming and reactive programming.

Principles of proactive programming

Highly effective programs for students with autism emphasize proactive strategies for reducing problem behaviors and teaching replacement skills. Proactive programs:

- Assume the problem behavior serves a purpose for the student and attempts to teach alternative and replacement skills that serve the same function

- Modify the antecedents and environmental controls
- Begin by determining the function of the maladaptive behavior for the student
- Seek replacement behaviors for the maladaptive behavior

Principles of reactive programs

Systematic reactive programs can effectively decrease the frequency and duration of problem behaviors. Unfortunately, most classrooms for students with autism focus entirely on reactive programming. Reactive programs:

- Wait for the maladaptive behavior to occur and then respond with a punishment
- Focus on the consequences of the behavior
- May ultimately reinforce the maladaptive behavior
- Do not significantly or permanently change maladaptive behaviors

Functional assessment

A comprehensive intervention program for students with autism will provide a careful balance between both a proactive and reactive program. This involves conducting a thorough functional assessment and developing an appropriate behavior intervention plan.

A thorough functional assessment is the first step in a proactive program. It begins the process of understanding the purpose of the student's behavior and what the student is trying to communicate. The goal of a functional assessment is to identify the purpose and effect of a target behavior by examining its function for the student.

An effective functional assessment is built on several assumptions:

- That the problem behavior serves a function for the student. A student exhibiting problem behaviors is using a functional approach to communication to achieve a specific outcome.
- Therefore, school personnel must conduct a functional assessment to thoroughly understand function of the behavior for the student.

- That if a student is repeating a problem behavior, then the consequence of the behavior has been reinforced for that student in the past. Each of us tends to repeat behaviors that are positively reinforced.
- That a student exhibiting problem behaviors often does not know the correct adaptive skills or has not been reinforced effectively for displaying appropriate adaptive behaviors.

Functional assessment made easy

Whether mandated through an IEP team or conducted as an informal assessment by the classroom staff, a functional assessment can be conducted efficiently and easily with the right tools.

Step 1: Define target behavior

First, define an observable and measurable target behavior. The problem behavior targeted for a functional assessment will vary with the student. The team may choose to target a behavior that can be easily corrected before moving to more challenging behaviors. Targeting lesser behaviors may build success for the student and staff and make changing more challenging behaviors easier.

If, however, behaviors are harmful to the student or others, the team may choose to work on several behaviors at once. All identified target behaviors must be clearly defined and measurable to ensure consistency across settings.

Step 2 : Information gathering

Collect information from a variety of sources. The team may interview teachers, parents, and related service personnel who work with the student.

Interview data focus on the antecedents and consequences of the behavior. Interview adults who have a significant relationship with the student and who can contribute to defining the target behavior and function.

Information may also be collected through direct observation. Observations focus on the frequency, duration, and intensity of the target behavior.

Observations should occur in the natural settings where the target behavior is exhibited. Direct observations also include an analysis of environmental factors that may contribute to the maladaptive behavior.

Physiological factors are the last area of data collection that may influence problem behaviors. Students with autism often have potential medical issues that are causing an increase in maladaptive behaviors. Physiological areas to be considered in a functional assessment include:

- Diet and nutrition
- Sleep patterns and fatigue
- Medication side effects
- Sickness
- Stress outside the classroom

It is important to carefully consider how these variables influence problem behaviors. If the student is hungry or thirsty and has no functional communication system, the outcome will be irritability and an increase in problem behaviors. The classroom team can effectively address these issues and reduce further problem behaviors.

Step 3: Developing a hypothesis

In this step, review the data and identify the function of the problem behavior. The function of problem behaviors varies with each student. The following are a few common functions and applicable questions to be addressed by the team:

Escape/Avoidance
- Is the task too difficult?
- Is the student bored?
- Does the behavior start when a request or demand is made?
- Does the activity take too long?
- Is the classroom too noisy?
- Does the behavior stop when the student is removed from the activity?

Attention
- Is the student receiving adequate attention for NOT displaying the problem behavior?
- Are other students receiving more attention?
- Is the student alone for long periods?
- Does the student exhibit the behavior when they are alone?
- Does the behavior occur to get a reaction?

Power/Control
- Is the student given choices in the classroom?
- Are there opportunities for the student to take a break?
- Does the behavior stop after the student receives a desired object?

Communication
- Does the student have a functional and reliable communication system?
- Is the student provided with the necessary equipment to communicate wants and needs?
- Does the behavior seem to be a way for the student to ask for help?

Stress/Frustration
- Is the student stressed?
- Does the student have adequate skills to release stress in an appropriate manner?
- Is the classroom environment chaotic?
- Does the student seem calm or relaxed after the problem behavior has stopped?

Self-stimulation or sensory stimulation
- Is the behavior part of the stereotypical pattern of behaviors?
- Is the environment producing adequate stimulation?
- Does the student have frequent opportunities for sensory integration?
- Does the student repeat the behavior when alone?
- Does the student appear unaware of his surroundings?

The multidisciplinary team examines the information collected and develops a written statement regarding the function of the behavior. A clear hypothesis statement is written in a positive manner, based on facts from information gathering. The following are examples of hypothesis statements:

- Morning circle is too long for Jonathan, and he bites other students to escape the task.
- Samantha refuses to complete her morning math work because she requires additional adult assistance. When the teacher is helping other students, Samantha attempts to run out of the room to get immediate attention from the teacher.
- When Stephen goes to the cafeteria with the fifth grade class, he pushes other students and runs down the hallway to be first in line and to avoid waiting with the other students.

Each hypothesis statement identifies the target behavior and provides an "informed guess" as to the function of the behavior for the student.

Key concept: functional communication—Students with ASDs often have severe deficits in expressive language and communication skills. Therefore, there is a strong need for alternative communication systems. Augmentative and alternative communication devices allow the student to communicate and respond to the environment. Problem behaviors will only persist or increase if the student is unable to communicate basic needs.

Step 4: Developing a behavior intervention plan

The behavioral intervention plan is a written document that includes:

- An operational definition of the target behavior
- Summary of the relevant data
- Written hypothesis statement stating the function of the behavior
- List of modifications to the environment
- Teaching replacement or alternative behaviors
- Criteria or outcome evaluation

- Consequence strategies: crisis intervention plan and reactive programming

Most school districts have developed appropriate forms to be used for a written behavior intervention plan. If no form is readily available, the teacher can easily create an individualized plan for use in the classroom.

The behavior intervention plan requires two main components: teaching replacement skills and modifying the environment. Teaching replacement skills or alternative behaviors assumes that the student's problem behavior is meeting a need for the student and that the student may not have the skills required for more adaptive behaviors. The replacement behavior, therefore, must be as effective and powerful as the maladaptive behavior.

For example, if Zachary receives immediate and intense attention from the teacher for biting another student, the new replacement behavior must also give Zachary the same immediate and intense attention from the teacher. Teaching Zachary to raise his hand and wait several moments for the teacher's attention will not be an effective alternative skill.

Key concept: teaching replacement skills—Teaching the desired replacement skill should result in:

- Meeting the same function or purpose for the student
- Teaching a skill that can be implemented across settings
- An efficient and effective alternative for the student

Teaching replacement behaviors to students with autism uses a variety of instructional techniques. While discrete trial instruction and incidental teaching are highly effective strategies in teaching replacement behaviors, the classroom staff can also implement other techniques including shaping, differential reinforcement, and token economies.

Reinforcement strategies

Since all people are motivated by positive reinforcement, using reinforcement strategies is a key element for teaching students with autism. Most typically developing students are reinforced through task completion and teacher praise, but students with autism are not typically reinforced through these internal methods. They require external motivation to maximize their learning and increase adaptive behaviors. Therefore, school personnel must identify appropriate reinforcers and use them effectively throughout the school day. Types of reinforcers include edibles (but use these seldom and only while other reinforcers are being developed), tangibles, social praise, and activities.

Guidelines for selecting reinforcers

Selecting reinforcers for students with autism is a continuous process that changes throughout the school year. Not all students are motivated by the same items. Selecting appropriate high-quality reinforcement involves:

- Observing the student in the classroom
- Completing a reinforcement survey
- Interviewing the student or other adults

The reinforcement interests of some students may be readily apparent, while reinforcing other students requires investigation. Some students may have little experience playing with certain toys and games and therefore must be taught to enjoy specific items or activities.

Avoid bribery

Reinforcement depends on the student's completion of a task or of his exhibiting a desired behavior. Therefore, reinforcement is NEVER to be used as bribery. For example, reinforcement would not be provided to a student in the middle of a tantrum. Nor would a student receive a high-quality reinforcer to entice him into working. Bribery teaches the student that he does not have to comply in order to achieve the desired outcome.

Reinforcement schedules

Reinforcement is provided to the student after the student has met the predetermined criteria for a task or has exhibited a desirable behavior. The rate of reinforcement will be based on the task and the individual skills of the student. A reinforcement schedule will assist the staff in determining the appropriate timing for reinforcement.

When you first teach a new skill or desired behavior, reinforcement will be immediate and continuous. This immediate and continuous reinforcement will ensure repetition of the desired behavior. As the student progresses with a newly acquired skill or behavior, the reinforcement schedule will be thinned and become more intermittent. An intermittent schedule is like a slot machine: the student receives the payoff at varying intervals and will not know in advance when a payoff will occur.

Delayed reinforcement is used in a token economy system where the tokens are earned and can be exchanged for the reinforcement at a later time.

Delayed reinforcement should be systematically scheduled to increase the desired behavior.

Inconsistencies with delayed reinforcement increase student frustration and trigger problem behaviors. Again, the goal of reinforcement is to help the student become naturally self-motivating.

Environment and curriculum modifications

Although teaching replacement skills to the student is a daily activity and an integral part of the behavior intervention plan, the classroom staff must also address environmental modifications. After completing a classroom inventory, the teacher must review the needs of each student. Although the overall classroom may be arranged appropriately, some students will have specific needs that must be addressed. Additional modifications, tailored where possible to the specific needs of each student, will help ensure on-task behavior and increased independence.

Specific modifications may include:

Level of support: The student may need more adult assistance to learn a new skill.

Time: The student may require more or less time to complete an assigned task. Some students may need more breaks in their schedule.

Level of difficulty: Be sure to create a curriculum that is neither too easy nor too difficult. Unchallenging repetitive tasks create boredom for the student and will likely increase maladaptive behaviors.

Reactive programming

Although the focus of teaching students with autism should be proactive programming, it is also essential to develop a reactive program. In a reactive plan, the team determines the steps that will occur after the maladaptive or problem behavior is exhibited.

There are several strategies available to school personnel to address behaviors after they have occurred. The multidisciplinary team should consider the least intrusive methods for decreasing the likelihood of problem behaviors. Response cost, extinction, and punishment are a few reactive techniques that may be used in a school setting.

Reactive programming can further decrease the frequency of problem behaviors and may help the team regain control in a crisis. In a well-designed behavior program, reactive procedures will be used minimally, and then only with respect for the student.

Response cost

A response cost technique reduces undesirable behavior by removing a reinforcer. A response cost program is designed to remove a reinforcer when the problem behavior occurs.

For example, the student may be highly reinforced by working on the computer. Therefore, the teacher has laminated the eight letters of the word COMPUTER and placed each individual letter on the student's desk. Each time the student exhibits the problem behavior, one letter is removed from the word COMPUTER. For every letter that remains at the end of the day, the student receives five minutes of computer time.

Other response cost programs may include point systems or marbles in a jar. Response cost systems do not teach replacement skills, and they focus only on the consequence of the problem behavior.

Extinction

Another reactive technique for problem behaviors is extinction. Extinction is the gradual decrease of the problem behavior as reinforcement is discontinued. Extinction attempts to reduce the problem behavior by eliminating the reinforcement that maintains the behavior.

Many teachers try to use "planned ignoring" in order to extinguish a problem behavior. Decreasing disruptive behaviors through planned ignoring will depend on the function of the behavior and the ability of the teacher to completely eliminate reinforcement. If the function of the behavior is attention, it is imperative to remove all attention from the student.

For example, a student who screams and tantrums for attention may still have his needs met if he receives attention not only from the adults, but also from the other students. Therefore, all positive attention must be removed before ignoring will extinguish the problem behavior.

Ignoring or paying little attention to problem behaviors can be an effective procedure in a reactive program. Caution must be taken not to completely ignore self-injurious behaviors and aggression because of the likelihood the behavior will escalate. In some cases, the staff must provide some minimal attention in order to secure the environment for the student and others. Minimal attention means:

- A calm and neutral voice
- Little or no eye contact
- Minimal physical restraint
- Reduced demands

Extinction is a planned reactive intervention and should be used only when the function of the behavior is reinforced through attention from others.

Aversions and punishment

I do not recommend using or implementing averse procedures in school settings for students with autism. Aversives can be characterized as intrusive procedures requiring corporal punishment, use of water sprays, performance of exercise, or the deprivation of necessary food and water. Aversives are not effective over time and may cause the student to fear the adult applying the punishment. School personnel must report any aversive treatment to the proper authorities.

- Even mild forms of punishment such as verbal reprimands and simple restitution should be used cautiously. Time out is often referred to as an effective punishment in a reactive program. Discretion must be used when implementing time out procedures. Time out means that the student receives no reinforcement. In the case of a typically developing student, being moved from the classroom to an isolated area may be considered time out from reinforcement. Unfortunately, this is not generally the case for students with autism. A student with autism will most likely perceive the time out area as reinforcing because:

- There are no demands being placed on him
- The function of his behavior is escape and avoidance
- He can initiate self-stimulatory behaviors that are highly reinforcing
- He may require a break or quiet area time

Time out from reinforcement must be carefully planned and used with caution to avoid reinforcing and increasing the problem behavior.

Crisis management

Despite careful planning and the development of active programming, school personnel may occasionally be faced with a crisis. Phases of a crisis cycle are:

- Phase 1. Calm; optimal; comfortable level; baseline
- Phase 2. Trigger
- Phase 3. Irritable; frustrated; demanding; anxious
- Phase 4. Peak
- Phase 5. Deescalation
- Phase 6. Recovery

School personnel must be very aware of the specific triggers for each student. Once a trigger has occurred for the student, it is important that appropriate and meaningful strategies be implemented to redirect the student to a preferred task. Encourage the use of previously taught stress management techniques. Also, be sure to control your own response to the trigger. Reduce any signs that you are agitated or stressed.

Practice, practice, practice

Crisis intervention is a serious undertaking. It requires multiple opportunities to practice the correct procedures. Because students are not in crisis every day, it is important for the staff to practice their crisis intervention skills. Practice role-playing different crisis scenarios. Have each staff member devise a plan and discuss the steps for intervention.

Conclusion

Again, reactive programming should occupy a small portion of the overall behavior program for students with autism. These procedures are only considered after other strategies have failed. If a crisis continues to occur for a particular student, teachers should reevaluate and reassess to determine the function of the behavior. The behavior intervention program for students with autism and Asperger's Syndrome should focus on teaching replacement skills and reinforcing appropriately displayed behaviors. Because many of these maladaptive behaviors are chronic, it may take the school team and parents many months to effectively teach a new skill. Therefore, it is important to focus on the process and celebrate the small changes.

You can contact Dr. Ernsperger by writing lorierns@netnevada.net.

Contributing Author Lori Ernspberger, Ph.D., Special Education, Indiana University—An expert in the field of autism and behavioral disorders, Dr. Ernspberger has over 17 years of experience as a public school teacher, administrator, and behavioral consultant. She owns and operates Autism and Behavioral Consulting, a firm based in Henderson, Nevada, that works with school district personnel and parents to provide effective educational programs and best practice strategies for students with autism and behavioral disorders. Dr. Ernspberger's book, *Keys to Success for Teaching Students with Autism*, has been very well received since its publication in 2003.

ADDRESSING MASTURBATION

Masturbation is a natural, biological behavior, which humans of all ages occasionally engage in. It can be a conscious, deliberate act, or it can be a behavior performed without thinking or even understanding its implications. Masturbation is regarded as a very private, sexual behavior. It's typically inappropriate to talk about it, and it's never appropriate to perform it in public. It's also not a behavior we usually think about with regard to others.

Early on, we learn the social rule that it's absolutely inappropriate to touch, rub, and generally stimulate our genital area in the presence of others. It's not a rule that we necessarily need to be taught. Young children may discover the pleasurable sensations that masturbation can produce, and they may continue to engage in it because they don't understand the social rules regarding masturbation. Eventually, most children correctly identify masturbation as a private matter and learn not to discuss it or perform it in public.

Students with special needs, particularly those with autism or mental impairment, are not likely to be embarrassed by masturbation or to understand the social and moral taboos attached to it. Sometimes negative attention merely exacerbates a situation, and a student will continue the inappropriate behavior. The student might enjoy the shocked reaction of others, or the negative attention when he or she masturbates in front of others. Teachers and parents often mistakenly believe that a child will eventually tire of masturbating and stop on his or her own. Sometimes that is true.

But masturbation is a pleasurable behavior, and it's unlikely that an individual will tire of it and give it up completely. Even when punished, or given natural consequences for masturbating, many students with special needs still continue to masturbate. Masturbation can become especially prevalent during adolescence. According to recent statistics, many teenagers masturbate. Ninety-five percent of all teenage boys occasionally masturbate. Seventy-five percent of teenage boys admit to masturbating on a regular basis. Also, twenty-five to forty-five percent of teenage girls masturbate. Most parents of teenagers are not aware of these statistics because neurotypical teenagers understand the social taboos of masturbation. They not only perform such behaviors in private, but keep this information to themselves and often hide the fact that they do, in fact, masturbate.

We need to realize that masturbation is a behavior that might not go away. As teachers and parents, it's important to approach masturbation with a calm, mature attitude. It will not help the situation if we get upset and angry about it. We start first by learning why a student is masturbating. Surprisingly, a child/student might not be masturbating for sexual gratification. There are other reasons for masturbation, especially with preadolescent children.

Dealing With Young Children Who Masturbate

Young children who masturbate often do so as a self-calming, comfort response. They are often unaware they are masturbating, or that they are doing anything wrong. If a young child is masturbating occasionally or pre-dictably, it's important to first *determine* why they are masturbating. For instance, they may have discovered masturbating one time when they were upset, or in need of sensory regulation, and the act of masturbating soothed them, calmed them, and even helped them to sleep. After that initial self-calming, they may have come to rely on masturbating to self-calm in a variety of situations.

A child could also have discovered masturbation when he or she was bored and subsequently found something to play with when putting hands into pants. So, for example, when he's bored, a young boy may find it fun and enjoyable to play with his penis. And after playing with his genitals, he finds that it feels good. So perhaps every time he's bored or seeking some enjoyment, his hands go down his pants.

When you know why a child is masturbating you will be able to find appropriate replacement behaviors for the inappropriate masturbation behavior. When a young child is masturbating, it's important to redirect him or her in a calm, matter-of-fact manner. Establish highly motivating replacement behaviors for the masturbating, such as a large motor activity, a squeeze toy, reading a book, hugging a stuffed animal, doing an activity that requires two hands, or sensory integration activities such as applying deep pressure.

Once they are able to choose more appropriate replacement behaviors, reward them for doing a good job keeping hands on the table or other appropriate place. Realize that preadolescent masturbating feels good and is comforting, but it is still more of an habitual behavior rather than one for sexual release.

Dealing With Adolescents Who Masturbate

When an adolescent is masturbating on a regular basis, it is often purposeful behavior and unlikely to stop. The adolescent is very likely getting sexual gratification from the masturbation.

Because of the sexual gratification, it is not likely you will be able to find a highly motivating replacement behavior for the masturbation. But because the student is a teenager, his or her masturbation will not be tolerated by society, as a young child's might; and furthermore, the masturbation behavior may risk his or her personal safety. In other words, a student may invite molesting and sexual abuse if he or she masturbates in public. In some cases, students have been physically abused if caught masturbating by other students or even other adults.

It is absolutely important that a student understand that masturbating is a very private behavior: no one should see it, no one should hear it, and no one should know about it.

Masturbating can only occur in very specific locations and conditions: when an individual is alone in his or her bedroom or bathroom with the door closed.

Parents need to accept the fact that their adolescent child is masturbating and allow him or her to masturbate in the privacy of his or her own bedroom and bathroom. If a teenager is not allowed to masturbate in appropriate, private locations such as bedroom and bathroom, then it is likely he or she will masturbate in very inappropriate places such as a playground, a public bathroom, at school, on the bus, etc. If you know a student or child is masturbating for sexual gratification, you need to address it directly.

Talk about what happens as a result of masturbation. Discuss erections and ejaculations, in the case of adolescent boys. Allow them to ask questions, and then answer them honestly. Talk about it with the adolescent until you know he or she fully understands what masturbation is and why it must be very private. The adolescent may want to establish his or her own private routine for masturbating. That's okay.

But again, remind them that it must be private and no one, not even mom or dad, wants to know about it.

The exception would be if there is pain, an unusual discharge, or something abnormal, like a lump. Pain may be the sign of an infection, such as a urinary infection, in which case the adolescent should tell parents and a doctor about the problem. We should not be private about something if there is pain and sickness.

At some point, other sexual topics may come up, such as dating, sexual intercourse, sexually transmitted diseases, birth control, and pregnancy. When you feel a student or child is able to understand these topics, then address them simply and directly. Let them know the facts and always ask and answer questions clearly.

You can write to the author, Mary Wrobel, at marywrobel@aol.com.

Contributing Author Mary Wrobel, speech-language pathologist and certified teacher—Ms. Wrobel is an autism consultant and presents at autism workshops in the U.S. (and soon in Canada). She graduated with a Master's degree from Western Illinois University in Macomb, IL, in 1980. Ms. Wrobel is the author of *Taking Care of Myself*.

8

EXCEPTIONAL INTELLIGENCE & MEASURING IQ

SAVANT SYNDROME— HOPE FOR THE FUTURE

George can tell you, almost instantly, which years in the next 50 that Easter falls on March 25. He can tell you the day of the week of any date over a 40,000-year span backward or forward. He and his identical twin brother trade 20-digit prime numbers for amusement, notes Oliver Sacks.[1] Yet George cannot multiply the simplest of numbers. George also remembers the weather for every day of his adult life. Unable to explain his incredible talents, George is content to say, "It's fantastic I can do that!" And it truly is.

Richard's swiss-oil crayon drawings are collected internationally. He has had no formal art training and is classified as legally blind. He began drawing at age three. At age 12, an art critic was "thunderstruck" by Richard's drawings, which he described as an "incredible phenomenon rendered with the precision of a mechanic and the vision of a poet." Some of Richard's drawings are in the collections of Margaret Thatcher and The Vatican. One, presented to Pope John Paul II, depicts thousands of pilgrims in Vatican Square. You can almost single out each of the persons on the drawing.

Tony is blind and autistic. He is also an incredible musician. He won a jazz contest as a teenager and was admitted to the prestigious Berklee College of Music in Boston, from which he then graduated Magna Cum Laude. He now plays 20 instruments and has produced four CDs that include many of his own compositions.

Joseph is a lightning calculator. He can multiply 341 by 927 in his head and quickly give you the answer: 316,107. He is fascinated with license plate numbers and remembers myriads of them only glimpsed at years earlier. His memory is so good that he can study a 36-number grid for less than two minutes and tell you what was in the grid, without making a mistake, in 43 seconds. He uses his memory in his work as a librarian. Joseph was one of the people Dustin Hoffman spent many hours with learning about autism and savant skills for his portrayal of an autistic savant, Raymond Babbitt, in the movie *Rain Man*.

Ellen is a musical virtuoso. A lover of opera, she memorized Evita within a week of hearing it. She also has a superior spatial sense and can keep time precisely without referring to a clock or other time piece. Since she is blind, she has never seen a clock. Her superior spatial sense is demonstrated by her ability to walk in any unfamiliar setting without running into objects, as if using some type of personal radar. She also has an extremely accurate memory and a preoccupation with rhythm that has been present since childhood.

These five remarkable individuals are persons with savant syndrome. They typify the musical, artistic, calendar calculating, lightning calculating, and spatial and mechanical skills that are so characteristically seen in savant syndrome, superimposed on autistic disorder, and always coupled with extraordinary memory. These special skills, linked with massive memory in persons with developmental disorders, including autistic disorder, is savant syndrome. And, just as these five individuals demonstrate the typical range of savant skills, they also demonstrate the 5:1 male–female ratio seen in savant syndrome.

More information about these special persons, and their equally special families, can be found in *Extraordinary People: Understanding Savant Syndrome*, a book first published 1988 and then reissued in an updated version in 2000.[2] There is more about these special persons as well on the savant web site at www.savantsyndrome.com.

Each story documents the emergence of special skills in a child, often at about age three or four, superimposed on symptoms and behaviors of autistic disorder. The special skills of these individuals are often in the areas of art, music, calendar calculating, mathematics, or mechanical and spatial skills. All are combined with prodigious memory. But the savant skills, rather than being frivolous, are in fact the child's way of communicating from their otherwise relative isolation, and the savant abilities become, by "training the talent," a conduit toward better language development, increased social and daily living skills, and overall independence.

What follows is a summary of where we are in understanding savant syndrome, today, where we've been in the past, the research directions in which we are proceeding, and, most important, how the special talents in the twice-exceptional child can be worked with and channeled toward fully actualizing abilities while at the same time lessening disabilities. Beyond that, a closer look at savant syndrome triggers a closer look at human potential overall; however, especially as the so-called "acquired savants" more recently described provide some hints at the hidden potential that may lie within us all.

Until we can understand and explain savant syndrome, we cannot fully understand and explain ourselves. And no model of brain function will be complete until it can fully incorporate and account for this remarkable juxtaposition of ability and disability in these extraordinary people. Beyond synapses and neurons, though, these stories also tell of the incredible power of the belief, determination, persistence, optimism, and love of family members for these special people and how this propels their potential. The stories provide uplifting examples of how it is not enough to care for the savant, and his or her mind. We must care about them, and their world, as well.

Where we have been

Savant syndrome, with its "islands of genius," has a long history. Benjamin Rush provided one of the earliest reports in 1789 when he described the lightning calculating ability of Thomas Fuller, "who could comprehend scarcely anything, either theoretical or practical, more complex than counting."[3] However, when Fuller was asked how many seconds a man had lived who was 70 years, 17 days, and 12 hours old, he gave the correct answer of 2,210,500,800 in 90 seconds, even correcting for the 17 leap years included. Actually, however, the first description of savant syndrome in a scientific paper appeared in the German psychology journal, *Gnothi Sauton,* in 1783. It described the case of Jedediah Buxton, a lightning calculator with extraordinary memory.[4]

The now-regrettable term *idiot savant* was coined by Down in 1887 when he presented 10 cases in colorful detail from his 30-year experience at the Earlswood Asylum.[5] These cases demonstrated the typical musical, artistic, mathematical, and mechanical skills, coupled with phenomenal memory, that have so unfailingly reoccurred in savant syndrome to the present day. Down meant no harm by that term.

At that time, "idiot" was an accepted classification for persons with an IQ below 25, and "savant," or "knowledgeable person," was derived from the French word *savoir*, meaning "to know." While descriptive, the term was actually a misnomer since almost all cases occur in persons with an IQ higher than 40. In the interest of accuracy and dignity, savant syndrome has been substituted and is now widely used. Savant syndrome is preferable to "autistic savant," since only about 50 percent of persons with savant syndrome have autistic spectrum disorder, and the other 50 percent have some other form of CNS injury or disease.

The first definitive work on savant syndrome was a chapter by Tredgold in his 1914 textbook, *Mental Deficiency.*[6] In 1978, Hill provided a review of the literature between 1890 and 1978 that included 60 reports involving over 100 savants.[7] That year, Rimland provided a summary of his data on "special abilities" in 531 cases from a survey population of 5,400 children with autism.[8] Treffert provided an updated review in 1988, which contained more detail on all of those earlier cases. Since that time, there have been six books on the topic and several review articles with extensive bibliographies.[9]

What we do know

The condition is rare, but one in 10 autistic persons show some savant skills. In Rimland's 1978 survey of 5,400 children with autism, 531 were reported by parents to have special abilities, and a 10 percent incidence of savant syndrome has become the generally accepted figure in autistic disorder.[8] Hermelin, however, estimates that figure to be as low as "one or two in 200."[10] The presence of savant syndrome is not limited to autism, however.

In a survey of an institutionalized population with a diagnosis of mental retardation, the incidence of savant skills was 1:2,000 (0.06 percent).[11] A more recent study surveyed 583 facilities and found a prevalence rate of 1.4 per 1,000, or approximately double the Hill estimate.[12]

Whatever the exact figures, mental retardation and other forms of developmental disability are more common than autistic disorder. So it turns out that about 50 percent of persons with savant syndrome have autistic disorder and the other 50 percent have other forms of developmental disability, mental retardation, or other CNS injury or disease. Thus, not all autistic persons have savant syndrome, and not all persons with savant syndrome have autistic disorder.

Males outnumber females in autism and savant syndrome

In explaining this finding, Geschwind and Galaburda, in their work on cerebral lateralization, point out that the left hemisphere normally completes its development later than the right hemisphere and is thus subjected to prenatal influences, some of which can be detrimental, for a longer period of time.[13] In the male fetus particularly, circulating testosterone, which can reach very high levels, can slow growth and impair neuronal function in the more vulnerably exposed left hemisphere, with actual enlargement and shift of dominance favoring skills associated with the right hemisphere. "Pathology of superiority" was postulated, with compensatory growth in the right brain as a result of impaired development or actual injury to the left brain.

This finding may account as well for the high male–female ratio in other disorders, including autism itself, since left hemisphere dysfunction is often seen in autism, as will be explained below. Other conditions, such as dyslexia, delayed speech, and stuttering, also with male predominance in incidence, may be manifestations of this same left hemisphere interference in the prenatal period.

Savant skills typically occur in an intriguingly narrow range of special abilities

Considering all the abilities in the human repertoire, it is interesting that savant skills generally narrow to five general categories: music, usually performance, most often piano, with perfect pitch, although composing in the absence of performing has been reported as has been playing multiple instruments (as many as 20); art, usually drawing, painting, or sculpting; calendar calculating (curiously an obscure skill in most persons); mathematics, including lightning calculating or the ability to compute prime numbers, for example, in the absence of other simple arithmetic abilities; and mechanical or spatial skills, including the capacity to measure distances precisely without benefit of instruments, the ability to construct complex models or structures with painstaking accuracy, or the mastery of map making and direction finding.

Other skills have been reported less often, including: prodigious language (polyglot) facility; unusual sensory discrimination in smell, touch, or vision, including synesthesia; perfect appreciation of passing time without benefit of a clock; and outstanding knowledge in specific fields such as neurophysiology, statistics, or navigation.[14] In Rimland's sample of 543 children with special skills, musical ability was the most frequently reported skill followed by memory, art, pseudoverbal abilities, mathematics, maps and directions, coordination, and calendar calculating.

Generally a single special skill exists, but in some instances several skills exist simultaneously. Rimland and Fein noted that the incidence of multiple skills appeared to be higher in savants with autism than in savants with other developmental disabilities.[15]

Whatever the special skill, it is always associated with prodigious memory. Some observers list memory as a separate special skill; however, prodigious memory is an ability all savants possess, cutting across all of the skill areas as a shared, integral part of the syndrome itself.

There is a spectrum of savant skills

The most common are splinter skills, which include obsessive preoccupation with, and memorization of, music and sports trivia, license plate numbers, maps, historical facts, or obscure items such as vacuum cleaner motor sounds, for example. Talented savants are those cognitively impaired persons in whom the musical, artistic, or other special abilities are more prominent and finely honed, usually within an area of single expertise, and are very conspicuous when viewed in contrast to overall disability. Prodigious savant is a term reserved for those extraordinarily rare individuals for whom the special skill is so outstanding that it would be spectacular even if it were to occur in a nonimpaired person. There are probably fewer than 50 prodigious savants known to be living worldwide at the present time who would meet that very high threshold of savant ability.

The skills tend to be right hemisphere in type. These (right hemisphere) skills can be characterized as nonsymbolic, artistic, concrete, and directly perceived, in contrast with left hemisphere skills, which are more sequential, logical, and symbolic and include language specialization.

The special skills are always accompanied by prodigious memory

Whatever the special abilities, a remarkable memory of a unique and uniform type welds the condition together. Terms such as automatic, mechanical, concrete, and habit-like have been applied to this extraordinary memory. Down used the term "verbal adhesion"; Critchley used the terms "exultation of memory" or "memory without reckoning";[16] Tredgold used the term "automatic"; and Barr characterized his patient with prodigious memory as "an exaggerated form of habit."[17] Such unconscious memory suggests what Mishkin and Petri referred to as nonconscious "habit" formation rather than a "semantic" memory system.[18] They proposed two different neural circuits for these two different types of memory: a higher-level cortico-limbic circuit for semantic memory and a lower level, cortico-striatal circuit for the more primitive habit memory that is sometimes referred to as procedural or implicit memory. Savant memory is characteristically very deep, but exceedingly narrow, within the confines of the accompanying special skill.

Savant syndrome can be congenital or it can be acquired following brain injury or disease later in infancy, childhood, or adult life

Recent reports of savant-type abilities emerging in previously healthy elderly persons with frontotemporal dementia is particularly intriguing.[19,20]

Savant skills characteristically continue, rather than disappear, and with continued use the special abilities either persist at the same level or actually increase.

In almost all cases, unlike the case of Nadia, there is no trade-off of special skills with exposure to more traditional schooling.[21] Instead, the special skills often serve as a conduit toward normalization with an actual improvement in language acquisition, socialization, and daily living skills.

No single theory has emerged thus far that can explain all savants

An important basic question surrounding savant syndrome is how do they do it? Numerous theories have been put forth, but no single overarching theory can explain all savants. The theories have included: eidetic imagery or the related but separate phenomenon generally called photographic memory; inherited skills; sensory deprivation and sensory isolation; highly developed rote memory; and compensation and reinforcement to offset lack of more general capacity or intelligence.

There are problems with each of these theories

For example, formal testing for eidetic imagery shows that phenomenon to be present in some but certainly not in all savants, and when present it may be more a marker of brain damage than an agent of savant abilities.[22, 23] Two studies, one with 25 savants and another with 51 subjects, showed relatives with special skills in some but certainly not all cases; another study of 23 relatives of carefully studied savants found only one family member with special skills.[24–26] Several investigators have shown that memory alone cannot fully account for savant abilities, particularly calendar calculating and musical skills.[27]

In recent years, several neuropsychological theories have also directly addressed the abundant reports of splinter and savant skills in the autistic population. "Weak central coherence" theory (WCC) cites a particular cognitive and perception style—focusing on details rather than the whole—as being present in persons with autism and postulates that such a style of information processing could be an important part of those persons with savant abilities. Not being distracted by more global patterns, the savant can focus on a single item or skill and perfect it.[28] Simon Baron-Cohen has advanced the "extreme male brain" theory of autism. This proposes that attributes of the male brain, systematizing and spatial skills, produce a special predilection for autism in males.[29–30] He finds such special systematizing skills and lack of social abilities and empathizing in persons with Asperger's Disorder particularly.[31]

However, the newer neuropsychiatric theories seem more to describe the autistic person than to explain him or her, and they do not account for the fact that of those with savant syndrome only 50 percent are autistic, while the remainder have other developmental disabilities, CNS disorders, or disease.

New findings

Left brain injury with right brain compensation

One theory that does provide an increasingly plausible explanation for savant abilities in many cases is left brain injury with right brain compensation. As pointed out above, the skills most often seen in savant syndrome are those associated with the right hemisphere, as described by Tanguay.[32] Rimland commented that in the autistic savant simultaneous, high-fidelity imagery and processing—right hemisphere functions—tend to be more prominent than the verbal, logical, and sequential processing more typically associated with the left hemisphere.[33]

In autism, left brain dysfunction has been demonstrated in a number of studies. As early as 1975, pneumoencephalograms demonstrated left hemisphere abnormalities, particularly in the temporal lobe areas in 15 of 17 patients with autism, four of whom had savant skills. Investigators in this study concluded that motor and language functions were "taken over" by the right hemisphere because of deficits in the left hemisphere.[34] A 1999 PET study showed low serotonin synthesis in the left hemisphere of persons with autistic disorder, and other studies have confirmed such left hemisphere deficits, as well.[35] Boddaert and coworkers demonstrated that five children with autism when at rest and when listening to speech-like sounds displayed a volume of activation that was greater on the right side and diminished on the left. The reverse was found among the eight children in the control group.[36] Escalante and colleagues demonstrated an atypical pattern of cerebral dominance and a history of early language disorder among individuals with autism when compared to both healthy participants and persons with normal acquisition of early language skills.[37]

With respect to savant syndrome, in 1980, Brink presented a case of a typically developing nine-year-old boy who was left mute, deaf, and paralyzed by a gunshot wound to the left hemisphere.[38] Following that injury, an unusual savant mechanical skill emerged, presumably from the undamaged right hemisphere.

Subsequent reports have likewise implicated left hemisphere injury, such as those in a musical savant and a mathematical savant with left hemisphere damage documented in both on neuropsychological tests and neuroimaging studies.[39, 40] Likewise, CT scans and neuropsychological test results for a prodigious musical savant described by Treffert showed left brain damage. Munoz-Yunta and coworkers report similar findings of left hemisphere damage and dysfunction in savant syndrome based on PET and magnetoencephalography techniques.[41]

A significant new discovery: the "acquired" savant

However, the most powerful conformation of the left brain dysfunction/right brain compensation theory in savant syndrome comes from a 1998 report by

Miller and coworkers. They described five previously nondisabled patients with frontotemporal dementia (FTD) who acquired new artistic skills with the onset and progression of FTD. Several of these individuals had no previous history of particular artistic ability.

Yet prodigious art skills emerged as the dementia proceeded. Consistent with characteristics and traits of savants, the modality of skill expression in these five, older adults was visual, not verbal; the images were meticulous copies that lacked abstract or symbolic qualities; episodic memory was preserved, but semantic memory was devastated; and there was intense, obsessive preoccupation with the artwork. Neuroimaging studies showed dominant (left) hemisphere injury and dysfunction.

The authors hypothesized that selective degeneration of the (particularly left) anterior temporal and orbitofrontal cortices decreased inhibition of visual systems involved with perception, thereby enhancing artistic interest and abilities. Kapur called this process "paradoxical functional facilitation" and speculated that this process accounts for unexpected behavioral improvement in discrete domains following brain injury.[42]

In an expansion of that work, Miller described seven additional FTD patients who acquired new visual or musical talents despite the progression of their dementia. The 12 FTD patients with these newly emerged savant-type talents were compared on SPECT imaging and neuropsychological testing to FTD patients without such talent. Nine of the 12 showed asymmetric left-sided SPECT deficits; one demonstrated bilateral abnormalities (left on MRI, right on SPECT); while two had asymmetric right-sided dysfunction (one of whom was left-handed).

The talented group performed better on tasks assessing right frontal lobe functions, but worse on verbal abilities. The authors conclude: "Loss of function in the left anterior temporal lobe may lead to the 'paradoxical functional facilitation' of artistic and musical skills. Patients with the left-sided temporal lobe variant of FTD offer an unexpected window into the neurological mediation of visual and musical talent."

These FTD cases are interesting additions to the earlier cases of newly "acquired" savant abilities such as Brink's case, already noted, following a gunshot wound to the left hemisphere. An internationally known, now adult, savant sculptor had his remarkable talent emerge following a childhood fall. Lythgoe and coworkers describe a 51-year-old male whose prolific drawing and sculpting skills unexpectedly emerged following a subarachnoid hemorrhage that affected principally frontal areas.[43]

SPECT Imaging in a nine-year-old artistic savant with autism

After finding left hemisphere dysfunction, particularly left anterior temporal dysfunction, in the 12 patients with frontotemporal dementia, Miller and coworkers performed neuropsychological and neuroimaging studies on a newly diagnosed nine-year-old artistic savant with autism.[44] This childhood artistic, autistic savant showed "striking parallels" to other artistic savants, particularly Nadia, with an obsession for one art medium (felt-tipped pen) and one type of subject (cartoon figures), and with extraordinary drawing skills and exceptional visual memory. MRI scan was normal. SPECT showed bilateral increased frontal perfusion with bilateral anterior temporal lobe hypoperfusion, which was worse on the left than on the right. This is the same site of dysfunction noted in the 12 elderly FTD patients with savant-type skills. These researchers conclude: "The anatomic substrate for the savant syndrome may involve loss of function in the left temporal lobe with enhanced function of the posterior cortex."

A gene for savant syndrome?

In the search for subgroups within the aggregate autism spectrum disorders, Nurmi and colleagues identified (among 94 multiplex families) 21 families as "savant skills positive" and 73 families as "savant skill negative."[45] The subset study of savant-skills positive families yielded significantly increased evidence for linkage to 15q11-q13 compared to savant-skills negative families. Interestingly, the presence of savant skills was the only factor that isolated a subgroup from the larger autistic spectrum disorders group. The authors note that Prader-Willi syndrome is due to a deletion on this same region of chromosome 15 (i.e., 15q11-13) and that some features (including puzzle skills, for example) of PWS and autism overlap. The researchers conclude that it is possible that a gene, or genes, in the chromosome 15q11-13 region "when perturbed contributes to predisposition to a particular cognitive style or pattern on intellectual impairments and relative strengths. Precisely how those skills are manifested in a given individual may be influenced by a variety of environmental, and possibly, genetic factors."

Prodigies and savant syndrome

There is emerging evidence that prodigies and savants may share certain underlying mental processes when carrying out their specialized, expert tasks. Event-related potentials (ERPs) can measure very early components of brain activity reflecting initial, "preconscious" stages of mental processing. This fast, low-level "preconscious" mental activity contrasts sharply with that seen when higher-level, "executive" functions are accessed during typical information processing. Birbaumer compared ERPs of a "human calculator"—a nonautistic arithmetic whiz—to same age, IQ matched, healthy controls.[46] Compared to controls, early on in the calculating process, the expert calculator showed evidence of "enhanced automatic low-level processing." Studies are now underway with autistic savant calculators to see whether this particular type of early, lower-level processing ("without reckoning") is the same as that used by the nonautistic "expert" calculator.

In a similar effort using PET, Pesenti and his team examined differences between a calculating prodigy and normal control subjects in the neural basis of mental calculations.[47] When completing less complex calculations in a typical manner, both the expert and nonexpert persons showed activation in the brain bilaterally but with a clear left-sided predominance for select regions. However when the "expert" completed complex calculations much more accurately and swiftly than controls, he "recruited" a system of brain areas implicated in episodic memory including right medial frontal and parahippocampal areas. Moreover, the expert utilized a unique method of exploiting the seemingly unlimited storage capacity of long-term memory in order to maintain the sequence of steps and intermediate results needed for the more complex calculations. On the contrary, the normal control group relied on the more limited span working memory system. Therefore, unique brain mechanisms are utilized by the expert when demonstrating this special skill. And, when doing these special skills, the prodigy is perhaps relying on some right brain capacities and some special memory recruitment, as may be the case for the savant.

An article by Kalbfleisch further explores the functional neural anatomy of exceptional talent and interfaces among talent, intelligence, and creativity in prodigies and savants.[48]

Repetitive Transcranial Magnetic Stimulation (rTMS)

Several investigators are exploring the use of rTMS to temporarily immobilize portions of left hemisphere function to see if, given Miller's work and some of the other left-sided findings summarized above, savant-type abilities emerge in healthy volunteers.

Snyder and Mitchell argue that savant brain processes occur in each of us but are overwhelmed by more sophisticated conceptual cognition.[49] They conclude that autistic savants "have privileged access to lower levels of information not normally available through introspection." Snyder and coworkers tested that hypothesis in 11 male volunteers using rTMS applied to the left frontotemporal region while carrying out two drawing tests and two proofreading tests.[50] rTMS did not lead to any systematic improvement in naturalistic drawing ability, but it did lead to "a major change in the schema or convention of the drawings of four of the eleven participants." Two of the participants noted improvement in their ability to proofread and recognize duplicated words.

In a similar study, Young and colleagues, using a wide variety of standard psychological tests and tasks specifically designed to test savant skills and abilities, showed that savant-type skills improved in five out of 17 participants during rTMS stimulation.[51] They conclude that savant-type skill expressions may be possible for some, not all, individuals, just as it appears to be the case in the disabled population. This group intends to carry out further studies using more efficacious and targeted stimulation.

These new studies suggest that savant syndrome may be due, at least in part, to "paradoxical functional facilitation" of the right hemisphere, allowing for new skills as a compensatory process. Increasingly, however, an alternative theory is advanced wherein these right brain skills are not necessarily newly developed but instead represent latent but dormant skills that are released from the "tyranny of the left hemisphere," or what is, more simply, left cerebral dominance in most persons.

Savants: past and present

Dr. Down's original 10 cases of savant syndrome. In his 1887 Lettsomian Lectures before the Medical Society of London, Down presented 10 cases encountered in his 30 years in practice that had particularly caught his attention. Each of these were individuals who, while mentally retarded, exhibited remarkable "special faculties." Down did not identify any of these special persons as autistic; that designation did not occur until Kanner's paper over 50 years later.[52] But a close reviewing of Down's entire lecture series reveals that he did, interestingly, specifically mention a group of individuals who differed in many ways from those with more typical mental retardation, a group he identified as "developmental" in origin. That is a term-developmental disability-now applied to autistic persons a century after Down's observations. Down's astute observations regarding this group of "developmental" cases is described in detail on the savant syndrome website at http://www.savantsyndrome.com in the articles section under the title of Dr. J. Langdon Down and Developmental Disorders.

Down's description of his 10 cases of "special faculties" in those 1887 lectures reads like descriptions of many savants over a century later. Each of his cases of developmental disability demonstrated some special skills combined with prodigious memory. That is savant syndrome. One of his patients, for example, had memorized verbatim *The Rise and Fall of the Roman Empire*. Other children drew with remarkable skill "but had a comparative blank in all the other higher faculties of mind." Still other children remembered dates and past events. Arithmetical genius was evident in some children, including lightning calculating.

Music and musical memory was also described among the special abilities. And there was yet another boy who was unable to use a clock or tell time in any conventional manner yet had perfect appreciation of past or passing time.

While not identified as such, in reading Down's careful and colorful accounts of his cases of "special faculties," it is clear that among the children were some with what would now be identified as autistic disorder, in which savant syndrome occurs with a distinctive frequency, as noted above. Among his cases one finds the typical artistic, musical, mathematical, and other enhanced abilities noted so often in the literature in the 118 years since Down's original observations.

Later cases, including those of Dr. Leo Kanner Tredgold, presented 20 additional cases 27 years later. His cases are a catalogue of the categories and skills—musical, artistic, mechanical, calendar, and mechanical/spatial—that are repeated so strikingly in all the subsequent cases to date.

The several hundred cases in the literature since Tredgold are summarized in a 1988 review article.[53] The 2000 edition of *Extraordinary People: Understanding Savant Syndrome* added additional cases. And the website www.savantsyndrome.com has added many new cases worldwide, as well.

Six of Kanner's original cases of Early Infantile Autism had specific musical abilities, and Kanner was struck by the overall heightened memory capacity of all 10 of these individuals. The identical twin calendar calculators first described by Horwitz have been extensively studied since that time.[54] The brothers have a calendar calculating range of 40,000 years, and they also remember the weather for each day of their adult life. Their ability to compute 20-digit prime numbers, inability to do simple arithmetic, and special abilities were described by Sacks and incorporated into some scenes in *Rain Man*.

Some well-known savants

Without doubt the best-known autistic savant is a fictional one—Raymond Babbitt—as portrayed by Dustin Hoffman in the Academy Award-winning movie *Rain Man*. The original inspiration for the savant portrayed in *Rain Man* is a 53-year-old male who has memorized over 8,600 books and has encyclopedic knowledge of geography, music, literature, history, sports, and nine other areas of expertise.[55, 56] He can name all the U.S. area codes and major city zip codes. He has also memorized the maps in the front of telephone books and can tell you precisely how to get from one U.S. city to another and then how to get around in that city street by street. He also has calendar calculating abilities, and more recently rather advanced musical talent has surfaced. Of unique interest is his ability to read extremely rapidly, simultaneously scanning one page with the left eye, the other page with the right. An MRI shows absence of the corpus callosum along with substantial other CNS damage. His history and savant abilities are described in detail on the savant website.

The phenomenal drawing ability of a British savant with autism has resulted in several popular art books published by him.[57, 58] His extraordinary memory is illustrated in a documentary film clip: after a 12-minute helicopter ride over London, he completes, in three hours, an impeccably accurate sketch that encompasses four square miles, 12 major landmarks, and 200 other buildings, all drawn to scale and perspective. A rather marked musical ability has surprisingly surfaced in this artist, as well.[59] Recently, an 11-year-old's artwork from the U.S. has gained international attention.[60]

The triad of blindness, autism, and musical genius continues to be conspicuously overrepresented and prominent throughout the history of savant syndrome, including Blind Tom at the time of the Civil War, Tredgold's case at the Salpêtrière, and several well-known present-day musical savants.[61] A Japanese musical savant's ability as a composer demonstrates decisively that savants can be creative: his 40 original pieces on two internationally popular CDs forcefully document that ability.[62] Smith describes in detail a remarkable language (polyglot) savant in *The Mind of the Savant*.[63]

However, female savants continue to be few. Self described the case of Nadia, which has triggered considerable debate about the possible "trade-off" of special skills for language and social skills acquisition. Viscott documented in detail, including psychodynamic formulations, a female musical savant whom he followed for many years.[64] Treffert described a blind, autistic musical savant who, along with her musical ability, demonstrated very precise spatial location abilities and precise time-keeping skills without access to a clock face or other time instruments.

Most reports continue to be anecdotal, single cases. However, Young traveled to a number of countries and met with 59 savants and their families, completing the largest study done on savants to date using uniform history taking and standardized psychological testing. Forty-one savants carried a diagnosis of autism and the remainder some other type of intellectual disability.

Twenty were rated as prodigious savants; 20 were rated as talented; the remaining 19 had splinter skills. The savants in this series of cases had the following elements in common: neurological impairment with idiosyncratic and divergent intellectual ability; language and intellectual impairments consistent with autism; intense interest and preoccupation with particular areas of ability; rule-based, rigid, and highly structured skills lacking critical aspects of creativity and cognitive flexibility; preserved neurological capacity to process information relating to the particular skills; a well-developed declarative memory; a familial predisposition toward high achievement; and a climate of support, encouragement, and reinforcement from families, case workers, teachers, caretakers, and others.

In a recent summary of work with savants, Nettlebeck and Young conclude that rote memory does not provide sufficient basis for savant skills; instead, such savant skills are based on extensive, rule-based knowledge confined to narrowly defined abilities that are imitative and inflexible. They conclude that savant skills do not represent separate forms of intelligence (outside the concept of overall intelligence) and that these skills depend on modular processing and memory structures that have been spared damage affecting other areas of the brain.

Rain Man the movie/Rain Man real life

Raymond Babbitt, the main character in the movie *Rain Man*, has become the world's best-known savant due to Dustin Hoffman's remarkably accurate and sensitive portrayal of savant syndrome in that film.

That 1988 movie, in its first 101 days, accomplished more toward bringing savant syndrome to public attention than all the efforts in the 101 years following Dr. Down's 1887 description of the disorder. A detailed description of the background and chronology of the movie, including the people Dustin Hoffman studied with as he prepared for his role, is described elsewhere. But several things warrant mention here.

First, the movie is not a documentary. Yet its accuracy added to its value as an informative and entertaining film. One indicator of that accuracy is that there was no six-day, cross-country "cure" of autism. The real change of character occurred in the brother, Charlie. This conveys the important message that in dealing with persons with disabilities, it is often we who need to accommodate their needs and special qualities—and not they who need to make all the changes required for them to live with us, side-by-side, in our communities. Third, as a gentle caveat, the audience needs to realize that Raymond Babbitt is a high-functioning autistic person, and not all autistic persons function at that high level; it is a spectrum disorder. Fourth, as a second caveat, the audience needs to realize that not all autistic persons are savants, and not all savants have autistic disorder.

The major message in the movie concerning the special qualities of the autistic savant is a welcome and positive one. The message raised public interest in both autism and savant syndrome. Few disabilities will receive the public focus and heightened visibility as autism and savant syndrome received as a result of *Rain Man*.

Training the Talent:

Successful education approaches

Etiologic considerations aside, what is the best approach to the savant and his or her special skills? Phillips framed the controversy in 1930 when he wrote: "The problem of treatment comes next. . . . Is it better to eliminate the defects or train the talent?"[65] Experience has given the answer—train the talent and some of the "defect" disappears. The special talent, in fact, becomes a conduit toward normalization: the unique savant skills promote better socialization, language acquisition, and independence. The special skills can be used to engage the attention of the savant. They can be used to help the savant express him- or herself. They can be used as channels for the expression of more useful abilities.

Clark developed a Savant Skill Curriculum using a combination of successful strategies currently employed in the education of gifted children (enrichment, acceleration, and mentorship) and autism education (visual supports and social stories), in an attempt to channel and apply in useful ways the often nonfunctional obsessive savant and splinter skills of a group of students with autism.[66] This special curriculum proved highly successful in the functional application of savant skills and an overall reduction in the level of autistic behaviors in many subjects.

Improvements in behavior, social skills, and academic self-efficacy were reported, along with gain in the communication skills of some subjects.

Donnelly and Altman note that increasing numbers of "gifted students with autism" are now being included in gifted and talented classrooms with nondisabled, gifted peers.[67] Discussing this, they outline some of the special approaches that are effective with gifted students with autism, including the use of an adult mentor in the field of their talent, individual counseling, and small group social skills training.

Some specialized schools are emerging, as well.

For example, Soundscape Centre in London recently began operating as the only specialized educational facility in the world uniquely dedicated to the needs and potential of persons with sight loss and special musical abilities, including musical savants.[68] Orion Academy (www.orionacademy.org) in Moraga, California, specializes in providing a positive educational experience for high school students with higher functioning Autism. Hope University (www.hopeu.com) in Anaheim, California, is a fine arts facility for adults with developmental disabilities. Its mission is to "train the talents and diminish the disability" through the use of fine arts therapy, including visual arts, music, dance, drama, and storytelling.

The Savant Academy (www.savantacademy.org) in Los Angeles, California, was established in 2003 to support the education of people with savant syndrome, including linguistic, mathematical, musical, and artistic savants. David Mehnert, the musician and teacher who established the Savant Academy, suggests specialized techniques to unlock hidden savant abilities, using music particularly as a pathway to special abilities. On the website, Mr. Mehnert provides more information about those techniques and provides, as well, some useful information about "myths" surrounding savant syndrome and about perfect pitch, an extremely important consideration when dealing with musical savants. More information about perfect pitch and teaching musical savants is also contained in a booklet by Susan Rancer, a Registered Music Therapist.[69]

Dr. Temple Grandin is well known as an international authority in her field of animal science. She is also well known for her books including *Thinking in Pictures* and *Animals in Translation*.[70,71] She is also autistic. Her recent book with Kate Duffy, *Developing Talents: Careers for Individuals with*

Asperger's Syndrome and High-Functioning Autism, is an excellent practical resource for discovering, nurturing and "training the talent," so that many persons on the autistic spectrum can experience the important experience of work and "the satisfaction of contributing to their families and their communities, of being independent and economically self-sufficient."[72] This book outlines methods of helping children "develop their natural talents" using "drawing, writing, building models, programming computers" and similar skills to help build a "portfolio" of skills they can apply in their search for a meaningful work experience. The book helps people on the autistic spectrum and their family members, teachers, counselors, and others better understand and develop the career planning process for these special persons with special skills.

Future directions

No model of brain function, including memory, will be complete until it can account for, and fully incorporate, the rare but spectacular condition of savant syndrome. While in the past decade, particularly, much progress has been made toward explaining this jarring juxtaposition of ability and disability, many unanswered questions remain.

However, interest in this fascinating condition is accelerating, especially since the discovery of savant-type skills in previously unimpaired older persons with FTD, and other "acquired" savant instances. This finding has far-reaching implications regarding buried potential in some or, perhaps, all of us.

Advanced technologies will help in those investigations. Images of brain structure are now integrated with studies of brain function using PET, SPECT, and fMRI. Diffusion Tensor Imaging (DTI) and direct Fiber Tracking now permit noninvasive tracking of white matter pathways within and among brain regions, better delineating the underconnectivity and overconnectivity problems perhaps causal in autism and savant syndrome itself.[73] Findings from all these newer techniques can then be correlated with detailed neuropsychological testing in larger samples of savants, comparing and contrasting those findings with data from both impaired and nonimpaired control groups, including prodigies. The interface between geniuses, prodigies, and savants is especially intriguing, and these studies can shed light on the debate regarding general intelligence *versus* separate intelligences. Some researchers suggest that savants provide a unique window into the creative process itself. From studies already completed, important information has emerged regarding brain function, brain plasticity, CNS compensation, recruitment, and repair.

But there is more to savant syndrome than genes, circuitry, and the brain's marvelous intricacy. Scientific interest aside, those with savant syndrome and their families, caregivers, teachers, and therapists have a great deal to teach us. Human potential consists of more than neurons and synapses. It also includes, and is propelled by, the vital forces of encouragement and reinforcement that flow from the unconditional love, belief, support, and determination of families and friends who not only care for the savant, but care about him or her, as well.

Savant syndrome remains a "challenge to our capabilities," as one person described it in an American Psychiatric Association paper in 1964, concluding that the real significance of savant syndrome lies in our inability to explain it. But savant syndrome is less now a "landmark to our ignorance" than at that APA meeting 41 years ago. More progress has been made in the past 15 years in better understanding and explaining savant syndrome than in the previous 100. And that important inquiry continues, with the prospect of us advancing further than ever before as we unravel the mysteries of these extraordinary people and their remarkable abilities and, in the process, learn more about our hidden potential, our possibilities, and ourselves.

You can contact Dr. Treffert by visiting www.daroldtreffert.com or calling (920) 921-9381. For more information, visit www.savantsyndrome.com.

References

1. Sacks O: The Twins New York Review of Books. 1987; 32:16–20.
2. Treffert D: Extraordinary People: Understanding Savant Syndrome. Omaha, NE, IUniverse.com, 2000. (Originally published New York, Harper & Row, 1989.)
3. Scripture, EW: Arithmetical prodigies Am J Psychol 1891; 4:1–59.

4. Gnothi Sauton oder Magazin der Erfahrungsseelenkunde als ein Lesebuch fur Gelehrte and Ungelehrte Edited by Mortiz, KP, Berlin, Mylius, 1783–1793.

5. Down JL: On Some of the Mental Affections of Childhood and Youth. London, Churchill, 1887.

6. Tredgold AF: Mental Deficiency. New York, William Wood, 1914.

7. Hill AL: Savants: mentally retarded individuals with special skills, in International Review of Research in Mental Retardation, vol 9, Edited by Ellis NR. New York Academic Press, 1978.

8. Rimland B: Savant capabilities of autistic children and their cognitive implications, in Cognitive Defects in the Development of Mental Illness. Edited by Serban, G. New York, Brunner/Mazel, 1978.

9. Nettlebeck T, Young R: Savant Syndrome. International Review of Research in Mental Retardation 1999 22:137–173.

10. Hermelin B: Bright Splinters of the Mind. London Jessica Kingsley Publishers, 2001.

11. Hill AL: Idiot savants: rate of incidence Percept. Mot Skills 1977; 44:161–162.

12. Saloviita T, Ruusila L, Ruusila U: Incidence of savant skills in Finland Percept. Mot Skills 2000; 91:120–122.

13. Geschwind N, Galaburda AM: Cerebral Lateralization:Biological Mechanisms, Associations, and Pathology. Cambridge, Mass, MIT Press, 1987.

14. Kehrer HE: Savant capabilities of autistic persons. ACTA Paedopsychiatrica 1992; 55:151–155.

15. Rimland B, Fein DA: Special talents of autistic savants, in The Exceptional Brain: Neuropsychology of Talent and Special Abilities. Edited by Obler LK, Fein, DA. New York, Guilford Press, 1988.

16. Critchley M: The Divine Banquet of the Brain. New York, Raven Press, 1979.

17. Barr MW: Some notes on echolalia, with the report of an extraordinary case J. Nerv Ment Dis 1898; 25:20–30.

18. Mishkin M., Petri H.L.: Memories and habits; some implications for the analysis of learning and retention, in Neuropsychology of Memory. Edited by Squire L.R., Butters N. New York, Guilford Press, 1984.

19. Miller BL, Cummings J, Mishkin F, Boone K, Prince F, Ponton M, Cotman C: Emergence of artistic talent in fronto-temporal dementia. Neurology 1998; 51:978–982.

20. Miller BL, Boone K, Cummings LR, Mishkin F: Functional correlates of musical and visual ability in frontotemporal dementia. British Journal of Psychiatry 2000; 176:458–463.

21. Selfe L: Nadia: A Case of Extraordinary Drawing Ability in an Autistic Child. New York, Academic Press, 1978.

22. Giray EF, Barclay AG: Eidetic imagery: longitudinal results in brain—damaged children. Am J Ment Defic 1977; 82:311–314.

23. Bender MB, Feldman M, Sobin AJ: Palinopsia. Brain 1968; 91:321–338.

24. Duckett J: Idiot-savants: Superspecialization in mentally retarded persons. Doctoral Dissertation, University of Texas in Austin; Department of Special Education, 1976.

25. Young R: Savant Syndrome: Processes underlying extraordinary abilities. Unpublished doctoral dissertation, University of Adelaide, South Australia 1995.

26. LaFontaine L: Divergent abilities in the idiot savant. Doctoral Dissertation, Boston University in Boston, School of Education, 1974.

27. Nettlebeck T, Young R: Savant Syndrome in International Review of Research in Mental Retardation, ed. CM Glidden. New York, Academic Press, 1999.

28. Frith U, Happe F: Autism: Beyond "theory of mind." Cognition 1994; 50:115–132.

29. Olliffe T, Baron-Cohen S: Are people with autism and Asperger's syndrome faster than normal on the Embedded Figures Test? Journal of Child Psychology & Psychiatry 1997; 24:613–620.

30. Heaton P, Hermelin B, Pring L: Autism and pitch processing: A precursor for savant musical ability? Music Perception 1998; 15:291–305.

31. Baron-Cohen S: The extreme male brain theory of autism. Trends in Cognitive Sciences 2002; 6:248–254.

32. Tanguay P: A tentative hypothesis regarding the role of hemispheric specialization in early infantile autism. Paper presented at UCLA Conference on Cerebral Dominance, Los Angeles 1973.

33. Rimland B: Infantile Autism: The Syndrome and its implications for a neural theory of behavior. New York, Appleton-Century-Crofts, 1978.

34. Hauser S, DeLong G, Rosman N: Pneumographic findings in the infantile autism syndrome. Brain 1975; 98:667–688.

35. DeLong R: Autism: New data suggest a new hypothesis. Neurology 1999; 52:911–916.

36. Boddaert N: Perception of complex sounds: abnormal pattern of cortical activation in autism. Am J Psychiatry 2003; 160:2057–2060.

37. Escalant-Mead P, Minshew N, Sweeney J: Abnormal brain lateralization in high-functioning autism. J Autism and Developmental Disorders 2003; 33:539–543.

38. Brink T: Idiot savant with unusual mechanical ability. Am J Psychiatry 1980; 137:250–251.

39. Steel J, Gorman R, Flaxman J: Neuropsychiatric testing in an autistic mathematical idiot-savant: Evidence for nonverbal abstract capacity. Journal of the American Academy of Child Psychiatry, 1984 3:469–487.

40. Charness N, Clifton J, MacDonald L: Case study of a musical "mono-savant:" A cognitive-psychological focus in The Exceptional Brain, eds. L. Obler and D. A. Fine. New York, Guilford, 1988.

41. Munoz-Yunta J, Ortiz-Alonso T: Savant or Idiot Savant Syndrome Rev. Neurol 2003 Feb; 36 Suppl 1:157–161.

42. Kapur N: Paradoxical functional facilitation in brain-behavior research: A critical review. Brain 1996; 119:1775–1790.

43. Lythgoe M, Pollak T, Kalmas M, de Hann M, Chong WK: Obsessive, prolific artistic output following subarachnoid hemorrhage. Neurology 2005; 64:397–398.

44. Hou C, Miller B, Cummings J, Goldberg M, Mychack P, Bottino B, Benson F: Artistic Savants Neuropsychiatry, Neuropsychology and Behavioral Neurology 2000; 13:29–38.

45. Nurmi EL, Dowd M, Tadevosyan-Leyfer O, Haines J, Folstein S, Sutcliffe JS: Exploratory sub-setting of autism families based on savant skills improves evidence of genetic linkage to 15q11–q13. Journal of the Academy of Child Adolescent Psychiatry 2003; 42:856–863.

46. Birbaumer N: Rain Man's Revelations. Nature 1999; 399:211–212.

47. Pesenti M, Zago L, Crivello F: Mental Calculation in a prodigy is sustained by right prefrontal and medial temporal areas. 2001 Nature Neuroscience; 4:103–107.

48. Kalbfleisch M: Functional neural anatomy of talent. Anatomical Record 2004; 277B:21–36.

49. Snyder A, Mitchell D: Is integer arithmetic fundamental to mental processing? Proceedings of the Royal Society of London Biological Science 1999; 266:587–592.

50. Snyder AW, Mulcahy E, Taylor JL, Mitchell D, Sachdev P, Gandevia SC: Savant-like skills exposed in normal people by suppressing the left fronto-temporal lobe. Journal of Integrative Neuroscience 2003; 2:149–158.

51. Young RL, Ridding MC, Morrell TL: Switching skills by turning off part of the brain. 2004 Neurocase 10:215–222.

52. Kanner L: Early Infantile Autism. Journal of Pediatrics 1944; 25:200–217

53. Treffert DA: The 'idiot savant': a review of the syndrome. Am Journal of Psychiatry 1988; 145:563–572.

54. Horwitz WA, Kestenbaum C, Person E, Jarvik L: Identical twins—idiot savants—Calendar calculators. Am J Psychiatry 1965; 121:1075–1079.

55. Peek F: The Real Rain Man. Salt Lake City, Utah, Harkness Publishers, 1996.

56. Treffert D, Wallace G: Islands of Genius. Scientific American 2002; 286:76–85.

57. Wiltshire S: Drawings. London, J.M. Dent and Sons, 1987.

58. Wiltshire S: Floating Cities. New York, Summit Books, 1991.

59. Sacks O: An Anthropologist on Mars. New York, Alfred Knopf,

60. Lehrman J: Drawings by an Artist with Autism. New York, George Braziller, Inc., 2002.

61. Miller L: Musical Savants: Exceptional Skill in the Mentally Retarded. Hillsdale, NJ, Lawrence Erlbaum Associates, 1989.

62. Cameron L: The Music of Light: The Extraordinary Story of Hikari and Kenzaburo Oe. New York, The Free Press, 1998.

63. Smith N, Tsimpli I: The Mind of the Savant: Language, Learning and Modularity. Oxford, Blackwell, 1995.

64. Viscott D: A musical idiot-savant. Psychiatry 1970; 33:494–515.

65. Phillips A: Talented Imbeciles. 1930 Psychological Clinics 18:246–255.

66. Clark T: The Application of Savant and Splinter Skills in the Autistic Population Through Curriculum Design: A Longitudinal Multiple-Replication Study. Unpublished Doctoral Thesis, The University of South Wales, School of Education Studies.

67. Donnelly JA, Altman R: The Autistic Savant: Recognizing and serving the gifted student with autism. Roeper Review 1994; 16:252–255.

68. Ockelford A: Sound Moves: Music in the education of children and young people who are visually impaired and have learning disabilities. London, Royal Institute for the Blind, 1988.

69. Rancer S: Perfect Pitch and Relative Pitch: How to identify & test for the phenomena: a guide for music teachers, music therapists and parents. Self—published. SusanRMT@aol.com.

70. Grandin T: Thinking in Pictures And Other Reports From My Life With Autism. New York, Vintage Books, 1995.

71. Grandin T: Animals in Translation: Using the Mysteries of Autism to Decode Animal Behavior. New York, Scribner, 2005.

72. Grandin T, Duffy K: Developing Talents: Careers for Individuals with Asperger's Syndrome and High Functioning Autism. Shawnee Mission, KS, Autism Asperger's Publishing Company, 2004.

73. Conturo T, Nicolas E, Cull T, Akbudak E, Snyder AZ, Shimony JS, McKinstry RC, Burton H, Raichle E: Tracking neuronal fiber pathways in the living human brain. Proc. Natl. Acad. Sci 1999; 10422–101427.

Contributing Author Darold A. Treffert, M.D.—Dr. Treffert is a clinical professor at the University of Wisconsin Medical School, in Madison, WI, and a member of the Behavioral Health Department at St. Agnes Hospital, in Fond du Lac, WI.

GENIUS MAYBE AN ABNORMALITY: EDUCATING STUDENTS WITH AUTISM

Editor's Note: This article was originally published in 2008 in the *Autism 101* 1st edition before the Asperger's Syndrome Diagnosis was subsumed within the broader ASD in the 2013 DSM-5 revisions. However, since the highly respected author Dr. Temple Grandin refers within the article to herself as having Asperger's Disorder, we have chosen to maintain all of the original references to AD. For readers who might be confused by this,be invited to replace Asperger's Disroder with 'ASD- High Functioning"

I am becoming increasingly concerned that intellectually gifted children are being denied opportunities because they are being labeled either with Asperger's Syndrome or with high-functioning autism. Within the last year, I have talked to several parents, and I was disturbed by what they said. One mother called me and was very upset that her six-year-old son had Asperger's Syndrome. She then went on to tell me that his IQ was 150. I replied that before people knew about Asperger's Syndrome, their child would have received a very positive label of intellectually gifted.

In another case, the parents of a teenager with Asperger's Syndrome called and told me that they were so concerned about their son's poor social skills that they would not allow him to take computer programming. I told his mother that depriving him of a challenging career in computers would make his life miserable. He will get social interaction through shared interests with other computer people. In a third case, a supersmart child was not allowed in the talented and gifted program in his school because he had an autism label. Educators need to become more aware that intellectually satisfying work makes life meaningful.

I am what I think and do

My sense of being, as a person with autism, is based upon what I think and do. I am what I think and do, not what I feel. I have emotions, but my emotions are more like those of a 10-year-old child or an animal.

My life has meaning because I have an intellectually satisfying career that makes life worth living. In my work designing livestock facilities, I have improved the treatment of farm animals and I have been able to travel to many interesting places. I have traded emotional complexity for intellectual complexity. Emotions are something I have learned to control.

It is essential that talented children labeled with either high-functioning autism or Asperger's Syndrome be trained in fields such as computer programming, where they can do intellectually satisfying work. As for many people with Asperger's Syndrome, for me my life is my work. Life would not be worth living if I did not have intellectually satisfying work.

I did not fully realize this until a flood destroyed our university library. I was attending the American Society of Animal Science meetings when the flood occurred. I first learned about it in a story on the front page of *USA Today*. I grieved for the "dead" books the same way most people grieve for a dead relative. The destruction of books upset me because "thoughts died." Even though most of the books are still in other libraries, there are many people at the university who will never read them. To me, Shakespeare lives if we keep performing his plays. He dies when we stop performing them. I am my work. If the livestock industry continues to use equipment I have designed, then my "thoughts live" and my life has meaning.

If my efforts to improve the treatment of cattle and pigs make real improvements in the world, then life is meaningful.

I have been reading with great satisfaction the many articles in magazines about Linux free software. People in the business world are not able to comprehend why the computer people give their work away. I am unable to think about this without becoming emotional. It is no mystery to me why they download their intellectual ideas into a vast, evolving, and continually improving computer operating system. It is because their thoughts will live forever as part of the "genetic code" of the computer operating system. They are putting themselves into the operating system—and their "intellectual

DNA" will live forever in cyberspace. As the program evolves and changes, the code they wrote will probably remain hidden deep within it. It is almost like a living thing that is continually evolving and improving. For both me and for the programmers who contribute to Linux, we do it because it makes our lives more meaningful.

Continuum of traits

There is a continuum of personality and intellectual traits from normal to abnormal. At what point does a brilliant computer programmer or engineer get labeled with Asperger's Syndrome? There is no black-and-white dividing line.

Simon Baron-Cohen, an autism researcher at the University of Cambridge, found that there were two times as many engineers in the family histories of people with autism. I certainly fit this pattern. My grandfather was an engineer who coinvented the automatic pilot for an airplane. I have second and third cousins who are engineers and mathematicians.

At a recent lecture, Dr. Baron-Cohen described three brilliant individuals with Asperger's Syndrome. There was a brilliant physics student, a computer scientist, and a mathematics professor. It is also likely that Bill Gates has many Asperger's Syndrome traits. An article in *Time Magazine* compared me to Mr. Gates. For example, we both rock. I have seen videotapes of Bill Gates rocking on television. Articles in business magazines describe his incredible memory as a young child.

There is evidence that high-functioning autism and Asperger's Syndrome have a strong genetic basis. G.R. DeLong and J.T. Dyer found that two-thirds of families with a high-functioning autistic had either a first- or second-degree relative with Asperger's Syndrome.

In the journal *Autism and Developmental Disorders*, Sukhelev Naragan and his coworkers wrote that educational achievement of the parents of an autistic child with good language skills were often greater than those of similar parents with normal children. Dr. Robert Plomin at Pennsylvania State University states that autism is highly heritable.

In my book, *Thinking in Pictures*, I devote an entire chapter to the links of intellectual giftedness and creativity to abnormality. Einstein himself had many autistic traits. He did not learn to speak until he was three years of age, and he had a lack of concern about his appearance. His uncut hair did not match the men's hairstyles of his time. Additional insights into Einstein are in *Thinking in Pictures* and other books in my reference list.

Genius is an abnormality?

It is likely that genius in any field is an abnormality. Children and adults who excel in one area, such as math, are often very poor in other areas. The abilities are very uneven. Einstein was a poor speller and did poorly in foreign languages. The brilliant physicist Richard Feynman did poorly in some subjects.

A review of the literature indicates that being truly outstanding in any field may be associated with some type of abnormality. Kay Redfield Jamison, from Johns Hopkins School of Medicine, has reviewed many studies that show the link between manic depressive illness and creativity. N.C. Andreason, at the University of Iowa, found that 80 percent of creative writers had mood disorders sometime during their lives. A study of mathematical giftedness, conducted at Iowa State University by Camilla Persson, found that mathematical giftedness was correlated with being nearsighted and having an increased incidence of allergies. I recently attended a lecture by Robert Fisher at Barrow Neurological Institute in Phoenix, Arizona. He stated that many great people had epilepsy, including Julius Caesar, Napoleon, Socrates, Pythagoras, Handel, Tchaikovsky, and Alfred Nobel. For additional information on the links between abnormality and giftedness, refer to the reference list.

Types of thinking

There appear to be two basic types of thinking in intellectually gifted people who have Asperger's Syndrome or high-performing autism. The highly social, verbal thinkers who are in the educational system need to understand that the thought processes of these people are different.

The two types are the totally visual thinkers like me; and the music, math, and memory thinkers described in Thomas Sowell's book *Late Talking Children*. I have interviewed several of these people, and their thoughts work in patterns in which there are no pictures. Sowell reports that in the family histories of late talking, music, math, and memory children, 74 percent of the families will have an engineer or a relative in a highly technical field such as physics, accounting, or mathematics. Most of these children also had a relative who played a musical instrument.

Every thought I have is represented by a picture. When I think about a dog, I see a series of pictures of specific dogs, such as my student's dog or the dog next door. There is no generalized verbal dog concept in my mind. I form my dog concept by looking for common features that all dogs have and no cats have.

For example, all of the different breeds of dogs have the same kind of nose. My thought process goes from specific pictures to general concepts, whereas most people think from general to specific. I have no vague, abstract, language-based concepts in my head, only specific pictures.

When I do design work, I can run three-dimensional, full-motion "video" images of the cattle handling equipment in my head. I can "test run" the equipment on the "virtual reality" computer that is in my imagination. Visual thinkers who are expert computer programmers have told me that they can see the entire program "tree," and then they write the code on each branch.

It is almost as if I have two consciences. Pictures are my real thoughts, and language acts as a narrator. I narrate from the "videos" and "slides" I see in my imagination. For example, my language narrator might say, "I can design that." I then see a video of the equipment I am designing in my imagination. When the correct answer pops into my head, it is a video of the successful piece of equipment working. At this point, my language narrator says, "I figured out how to do it." In my mind there is no subconscious. Images are constantly passing through the computer screen of my imagination. I can see thought processes that others have covered up with language. I do not require language for either consciousness or for thinking.

When I learned drafting for doing my design work, it took time to train my visual mind to make the connection between the symbolic lines on a layout drawing and an actual building. To learn this, I had to take the set of blueprints and walk around in the building, looking at the square concrete support columns, seeing how the little squares on the drawing related to the actual columns. After I had "programmed" my brain to read drawings, the ability to draw blueprints appeared almost by magic. It took time to get information in, but after I was "programmed," the skill appeared rather suddenly.

Researchers who have studied chess players state that the really good chess players have to spend time inputting chess patterns into their brains. I can really relate to this. When I design equipment, I take bits of pictures and pieces of equipment I have seen in the past and reassemble them into new designs. It is like taking things out of the memory of a CAD computer drafting system, except I can reassemble the pieces into three-dimensional, moving videos. Constance Milbrath and Bryan Siegal at the University of California found that talented autistic artists assemble the whole from the parts. It is "bottom up thinking," instead of "top down thinking."

Teachers and mentors

Children and teenagers with autism or Asperger's Syndrome need teachers who can help them develop their talents. I cannot emphasize enough the importance of developing a talent into an employable skill. Visual thinkers like me can become experts in fields such as computer graphics, drafting, computer programming, automotive repair, commercial art, industrial equipment design, or working with animals.

The music-, math-, and memory-type children can excel in mathematics, accounting, engineering, physics, music, and other technical skills. Unless the student's mathematical skills are truly brilliant, I would recommend taking courses in library science, accounting, engineering, or computers. Learning a technical skill will make the person highly employable. There are few jobs for mediocre mathematicians or physicists.

Since social skills are weak, the person can make up for them by being so good at something that they will be attractive as employees. Teachers need to counsel individuals to go into fields where they can easily gain employment. Majoring in history is not a good choice because obtaining a job will be difficult. History could be the person's hobby instead of the main area of study in school.

Many high-functioning autistic and Asperger's teenagers get bored with school and misbehave. They need mentors who can teach them a field that will be beneficial to their future. I had a wonderful high school science teacher who taught me to use the scientific research library. Computers are a great field because being weird, or a "computer geek," is okay. A good programmer is recognized for his/her skills. I know several very successful autistic computer programmers. A bored high school student could enroll in programming or computer-aided drafting courses in a local community college.

To make up for social deficits, the autistic person needs to become so good at their work that its brilliance is recognized. People respect talent. They need mentors who are computer programmers, artists, draftsmen, etc., to teach them career skills. I often get asked, "How does one find mentors?" You never know where a mentor teacher may be found. He may be standing in the checkout line in a supermarket. I found one of my first meat industry mentors when I met the wife of his insurance agent at a party. She struck up a conversation with me because she saw my hand-embroidered western shirt. I had spent hours embroidering a steer head on the shirt. Post a notice on the bulletin board at the local college in the computer science department. If you see a person with a computer company name badge, approach him and show him work that the person with autism has done.

Sell your work, not your personality

Since people with autism and Asperger's Syndrome are inept socially, they have to sell their work instead of their personalities. I showed my portfolio of pictures and blueprints to prospective customers. I never went to the personnel office. I went straight to the engineers and asked to do design jobs.

Another approach is to put up a web page that showcases work in drawing or programming. Freelance work is really great. It avoids many social problems.

I can go in and design the project and then get out before I get social problems.

There have been several sad stories where an autistic draftsman or technician has been promoted to a management position. It was a disaster that ended up in the person being fired or quitting. Employers need to recognize the person's limitations. An excellent draftsman, commercial artist, technician, or computer programmer may lose their career when promoted to management. These people should be rewarded with more pay or a new computer instead of management jobs.

People with autism and Asperger's Syndrome need concrete, well-defined goals at work. For example, the job is to design a better speech recognition program. When one project is finished, they should be given another project with a well-defined goal. If too many projects are thrown at them all at once, they will become confused. Let the person with autism or Asperger's Syndrome finish the first project before he/she is given another. The projects can be really hard, but they must have a well-defined goal.

Teaching citizenship

Since people with autism and Asperger's Syndrome are emotionally immature, they must have basic morality reinforced when they are small children. When I was little, I was taught in a concrete way that hurting other people, stealing, and lying were bad. At age 8, I stole a toy fire engine, and my mother made me give it back. She told me, "How would you like it if someone stole one of your model airplanes?" She also told me that you do not hit other kids because I would not like it if they hit me. It was the Golden Rule: "Do unto others as you would want them to do unto you." Some Asperger's Syndrome children and adults have done some bad deeds because the basic rules were not taught to them. I live a rule-based life, and I have a rule system I still use today.

Anxiety problems

For many people with autism and Asperger's Syndrome, anxiety and nervousness is a major problem. This is discussed in detail in my book *Thinking in Pictures*. Anxiety problems worsen with age. My anxiety became unbearable in my early thirties. It was like a constant state of stage fright. At times, my nervous system was so aroused that I felt as if a lion were stalking me, but there was no lion. I have talked to several people with autism who quit good, high-paying jobs in graphic arts when anxiety and panic attacks made going to the office impossible.

Many people with autism or Asperger's Syndrome need medication to control their anxiety. I have been taking antidepressants for almost 20 years. My career would have been ruined if I had not started taking antidepressants to control my anxiety. I know many autistic and Asperger's adults who are taking Prozac or one of the other Serotonin reuptake inhibitors. People need to be counseled that medications such as Prozac can improve their lives.

The anxiety is due to biological problems in the nervous system. Recent brain research is showing that there is immature development in certain parts of the brains of people with autism. Autopsies of brains of people with autism show that there are biological abnormalities that occur when the fetus is developing. Antidepressant medication helps reduce anxiety caused by biological problems in the nervous system.

You can learn more about Dr. Grandin and her work at http:/ www.grandin.com.

References

1. Andreason, N.C. 1987. Creativity and mental illness prevalence rates in writers and first-degree relatives. American Journal of Psychiatry 144: 1288–1292.
2. Bailey et al. A clinicopatholic study of autism. Brain. 121: 889–908 (Brain Study).
3. Kemper, T., and Barman, M. 1998. Neuropathology of Autism. Journal of Neuropathology and experimental Neurology. July, (Brain Study)
4. Cranberg, L.D., and Albert, M.C. 1988. The Chess Mind, In L.K. Obler and D. Fein, Editors. The Exceptional Brain. Guilford Press New York. Pp. 156–190.
5. Delong, G.R., and Dwyer, J.T. 1988. Correlation of family history and specific autistic subgroups: Asperger's syndrome and bipolar affective disease. Journal of Autism and Developmental Disorders 18: 593–600.
6. Gleik, J. 1993. Genius: Richard Feynman and modern physics. Little Brown, New York.
7. Grandin, T. 1995. Thinking in Pictures. Doubleday, New York. Now published by Vintage Press Division of Random House.
8. Grandin, T. 1995. How people with autism think. In: E. Schopler and
9. G.B. Mesibov, Editor. Learning and Cognition in Autism. Plenum Press, New York.
10. Grant, A. 1885. Charles Darwin. Appleton, New York.
11. Grant, V.W. 1968. Great Abnormals. Hawthorn, New York.
12. Highfield, R., and Garter, P. 1993. The private lives of Albert Einstein. St. Martin's, New York.
13. Kevin, G. 1967. Inspired Amateurs. Books for Libraries Press, Freeport, New York.

14. Kincheloe, J.L., Steinberg, S.R., and Tippins, D.J. 1992. The Stigma of Genius. Hollowbrook, Durango, Colorado.

15. Landa, R., Piven, J., Wzorek, M.M., Gayle, J.O., Chase, G.A., and Folstein, S.E. 1992. Social language use in parents of autistic individuals. Psychological Medicine 22: 245–254.

16. Milbrath, C., and Siegol, B. 1996. Perspective taking in the drawings of a talented autistic child. Visual Arts Research, School of Arts and Design, University of Illinois, Urbana, Illinois USA. Pp22: 56–75.

17. Myerson and Boyle. 1941. The incidence of manic-depressive psychosis in certain socially prominent families. P. 20. In K.R. Jamison, 1993. Touched with Fire. The Free Press, New York.

18. Narayan, S., Moyer B., and Wolf, S. 1990. Family characteristics of autistic children: a further report. Journal of Autism and Development Disorders 20: 523–535.

19. Pais, A. 1994. Einstein lived here. Oxford University Press, New York.

20. Patten, B.M. 1973. Visually mediated thinking: a report of the case of Albert Einstein. Journal of Learning Disabilities 67: 15–20.

21. Persson, C.B. 1987. Possible biological correlations of precocious mathematical reasoning ability. Trends in Neuroscience 10: 17–20.

22. Plomin, R., Owen, M.J., and McGuffn, G. 1994. The genetic basis of complex human behaviors science, 264: 1733–1739.

23. Sowell, T. 1997. Late Talking Children, Basis Books, Division of Harper Collins, New York.

Contributing Author Temple Grandin, Ph.D., Animal Science, University of Illinois—One of the most world's most accomplished and well-known adults with autism, Dr. Grandin is a prominent speaker and writer on this subject. In her book *Thinking in Pictures*, Dr. Grandin delivers a report from the country of autism. Writing from the dual perspectives of a scientist and an autistic person, she tells us how that country is experienced by its inhabitants and how she managed to breach its boundaries to function in the outside world. What emerges documents an extraordinary human being, one who gracefully and lucidly bridges the gulf between her condition and our own. Dr. Grandin is also a gifted scientist who has designed livestock handling facilities used worldwide and is an associate professor of Animal Science at Colorado State University.

MEASURING IQ AND THE MYTH OF MENTAL RETARDATION

Note: This article is based on, and includes excerpts from, the book *Challenging the Myths of Autism* (2011) by Jonathan Alderson

Ahmad's mother sat across from me in her tiny living room. The furnishings were sparse. The room was bare. She had been forced to hide any precious decorations, picture frames, trinkets, vases, and keepsakes out of reach for her son's safety because of his extreme hyperactivity. He bounced across the floors, onto chairs and the sofa, for hours. It was our first meeting. She told me the details of her struggle with the Ontario health system that took 18 months to diagnose her son. They finally told her he had severe autism. She didn't flinch as she told me this—it seemed matter of fact. But the assessment report went further. She looked down and clearly felt some emotion as she shared that Ahmad was also labeled Mentally Retarded (MR). It upset her to say this out loud. At just four years old, her son was written off as "uneducable." She told me what she had read about the low expectations for any meaningful development. The MR diagnosis was a curse in her mind. Ironically, autism seemed somehow more hopeful.

Many parents lose hope when the MR label is tacked onto an ASD diagnosis. They recognize their child will be judged twice. An MR diagnosis can mean better services, but parents also realize society's negative judgments and the limitations they impose.

The stereotype that all people diagnosed with autism are math geniuses or savants exists side-by-side with the commonly cited statistic that 70–90 percent of people with ASD have an IQ score under 70. Research says most are mentally retarded. A 2010 article in the India Express News Service reported that "most government hospitals in the state are still signing the health certificates of autistic patients as 'mentally–retarded.'" In 2003, Dr. Laura Schreibman presented a lecture at the University of California at San Diego (UCSD) claiming to parents in the audience as fact that autism is commonly accompanied with mental retardation, saying, ". . . we know that probably about 75–80 percent of these individuals have some degree of mental retardation and in many of them it is severe."

Yet parents and autism therapists alike attest to the wide range of intelligence that the ASD population demonstrates. In my own practice of designing and directing autism treatment programs for more than 20 years, I also have seen a wide range of levels of intelligence in the children I meet. I've also learned that since many of the children are nonverbal or only somewhat verbal, they are not necessarily able to express and demonstrate their intelligence.

Working with one young girl, I also learned first-hand that there are often physical disabilities that limit a person's ability to share and express their innate intelligence. Sadie had cerebral palsy and was confined to a wheelchair. She also had a diagnosis of autism. She had poor eye contact and spent a lot of the day slumped in her wheelchair, unmotivated to interact with others. She had been assessed with a low IQ. She could say a few words but only inconsistently, sometimes mouthing the words silently.

Our team's first goal was to find toys and activities that would interest this little girl. We weren't trying to teach her anything yet, except that we were user-friendly and were interested in whatever she was interested in. We presented a whole range of choices including physical play like tickle and wheel-chair dancing. Sadie showed us quickly that she could understand most of what we were saying. When she was motivated by something, she did her best to gather energy and, with great effort, try to play with us. She was gentle and genuinely sweet. The best reward for our efforts was the huge smile she beamed when she liked an activity, arching her head back looking right into our eyes.

After the first two days of sessions, we felt we had made a connection with Sadie. She was watching us with her eyes more and more. She seemed happier, but we still weren't certain about her cognitive abilities. What kind of intelligence did she have? Could she learn to speak, for example? Then, during a therapy session on the third day, a therapist heard Sadie say several words very clearly. "I heard her say, 'again,' three times," he blurted out after the session. I asked him to describe in detail how it happened and what it sounded like. He had been singing the "head-shoulders-knees-and-toes" song along with the actions. She was moving her body too as much as she could and was looking straight at him the entire song. When he finished singing, she said, "Again!" in a breathy, very soft voice. We played the game again in the following session so that our senior therapist could see for himself. What other clues could we observe? Then he saw it. Each time he heard Sadie whisper a word, she was sitting more upright. At the peek of a game, her body was less slumped in the wheelchair, and she held her head up straighter. "That's it!" He thought, "She's in a better position to make vocal sounds." When she wasn't slumped on her diaphragm, her airway was obviously more open.

Working with another staff, the senior therapist kneeled down in front the wheelchair. He told Sadie he had an idea that might help her be able to talk to us more easily. He asked her if they could help her sit up straighter by holding her under her arms. She nodded and smiled yes. Once her upper body was upright, he asked her to tell him how that felt. She mouthed a word but no sound came out. From his position kneeling in front, he studied her behavior very closely and noticed she hadn't taken a breath before speaking. Even though her airway was more open now, for some reason she wasn't taking a breath before trying to speak. Her breath control—the breathing-talking cycle—wasn't coordinated. He reached forward and put his hand lightly on her diaphragm—"Take a breath, Sadie," he coached. She followed his cues and took a deeper breath. "How does that feel now?" he asked. "Good." she answered clearly. It wasn't a whisper, either. And for the next few minutes, with the other therapist supporting Sadie to sit up, he reminded her to take a breath each time before she spoke. "How do you like the games we're playing with you?" he asked. "Fun!" she said out loud. Her parents stood nearby with tears rolling down their cheeks. Sadie was talking. With more breath-control training and posture strengthening, Sadie would go on to show, and tell, her family and teachers how smart she really was. Needless to say, along with her posture, her IQ scores surged upward.

Unfortunately, the MR label is now strongly associated with autism. It stereotypes an entire population that, as it turns out, has remarkably varied patterns of intelligence—arguably a wider range than the neurotypical population. The stereotype has negative implications and leads to false conclusions. The stereotype continues to be promoted by physicians, researchers, and popular media alike. The myth lives strong, and I wanted to investigate where it originally came from and why it persists to then hopefully be able to debunk it.

When I wrote about what I call "the myth of mental retardation" in my book *Challenging the Myths of Autism* (HarperCollins, 2011), I discovered a fascinating history that is full of researchers' mistakes and carelessness.

Autistic children were once considered bright with above-average intelligence. Psychologists explained that the intelligence just wasn't obvious because of social and communication delays. Back then, in 1943, when the famous Austrian physician Leo Kanner first popularized the diagnosis of autism, he wrote in detail about his young autistic patients' cognitive strengths: "The astounding vocabulary of the speaking children, the excellent memory for events of several years before, the phenomenal rote memory for poems and names, and the precise recollection of complex patterns and sequences, bespeak good intelligence" (p. 247). Unfortunately, this positive association didn't last long. Intelligence scores in autism began spiraling downward.

Meredyth Goldberg Edelson, Professor at Williamette University in Oregon, synthesizes clearly the birth of the association between mental retardation and autism. Piecing together more than 200 sources, Goldberg Edelson provides a concise history of the shifting reported prevalence rates of MR in autism over the past century. Basically, she plots a history in which autism was first thought of as high intelligence, then it shifted to be associated with ever lowering IQ scores for about 50 years from the 1950s to early-2000s. Only recently are we rediscovering and acknowledging the intelligence of people with autism.

It's absolutely true that many children diagnosed with autism have scored below 70 on the IQ, but how accurate are intelligence tests for children with language delays? If a person doesn't have language skills to actually answer the test questions or even just to understand the questions being asked in the first place, how valid is the test for this group?

Not all intelligence tests are the same. There is a variety of tests that measure intelligence in different ways. Some tests are more popular, but none can claim to be the definitive measure of intelligence. Dr. Meredyth Goldberg Edelson first became interested in the question of intelligence in autism when she tested about 300 children diagnosed with autism. But instead of using the conventional Stanford-Binet, she used the Test of Non-verbal Intelligence (TONI) and found consistently higher scores than what previous tests had shown. The kids in her group on average scored around 90 (an IQ score that is about average in the general population). Of the 297 children in her study, only 19 percent scored in the mental retardation range—vastly lower than the myth of 70–90 percent. The kids scored higher, she believes, because the TONI doesn't require verbal responses. How valid are tests that require verbal responses for people with language disorders and attention deficit disorders? she wondered.

Professor Laurent Mottron at the University of Montreal and his colleague Michelle Dawson are two of the pioneers trying to answer this question. They argue that the most commonly used tests like the Stanford-Binet and the Wechsler Scales are too dependent on good verbal ability. Test takers have to sit and listen to many of the questions read out loud and then are required to answer verbally. People with a communication disorder aren't able to verbally answer the questions. They fail even though they might know the answers. In other words, these types of verbal-based tests measure communication skills as much as they do intelligence. Therefore, some argue, the tests aren't valid for nonverbal children. Writing for *Newsweek*, Sharon Begley interviewed Michelle Dawson and documented her view that "Testing autistic kids' intelligence in a way that requires them to engage [verbally] with a stranger is like giving a blind person an intelligence test that requires him to process visual information." Since language delay and communication disability are part of the diagnosis of autism, we should use tests that are sensitive to measuring intelligence that aren't limited or influenced by the known language barriers.

Mottron and Dawson did just this. They used Raven's Progressive Matrices, a test that is more nonverbal and visual-oriented. This test measures what is called "fluid intelligence." Thirty-eight children with autism were tested on the Raven's Progressive Matrices as well as on the commonly used Wechsler Scales of Intelligence (WISC). On average, their scores on the "fluid intelligence" test were 30 percentile points higher than on the WISC. This could make the difference between an MR score of 70 and average intelligence of 100. An important difference, indeed.

Thankfully, a new generation of investigators is taking a closer look and using new testing tools. Currently, the leading experts on IQ and autism are reporting higher IQ scores once again. Based on these ideas, I propose a possibility-promoting (rather than a limiting) recharacterization of intelligence and autism:

There is a wide range of intelligence in autism. Like in the neurotypical population, intelligence in autism stretches from Savant to bright to average to mental retardation and points in between. When we expand our definition of what we call intelligence we begin to see more skills, abilities, strengths, and talents. When we limit intelligence just to IQ, we limit ourselves and those we test. There are many different kinds of intelligence including spatial, musical, interpersonal, and logical-mathematical, among others. There are benefits to each different type of intelligence and a role for each in society. Diversity of intelligence strengthens families, companies, and communities. There may be some unique types of intelligences in the autistic population because of differences in sensory perception and differences in thinking processes. We can learn more about these differences, understand their contributions, and create a place in our expanding definition of human intelligence. Many people with autism communicate in different ways, so their intelligence may not be measurable or visible by neurotypical standards. Like everyone, people on the spectrum appreciate having their intelligence recognized, supported, and acknowledged rather than having their differences listed to be fixed. As parents, friends, family, neighbors, employers, educators, therapists, and policy makers, the onus is on us to actively look for expressions of intelligence in all its forms, and to support it to develop and shine.

And as for Ahmad . . . his mother and his therapist team were receptive to this reframing and to the possibilities it opened up of discovering Ahmad's intelligence. Despite his nonverbal autism diagnosis, he is sitting at the dining table and feeding himself for the first time at nine years old; he is less hyperactive; and he demonstrates his good intelligence to us every day. Recently, he surprised us by learning a kids' playground "see see my playmate" clapping game and doing it without a hitch at top speed. He remembers physical exercise routines we teach him, and one of the therapists found out that Ahmad is pretty good at giving shoulder rubs. After giving Ahmad a nice shoulder massage, the therapist turned around, and Ahmad gently rubbed the therapist's shoulders for a few minutes. What fun!

Jonathan Alderson, Ed.M., is an autism treatment specialist and founder of the innovative integrated Multi-Treatment Intervention Program (www. IMTI.ca). A graduate of Harvard University, with experience as a curriculum specialist coordinator with Teach for America, he trained at the Autism Treatment Center of America in Massachusetts and worked as administrator and senior family trainer in their Son-Rise Program. He has worked with over 3,000 children and families. Now based in Toronto, he is a contributor for the Huffington Post, a member of the Seneca College behavioral Sciences Advisory Committee and founding cochair of the Young Professionals for Autism Speaks Canada Advisory Board. He has lectured on his multidisciplinary approach to autism treatment throughout Canada, the USA, England, Ireland, Holland, Spain, Australia, Israel, and Mexico. He is the author of *Challenging the Myths of Autism*, which has inspired educators and parents to consider a radical reframing of how we think about and treat people diagnosed with autism. His book has been honored with the Mom's Choice Gold Award, the American Non-Fiction Authors' Association Silver Award, and the 2012 International Book Award for Best Parent-Resource.

9

GUIDING ADOLESCENCE AND ADULTS WITH AUTISM

PREPARING FOR ESSENTIAL TASK OF THE REAL WORLD

What's so special about adolescence?
"The period of life beginning with puberty and ending with complete growth and physical maturation."
—Stedman's Medical Dictionary, 1995

Bookstores and libraries are full of books that try to help parents and professionals understand adolescence. Almost every newspaper or magazine includes a story about yet another challenge that confronts adolescents in the twenty-first century. Why is it that so many of us look to the experts for advice in negotiating this phase of our youngsters' lives when this is the time of life that we remember best? Perhaps it is the complexity of physical, social, and emotional development. Perhaps it is our own memories of "the best and worst of times." Perhaps it is the signal that our children will be adults before we know it. And, although the books and experts may differ in their conclusions and advice, they share at least two conclusions about adolescence in general:

- Adults need to be sharp to understand what's going on. No two adolescents are the same, and there is no one-size-fits-all strategy for parenting or teaching.
- Adolescent brains are undergoing remarkable growth and change. These changes prepare the adolescent for the increasingly abstract and complex demands of the adult world. During this time, even the most typical of adolescents may process information in unique, often perplexing ways.

Is it any wonder, then, that parents and professionals are even more confused by the thoughts, feelings, and behavior of adolescents with autism spectrum disorders? This chapter aims to shed light on some of the confusion. By no means, though, can one chapter answer all the questions. Instead, the goal is to provide food for thought and to point parents and professionals in the direction of additional answers. (You will find references at the end of this chapter. My own ideas are expressed in greater detail in my book *Asperger's Syndrome and adolescence: Helping preteens and teens get ready for the real world.*)

Adolescence meets autism spectrum disorder (ASD)

The advantages of ASD during adolescence

Although we don't often think of it, adolescents with ASD often bring with them a host of characteristics that can protect them from some of the social/emotional conflict and chaos of adolescence. These characteristics can also spare parents a few headaches, as they limit exposure to the more reckless aspects of adolescent life. They include:

- Belief in, and need for, rules, which allows the adolescent to behave well, at least as long as he/she knows the rules—more about this later.
- A preference for telling the truth, which virtually ensures that the adolescent with ASD will confess any transgression.
- Black-and-white thinking, which makes it less likely that the adolescent will try to look for the loopholes in the rules or directions that adults have given.
- Reduced concern for what others think and popularity, which can decrease susceptibility to negative peer pressure and fads.
- Ability to focus on things that matter, especially one's passions and preoccupations, which can lead to productivity and discovery.
- Special talents and interests, which can be sources of new ideas and ways to connect with others, and which can support strategies for coping.

When he or she studies, lives, or works with people who understand his/her strengths and challenges, the adolescent with ASD can be an active and exemplary participant. The strategies that the adolescent uses to reduce unpredictability and anxiety also tend to prevent the risky behaviors that tempt typical peers. And, when engaged in a pursuit that interests them, adolescents with ASD are among the most conscientious and productive of workers. As Temple Grandin has often commented, people with ASD get more done because "the rest of you just stand around chatting all the time."

A real-life example: Thirteen-year-old Marc attended a school that placed a high premium on personal and community responsibility. When several of the boys in his grade became involved in a scheme to sell their parents' prescription drugs, most of their friends looked the other way. They didn't want to risk being called a "snitch" (or worse). Marc heard about the scheme and quickly realized that it violated many school and community rules. He immediately went to the school principal and gave names and details of the scheme. Marc's parents and teachers praised him for averting what could have been disastrous for the entire school community.

The disadvantages of ASD during adolescence

While many of the characteristics of ASD make it easier for the adolescent to follow rules and persist in problem solving, each of these characteristics can also have its drawbacks. Black-and-white thinking may keep a student on the right side of the school rules but doesn't help much in the world of adolescent friendships. Similarly, persistence in pursuing special interests can get in the way of completing schoolwork in other subjects.

In addition, adolescents with ASD typically struggle with one or more of the following concerns:

- Poor regulation of the Four As (Alertness/Arousal, Attention, Activity, Affect), which can lead the adolescent to break many of the rules that he/she holds most dear. For example, when surrounded by lots of people, Sally becomes so "revved" that she can't pay attention to the person who is talking with her. She also begins to rock back and forth (activity) to help settle down her nervous system (alertness or arousal). If she has to stay in the situation, she's likely to feel increasingly overwhelmed and to display emotion (affect) in ways that are not suitable for the situation.

- Clumsiness, which can lead the adolescent with ASD to stand too close to others, to display awkward body language, and to have trouble negotiating the crowded hallways of school or malls. And in a culture that places extraordinary value upon athletic skills, the adolescent with poor motor skills may not know how to fit in.

- Difficulties in seeing the forest for the trees, which can pose the risk that the adolescent will get stuck on details and miss the big picture. It's not at all unusual for a very bright adolescent with high functioning ASD, for example, to recite every detail in a movie without knowing what the movie is about. And, since social interaction is so often a matter of big picture, they are likely to engage in "socially penalizing behavior," a term coined by Elsa Abele, an expert in social communication.

- Inefficiencies in social communication, which are probably universal for adolescents with ASD. These inefficiencies can range from severe challenges in oral expression to milder difficulties in understanding the subtleties of adolescent humor and slang. Regardless of the severity, these inefficiencies make it difficult for the adolescent with ASD to know what other people mean. They can miss the point in academic lessons (and study the wrong things) or fail to heed the indirect directions and warnings of peers and adults (for example, "Don't you think your sister would like a turn on the computer?"). Inefficiencies in social communication are likely to affect every aspect of daily life.

- Problems in perspective-taking (Theory of Mind), which tend to go hand in hand with inefficient social communication.

How can we make inferences about another person's feelings unless we can read verbal and nonverbal communication? And how can we adjust our own behavior to create a desired impression unless we know something about what the other person likes, dislikes, feels, and thinks? Over and over again, I am dismayed by how difficult it is for bright adolescents with autism to answer the question "What is (person's name) like?" Even when the adolescent can describe the person's physical characteristics, possessions, and behavior, he/she is unable to predict the person's reaction or preferences. Without adequate Theory of Mind, the adolescent is unable to behave empathically or respectfully.

- Challenges in problem solving, which are common, even for the most intellectually gifted individual with ASD. Many of these difficulties are associated with limited ability to identify what is salient (or important) in a situation. Without efficient salience determination, the adolescent is unlikely to know what to look or listen for and, unfortunately, to fail to filter out irrelevant thoughts or actions. Another obstacle to problem solving is poor generalization. Often, the adolescent with ASD does not see the similarity between the current task and previous situations. Instead of applying the skills that worked so well last time, he or she starts over from the beginning.

- Inexperience in social situations, which is a frequent contributor to the everyday functioning of the adolescent with ASD. While everyone else learned "playground politics" (Stanley Greenspan's term) in the sandbox at preschool, the child with an ASD had too many motor or sensory challenges to tolerate the playground. While peers had play dates and sleepovers, the child with ASD still communicated too inefficiently for parents to trust him/her with another family.

Hanging out at the mall, going to the movies, or sitting around gossiping are seldom on the list of favorite activities for children with ASD. Hence, the individual with ASD enters adolescence without the information necessary to manage a growing body, a questioning mind, and ever-changing emotions.

A real-life example: for the first time in her life, 17-year-old Anne had some friends. Girls in the art club recognized Anne's drawing talents and were receptive to her lengthy descriptions of animé characters (her special interest). Over a weekend, Anne's parents told her that she had earned the privilege of going to the anime convention in a nearby city. Eager to tell this exciting news to her friends, Anne went to school on Monday morning and spied her friends at the end of the hall. Two girls were huddled around a third girl, who was obviously upset, according to an observant teacher. Anne was so intent upon her desire to share her news that she totally missed the big picture that a friend was in distress.

When she bounded up to the girls and shouted out her exciting news, the other three looked at her with disdain. Why didn't she know that a friend was upset?

Six essential tasks and how to master them

Partnership—a necessary first step

Remember that the one of the tasks of adolescence is to learn to be as independent as possible. Doesn't it make sense, then, that the adolescent with an ASD should be a working partner in the process?

The first step in any intervention program is to ensure that you and your working partner (the adolescent) have a mutual understanding of the goals and how to try to reach them.

Task 1: Adaptive self-management of thoughts, feelings, and behavior

Adaptive self-management refers to a person's ability to regulate alertness, attention, activity, and affect (emotion) efficiently enough to support active participation in everyday life. As suggested above, poor self-regulation is one of the most common challenges faced by individuals with ASD. Adults with ASD, such as Temple Grandin, confirm that challenges in self-regulation are among significant obstacles to success in the world of work. As she stated matter-of-factly in one presentation, "If you throw your computer monitor out the window when you're mad, you'll get fired." Others, such as Stephen Shore and Jerry Newport, explain that self-regulatory challenges (especially sensory sensitivities) can have a dramatic effect upon dating and relationships.

There is no doubt that adolescents with ASD try hard to manage their sensations, thoughts, and feelings. Their repetitive behaviors, need for routine, and single-minded focus on preferred topics are examples of these efforts. The problem is that their self-regulatory strategies are frequently inefficient or inappropriate to the situation.

Many individuals with ASD must deal with extremely high stress levels. The accumulation of sensory assaults, language and social demands, and flexibility requirements taxes the person's capacity to manage. At a certain point, an apparently small thing can lead to a meltdown. Observers often wonder why the person with ASD is overreacting to something so trivial. It's important to realize that the individual is not reacting to that last event, but, more likely, the event is the straw that broke the camel's back.

A real-life example: Rick is a 14-year-old in Grade 8. Although his nonverbal problem-solving skills are quite impressive, his language skills are similar to those of a child in Grade 1. Rick converses well one-on-one with people who know how to adjust their language to his skills. But when another person enters the conversation or when the language level gets too complicated, Rick gets anxious and begins to quote Disney videos. The benefit of Rick's "scripting" is that it takes him away from an anxiety-provoking situation. A disadvantage is that he is unavailable for appropriate interaction with other people. Rick also gets stuck in his scripting and is unable to understand and follow the directions of his parents and teachers. If adults insist on compliance, Rick is likely to yell out, "NO! You can't make me!" and run from the room. In other words, Rick's stress levels are so high they have prompted a fight or flight response.

Of course, it's impossible to eliminate all of the stress in life. And occasionally everyone has trouble coping with the last straw. The key to self-management is to reduce stress and strain before it reaches unmanageable levels. This is accomplished by two types of interventions: modifications of environment and routine, and preventive stress management. Over the course of adolescence, it's important to shift more and more of the responsibility for these interventions to the person with ASD. It is this shift that allows the adolescent or young adult to function with maximum independence.

Modifications of environment and routines

- Create spaces that support the adolescent's sensory needs. For example, a student with hypersensitive hearing is likely to need a quiet home base or retreat space at school and at home, for study or for regrouping.
- Carefully consider the sensory load associated with places like the school bus or cafeteria. The convenience associated with bus transportation or a hot lunch might not be worth the costs of sensory overload or exposure to teasing.
- Allow access to music, snacks, and other sensory tools that enhance concentration and reduce stress. It may actually help to listen to music while doing homework or to eat a crunchy snack before a class that requires a lot of listening.
- Experiment with clothing and hygiene routines that reduce irritation but do not create socially penalizing situations. One adolescent girl was constantly adjusting her bra, drawing stares from other people. At the suggestion of her counselor, the girl and her mother went to a department store with experienced saleswomen. Although the girl detested the hour or so of bra fittings, the result was the discovery of a style that fit comfortably. After several washings, the bras were comfortable and the adjustments ceased. A young man was hypersensitive to the feel of a toothbrush in his mouth. His occupational therapist suggested that he brush his teeth while in the shower. Voilà! Problem solved! (By the way, the same young man later discovered that he could shave in the shower with similarly positive results.)
- Make sure that the adolescent has a sleep routine. This includes falling asleep at a reasonable time and awakening at the time needed to get ready for school or work. Consult a physician if this is not possible.

Direct teaching of stress management

- Teach the adolescent to monitor physical and emotional signs of stress. The Alert Program (also known as "How does your engine run?") by Williams and Shellenberger can teach individuals how to recognize their level of alertness/arousal and choose suitable remedies to perk up or settle down their nervous systems.

- Experiment with relaxation strategies that fit the adolescent's learning profile. For example, Cautela's book on relaxation techniques is particularly helpful for adolescents with cognitive challenges. On the other hand, an adolescent with better verbal skills might enjoy meditation or autogenic relaxation training. (See the reference by Goldbeck and Schmid, 2003.) For students with adequate imitation skills, yoga can be extraordinarily helpful. A helpful hint: adolescents are more likely to accept these strategies if they are presented to an entire class!

- Develop a regular exercise routine, adapted to the student's sensory and motor profile. Adolescents with ASD are often more comfortable with nonball sports and with exercise that does not require special (uncomfortable) clothing or equipment. Running, swimming, skiing, weight training (for those older than 14), and martial arts (with a sensitive teacher) are examples of exercise regimens that have been successful for individuals with ASD. Remember, research has demonstrated that exercise is superior to medication and other therapies as an antidepressant!

- Consider involvement in the arts, as a participant or as a spectator. Music, visual arts, and drama have multiple payoffs. From a regulatory status, they can be remarkably efficient. They have the added benefit of exposing the adolescent to other people who tend to be more accepting of diversity.

- Help the adolescent learn to use special talents and interests as stress management strategies. For example, an adolescent who likes to make clay figures might add a half-hour of sculpting time to his morning or evening routine.

- If special interests are not developmentally or socially appropriate, use them as starting points. For example, one middle schooler was obsessed with PokeMon long after his peers had moved on to other card and electronic games. His school counselor countered the boy's resistance to the other games by setting up an incentive system: for every half-hour spent playing a game of his peer's choice, he earned a half-hour of playing PokeMon with the counselor.

The benefits of music: When I extolled the self-regulatory virtues of music during one workshop, an occupational therapist provided additional information about why playing an instrument (especially a horn) is so efficient. Not only does playing require the individual to breathe in a controlled way, but it also requires the musician to use hands together at the midline of the body, an action that we know to be organizing for the nervous system.

Task 2 : Functional and portable communication

Functional and portable communication means that the individual is able to convey needs, desires, thoughts, and feelings to anyone anywhere. All too often, we hear parents or professionals say, "But I know what he means." That's terrific, but it doesn't do much good if you're not with the individual with ASD. While the type of communication is going to vary with the individual (whether it is speech, gestures, or augmentative systems), everyone needs to be able to convey the following communicative intents:

- Joint attention: the ability to share a mutual focus with another person, whether nonverbally or verbally.
- Desire or need for an item or activity.
- Dislike for an item or activity.
- Initiation of social attention or interaction.
- Continuation of social interaction: reciprocity or two-way communication.
- Desire for "space" or to be left alone.
- Request for information or clarification.
- Comments upon the words or actions of others.
- Communicative repair: for example, "Oh, I didn't mean that I wanted you to go away. I just meant that I need to think a minute."

- Negotiation.
- Conflict resolution.

While most of us assume that these skills can be problematic for adolescents with greater communicative challenges, we may not realize that those with Autism typically need just as much help (though perhaps in a different way).

A real-life example: After several weeks of successful employment in a used book store, 19-year-old Sam suddenly stopped going to work. He wasn't ill. He was just too overwhelmed to go. After a lengthy discussion in my office, the problem surfaced. Sam's boss had given him a "punch list" of things to do when there were no customers in the store. When he got to the task of "straighten the books on the shelf," Sam didn't know what was meant. "You can't straighten used paperbacks. They're too floppy," Sam thought.

Sam's confusion made him anxious, and his anxiety made him flee. Once he left, he was too embarrassed to call his boss. The bottom line: Sam hadn't mastered the communicative skill of seeking clarification. No one had thought to teach him.

- By adolescence, individual therapy only within the office of the speech/language pathologist (SLP) is often insufficient. Some of the most effective intervention I have observed occurred when the SLP observed in the real-life setting, practiced the requisite skill with the adolescent one-on-one or in a small group, and then assisted the adolescent in generalizing the skill back to the real-world setting. It's also essential to work first on skills that are critical and/or meaningful for the adolescent's success. Of equal importance is the recognition that communication training is not just Coach peers regarding the communication strengths and challenges of the adolescent with ASD.

Direct teaching of skills

- Always start with the skills that the adolescent needs or wants most. For example, 16-year-old Melanie had absolutely no interest in working on social communication until she noticed that the other girls on the track team passed the time between events by chatting. She came to the next session asking for help with learning conversation starters. All of a sudden, she was quite motivated to work on social communication.

- Teach skills within a meaningful context, whenever possible. Alex's team wanted him to learn socially appropriate mealtime manners and conversation. Yet his sensory sensitivities were such that he couldn't tolerate the lunchroom, and he ate lunch in the classroom with his assistant. Alex had very little to say until the team decided to bring in peers during lunchtime. All of a sudden, Alex was intrigued with social interaction. And the peers let him know when he "grossed them out" by chewing with his mouth open or belching loudly. They were much more successful in modifying Alex's mealtime behavior than the adults had been.

- When necessary, teach scripts for specific social situations. Many of the adolescents I know follow Temple Grandin's suggestion of using "mental videos" to remember what to say in certain situations.

- Be sure to teach slang, including when to use it and when to avoid using it. In adolescence, this also includes teaching when/when not to curse.

- Teach code switching. In other words, make sure that the adolescent knows which topics, words, and tone of voice can be used in different situations.

- For students who learn well from videos, use favorite movies or TV shows to illustrate target skills. Videos are particularly helpful in teaching about nonverbal skills, such as body language, facial expressions, and personal space. Don't hesitate to videotape peer models engaging in the communicative behaviors that you'd like the adolescent to acquire.

- Refer to references by Freeman and Dake, McAfee, Garcia Winner, and Gutstein for lesson plans and more ideas.

Task 3: Social cognition/awareness (or "Theory of Mind")

A real-life example: For what seemed like years, Corey's parents and team had been trying to teach him to be empathic. But he just wasn't able to step out of his own shoes long enough to take another person's point of view. Then, in Grade 8, he came to his therapy session saying that he thought I would be proud of him. He went on to describe a situation at his locker earlier that day. One of the top three girls in the eighth grade had been at her locker a few doors down. When she bent over, Corey was able to see down the neckline of her tank top. When asked what he did next, Corey said, "I turned and went into my classroom." I asked why he had chosen that action.

Corey said, "I didn't think she would want to know that I saw."

Understanding of the mental states of others allows us to follow directions, avoid hurt feelings and other interpersonal scrapes, and form friendships and close relationships. Difficulties with social awareness and Theory of Mind also predispose the adolescent to sound rude and disrespectful to listeners who do not understand ASD. Social awareness also underlies the behavioral adjustments that we make from one situation to another and from one person to the next. To parents, poorly developed social cognition/awareness leads to the concern that their child will never develop empathy.

For many individuals with ASD, empathy and social awareness are learned in a logical or scripted format. For example, the work of Simon Baron-Cohen (e.g., *How to Teach Children with Autism to Mind Read*) provides a series of pictures and formulas that explains what makes a person feel a certain way. Parents sometimes say that they don't want their son or daughter to merely behave in a considerate or empathic way, but also to feel empathy. I typically reply that I hope that the adolescent will eventually feel empathy, but in the meantime we need to make sure that he or she acts emphatically and avoids social penalties.

Modifications and accommodations

- Make sure that peers and adults understand that the adolescent's social errors are likely to be a result of naïveté and social incompetence, not disrespect. Otherwise, the adolescent with ASD will receive negative disciplinary consequences that follow school policy but do little to teach adaptive replacement behaviors.

- Use the principles of applied behavior analysis and functional assessment to understand when, where, and with whom the adolescent makes social and behavioral errors. Functional assessment of behavior can point us toward the supports that will increase the adolescent's understanding of the situation and the new behaviors that should be taught.

- "Make the implicit explicit," as my SLP colleague Nancy Cegalis states. Be very clear about behavioral expectations and the social and emotional consequences of the adolescent's actions and words. For example, after overlooking the shrill ear-splitting (but gleeful) repetitive vocalizations of their 13-year-old daughter when she was ill with allergies, Suzy's parents decided they needed to address this socially penalizing behavior once she felt better. They started with a social story that explained that loud shrieks hurt people's ears and made them unhappy. The social story ended with a picture of a person gesturing "Sh-h-h." Suzy was then reinforced each time she responded positively to the reminder of "That hurts my ears. Sh-h-h."

Direct teaching of the "rules of the social road"

- Teach manners and social conventions. Even if the adolescent doesn't understand the reasons, make sure that he or she knows how to behave in common situations. Social stories are excellent ways to teach social conventions. Videos are also quite helpful. Alex Packer's book is a humorous guide to manners for all adolescents. Remember, though—no nagging! Adolescents with ASD are as immune to nagging as their typical counterparts.

- Talk about photos or magazine pictures that illustrate mental states. Draw arrows to the facial expressions, body language, and background details that give clues. Then speculate about the emotions and reasons for it. (Dr. McAfee provides a number of wonderful suggestions about this in *Navigating the social world*.)

- Make a chart of "passions and peeves" for family members. Talk about what each person likes and dislikes. Record it on a giant poster board. Then talk about what a person could do to please Mom when she's had a frustrating business trip or what to avoid when Dad is feeling stressed.

- Teach discretion. For a more verbal adolescent, use a concentric circles chart (some call this a Circle of Friends) with the adolescent at the center to illustrate which topics can be talked about at different levels of closeness. A less verbal adolescent may need a simpler format, such as a two-column chart with headings "Private" and "Public." Then use sticky notes or pictures to document what can be said or done in private *versus* public contexts.

- Read books or watch movies with the adolescent and talk about the emotions of the characters. Books or videos are often more helpful than verbal discussions because they can be reviewed again and again to assist understanding.

Task 4: Emotional competence

Emotional competence refers to the ability to recognize, understand, express, and modulate (or control) feelings. As discussed above, recognition and regulation of emotion is essential to behavior management. All too often, adolescents with ASD don't recognize their emotions until they have already acted upon them. Another significant challenge for a number of adolescents with ASD is the emergence of anxiety and/or depression. Emotional competence rests upon prevention of anxiety and depression as well as the recognition and understanding of feelings in the moment.

Modifications and accommodations

- Practice "low and slow." As soon as the adolescent begins to get agitated, we need to settle ourselves down. Lower the volume

and pitch of our voices. Slow down our rate of speech. Allow
plenty of processing time. Slow our breathing and actions.
Loudness, finger-pointing, and threats (such as "Do you want
a time out?!") only increase the level of the fight or flight
response that the adolescent experiences.

- Help the adolescent use adaptive self-management strategies
  preventively. See the section on Self-management for suggestions.
- Use visual schedules and subschedules to ensure that the
  adolescence knows what to expect. These may include pictures,
  words, and/or high tech (such as a PDA). The key element is
  that of predictability.
- Predict glitches (or unexpected events). Whenever you introduce
  a schedule of any kind, remind the adolescent that something
  unexpected may happen. Social stories can help explain glitches.
- Use social stories and other visual supports to explain a situation
  and expected behavior in advance. Provide information
  regarding what will happen, how other people are likely to
  feel and act, and how the adolescent can act in order to be
  most comfortable. For adolescents with substantial regulatory
  challenges, include a safe exit strategy, such as "If you get
  overloaded by all the talking, you can go to Uncle John's study
  and play Game Boy."

Consult the adolescent's physician if anxiety, sadness, hopeless or repetitive
thoughts, and behaviors interfere with daily functioning. While medication
is not a cure-all, it may take the edge off the emotions long enough for the
adolescent to benefit from other interventions.

Direct teaching of skills

- Ensure that the adolescent has a repertoire of remedies for
  settling down and perking up his/her mind and body. See the
  section on Self-management for suggestions.
- Use a Feelings Chart to help the adolescent make connections
  between the physical signs of the emotion, the "name" of the

emotion, a possible reason for the feeling, and an adaptive remedy if needed. This may start with something like "You're frowning, grinding your teeth, and yelling. You look like you're angry." (For less verbally skilled individuals, present this in photo or picture form.) Avoid asking "why" questions, as these tend to be disorganizing. Instead, for the more naive adolescent, say something like, "I wonder if you're angry because we ran out of chocolate ice cream." For the more sophisticated adolescent, try, "You're mad because . . . ." and wait. Once the adolescent knows a reason for the feeling, you can move on to "What can you do about it?" or "You feel angry. Do you want to . . . . or . . . ?" Keep the Feelings Chart and a menu of possible remedies handy for quick reference when a similar situation arises again. See my book for more ideas.

- For the adolescent with intrusive or repetitive thoughts and actions (obsessions or compulsions), work with the team to complete a functional assessment of the behavior before trying to eliminate it. Repetitive thoughts and actions often serve a self-soothing function. If we try to take these away without replacing them with an adaptive alternative, the adolescent is likely to develop a new troublesome behavior. Once you know the function of the behavior, you can work with the team to create a positive behavioral support plan.

- Reinforce every instance of adaptive coping. For example, Ed had begun to make threatening gestures and comments whenever his mother interrupted his activity with a direction to do something different. Both of them were quite shocked when he actually hit her one day. Ed then agreed that he needed to learn another strategy for coping with disappointment. We agreed that turning around and walking away was a good first step, although his parents hoped that he could eventually follow their directions immediately. In the first phase of teaching coping, Ed's parents noted on a point sheet each time he accepted a direction without threatening behavior (and gave him triple points for complying immediately). They also commented (after he had calmed down) about times when he started to threaten but then stopped himself. Within several weeks, Ed's threatening behavior was eliminated.

- Help the adolescent use special interests and talents as coping mechanisms.

A real-life example: Bart had already learned that his interest in music could help him connect with peers in the band. The new peers helped him branch out in his musical tastes, trying types of music that he had previously rejected. Soon Bart learned that he could choose music according to the mood he needed to be in—cool jazz to settle himself down for studying or Canadian Brass to perk himself up when he was dragging. By the way, Bart also parlayed his encyclopedic musical knowledge into a part-time job as a DJ!

Task 5 : "Showing what you know"

As a psychologist who evaluates children and adolescents with ASD, I often find that the individual is inefficient at demonstrating knowledge on demand. My own observations of the student or observations by parents and professionals often suggest that the adolescent can provide much more information when the idea "just comes" than when asked directly. But the real world of work and relationships can seldom wait for the solution to "just come." This makes it critical for us to ensure that the adolescent can access information and skills on a bad day as well as on a good day, in an unfamiliar context as well as in a familiar one.

While the specific information or skill to be accessed is going to depend upon the adolescent's cognitive and communicative abilities, there are several strategies that are helpful to everyone.

Modifications, accommodations, and direct teaching

- Remember the Hanes underwear slogan of many years ago: "You can't think right when your underwear's too tight."

Lesson to be learned: our bodies and minds have to be well regulated for us to learn and problem solve.

- Teach the adolescent how to follow a schedule or list of activities. Ideally, the adolescent should be able to make a transition from one task or activity to another with a minimum of interfering behavior or redirection.

- Always identify the purpose of an activity or task. This will allow the adolescent to focus more easily upon salient aspects and to ignore irrelevant aspects.

- Whenever possible, help the adolescent activate prior knowledge about a topic or skill. Individuals with autism often have difficulty with generalization, largely because they don't automatically recognize the similarity between a current situation and one that went before.

- Use task cards to improve independent functioning. A task card is like a recipe in that it lists the necessary materials and then the steps required for completing a task. Task cards can employ photos, pictures, words, or a combination. Once an adolescent can complete a task with adult supports, gradually withdraw the assistance until the student is entirely independent. Keep a notebook of task cards. After several are mastered, simply list the task on the daily schedule and have the student find the necessary task card and materials.

- Teach the adolescent how to find information. Every adolescent should be able to seek information or assistance, whether in a book or online, or from another person. Many teachers use task cards to help the student remember how to seek certain types of information.

- Use templates to help the adolescent express information. For a student who is struggling with oral expression, sentence strips such as those in the Picture Exchange Communication System (PECS) assist in the expression of complete thoughts. For more verbal adolescents, use story grammar templates (Who? Where? When? What happened? How did everyone feel?)

to remind them what information is necessary when telling someone else about an event. Adolescents with more advanced written expression skills will also benefit from the use of paragraph or essay templates to organize their work.

Task 6: Safety and life skills

Unfortunately, few adolescents with ASD are able to generalize efficiently from skills taught in books to real-world situations. I like to use video modeling, social stories, power cards, and task cards to preteach rules and skills and then to go with the adolescent into the real world for additional practice.

A real-life example: Stan had two goals that he wanted to achieve by his eighteenth birthday, only a few months away. He wanted to register to vote and he wanted to order his own meal at our traditional birthday lunch at the local house of pizza. For several years, Stan was too anxious to order. More recently, his speech was still unintelligible to "outsiders." For several weeks before his birthday, Stan used the menu to read aloud his selection. He then practiced in front of his mother and in front of me. We role-played what he could do when the restaurant worker didn't understand him. He decided to do a quick relaxation exercise before going into the restaurant. We agreed that writing down his order could be his last resort.

After preteaching and practice, Stan successfully ordered. Later that day, he also secured his voter registration card!

Teaching safety and life skills to adolescents with ASD is just like teaching anything else: we have to identify the steps, teach each step systematically with visual supports, use task analysis to problem-solve when there are glitches, and plan for generalization. There are a number of tools on the market that can save you the effort of reinventing the wheel, including Wrobel's 2003 book on hygiene and personal care.

Jerry and Mary Newport's book on sexuality also provides a number of helpful lessons regarding safety in dating and relationships. The most important point is that safety and life skills must be taught directly, even to the most gifted of adolescents with ASD.

A few other important issues

Disclosure and self-advocacy

The decisions about what, when, and whom to tell about ASD are ultimately left to the adolescent and his/her family. Individuals who are more severely affected by autism usually face fewer questions about disclosure, because their challenges are more visible. Adolescents with high functioning Autism often face a more difficult choice, however.

A real-life example: Madeleine had an Individual Education Plan (IEP) throughout school. When she went to art school for college, she insisted that she wanted to try it on her own. Madeleine did not register with the college learning support center nor did she admit to professors that she had high functioning Autism. Madeleine managed quite admirably with most of her coursework. Two art professors became quite impatient with her slow pace, however. At first, Madeleine tried to explain it as her "learning style." The professors were not sympathetic, though, and Madeleine fell further and further behind. Finally, Madeleine went to the learning support center with her high school IEP, revealed that she has Autism, and enlisted the assistance of an advisor there. The advisor helped Madeleine explain AS to the professors, and their attitudes became more supportive.

Ultimately, disclosure and self-advocacy are tools to secure supports necessary for success in the real world. Early in adolescence, parents and other adults are likely to take the lead in advocating for these supports. Ideally, over the course of adolescence, the individual with ASD becomes more skilled in asking for what he or she needs. This process is described quite eloquently in essays written by individuals with ASD and published in books edited by Dawn Prince-Hughes (2002) and Stephen Shore (2004).

Employment

Employment success for individuals with ASD varies widely, but all too many are underemployed or unemployed. Fortunately, there are some excellent resources about career development and employment. Please refer to books by Meyer (2001) and Grandin & Duffy (2004) for suggestions. But, remember, employment success is likely to rest more upon adequate self-management and communication skills than upon technical skills or information.

Supported living

Certainly we all hope that our adolescents will mature into adults who can live independently. When this is not the case, states and provinces have a variety of programs to assist adults with living as independently as possible. What isn't so well known, though, is that these programs are often overwhelmed with referrals. Don't wait until your son or daughter is an adult to look into this. Talk with your local developmental disabilities agency early in adolescence. It's better to have a spot and not need it than the other way around.

Medication

It is commonly accepted that there is no medication for autism per se. It is also accepted that medications are often helpful for some of the troubling aspects of ASD. In adolescence, medications are used most frequently to address anxiety, depression, repetitive behaviors, and poor impulse control. Discussion of the use of medication is beyond my expertise. Please refer to books by Tsai (2002) and Volkmar and Wiesner (2004) for comprehensive information.

Psychotherapy and other supports

Many adolescents with ASD are not able to take advantage of traditional insight-oriented psychotherapy, but appropriate services from psychologists, psychiatrists, clinical social workers, and other psychotherapists can be very useful in:

- Evaluating and explaining the adolescent's developmental profile
- Developing the working partnership
- Conducting functional assessments of behavior and creating positive behavioral support plans
- Teaching self-management, social cognition, and communication skills

- Providing cognitive behavioral interventions to address anxiety, depression, obsessive-compulsive behaviors, and other problems
- Providing support for parents, siblings, and educational teams
- In addition to the supports derived from psychotherapy, many adolescents with ASD will benefit from social skills groups, occupational and/or physical therapy, and recreational therapy. Ideally, each of these interventions will be a part of coordinated program.

One last take-home message

We often worry about what will happen to our children when they grow up, especially when the child has a disability. As we look to the future of our children, though, we must remember the words of Ralph Waldo Emerson (1878): "What is a weed? A plant whose virtues have not yet been discovered."

I wish you the best of fortune in the discovery of your adolescent's virtues.

References

NOTE: References marked AS-AD are particularly focused upon adolescents with the formerly known Asperger's Syndrome.

American Academy of Child and Adolescent Psychiatry (1999). Practice parameters for the assessment and treatment of children, adolescents, and adults with autism and other pervasive developmental disorders. *Journal of the American Academy of Child and Adolescent Psychiatry*, 38, 32S-54S.

Andron, L. (2001). *Our journey through High Functioning Autism and Asperger's Syndrome: A Roadmap*. London: Jessica Kingsley Publishers. (AS-AD)

Attwood, T. (1998). *Asperger's Syndrome: A guide for parents and professionals*. London: Jessica Kingsley Publishers. (AS-AD)

Baker, L.J., & Welkowitz, L.A. (2005). Asperger's *Syndrome: Intervening in schools, clinics, and communities*. Mahwah, NJ: Lawrence Erlbaum Associates.

Bashe, P.R., & Kirby, B.L. (2001). *The OASIS guide to Asperger's Syndrome*. New York: Crown Publishers.

Bolick, T. (2001). *Asperger's Syndrome and adolescence: Helping preteens and teens get ready for the real world.* Gloucester, MA: Fair Winds Press. (AS-AD)

Bothmer, S. (2003). *Creating the peaceable classroom.* Tucson, AZ: Zephyr Press.

Cautela, J., & Groden, J. (1978). *Relaxation: A comprehensive manual for adults, children, and children with special needs.* Champaign, IL: Research Press Company.

Cohen, D.J., & Volkmar, F.R. (Eds.) (1997). *Handbook of autism and pervasive developmental disorders* (Second edition). New York: John Wiley & Sons. (AS-AD)

Cumine, V., Leach, J., & Stevenson, G. (1998). *Asperger's Syndrome: A practical guide for teachers.* London: David Fulton Publishers. (AS-AD)

Debbaudt, D. (2002). *Autism, advocates, and law enforcement professionals.* London: Jessica Kingsley Publishers.

Ducharme, J.M., & Drain, T.L. (2004). Errorless academic compliance training: Improving generalized cooperation with parental requests in children with autism. *Journal of the American Academy of Child and Adolescent Psychiatry,* 43, 163–171.

Duke, M.P., Nowicki, S., & Martin, E.A. (1996). *Teaching your child the language of social success.* Atlanta: Peachtree Publishers. (AS-AD)

Faherty, C. (2000). *Asperger's—What does it mean to me?* Arlington, TX: Future Horizons.

Fouse, B., & Wheeler, M. (1997). *A treasure chest of behavioral strategies for individuals with autism.* Arlington, TX: Future Horizons, Inc.

Freeman, S., & Dake, L. (1997). *Teach me language: A language manual for children with autism, Asperger's syndrome and related developmental disorders.* Langley, BC, Canada: SKF Books.

Fullerton, A., Stratton, J., Coyne, P., & Gray, C. (1996). *Higher functioning adolescents and young adults with autism.* Austin, TX: Pro-Ed. (AS-AD)

Gagnon, E. (2001). *Power cards: Using special interests to motivate children and youth with Asperger's Syndrome and autism.* Shawnee Mission, KS: Autism Asperger's Publishing Co.

Gilpin, R. W. (1993). *Laughing and loving with autism.* Arlington, TX: Future Horizons. (and its sequels)

Goldbeck, L., & Schmid, K. (2003). Effectiveness of autogenic relaxation training on children and adolescents with behavioral and emotional problems. *Journal of the American Academy of Child and Adolescent Psychiatry,* 42, 1046–1054.

Grandin, T. (1995). *Thinking in pictures.* New York: Doubleday. (and other books by Dr. Grandin)

Grandin, T., & Duffy, K. (2004). *Developing talents: Careers for individuals with Asperger's Syndrome and high functioning autism.* Shawnee Mission, KS: Autism Asperger's Publishing Co.

Gray, C. (2000). *The new social story book: Illustrated edition.* Arlington, TX: Future Horizons.

Gutstein, S. E. (2000). *Autism Aspergers: Solving the relationship puzzle.* Arlington, TX: Future Horizons.

Haddon, M. (2003). *The curious incident of the dog in the night.* New York: Doubleday.

Heinrichs, R. (2003). *Perfect targets: Asperger's Syndrome and bullying.* Shawnee Mission, KS: Autism Asperger's Publishing Co.

Hoeksma, M.R., Kemner, C., Verbaten, M.N., & van Engeland, H. (2004). Processing capacity in children and adolescents with pervasive developmental disorders. *Journal of Autism and Developmental Disorders,* 34, 341–354.

Howlin, P., Baron-Cohen, S., & Hadwin, J. (1999). *Teaching children with autism to mind-read:* A practical guide. Chichester: John Wiley & Sons.

Jacobsen, P. (2003). *Asperger's Syndrome and psychotherapy: Understanding Asperger's Perspectives.* London: Jessica Kingsley Publishers.

Kashman, N., & Mora, J. (2002). *An OT and SLP team approach: Sensory and communication strategies that work.* Las Vegas: Sensory Resources.

Klin, A., Jones, W., Schultz, R., Volkmar, F., & Cohen, D. (2002). *Defining and quantifying the social phenotype in autism.* American Journal of Psychiatry, 159, 895–908.

Klin, A., Volkmar, F.R., & Sparrow, S.S. (Eds.) (2000). *Asperger's Syndrome.* New York: Guilford. (AS-AD)

Kluth, P. (2003). *"You're going to love this kid!" Teaching students with autism in the inclusive classroom.* Baltimore: Paul H. Brookes.

Levine, M. (1990). *Keeping a head in school.* Cambridge, MA: Educators Publishing Service. (AS-AD)

Levine, M. (1999). *Developmental variation and learning disorders* (Second Edition). Cambridge, MA: Educators Publishing Service, Inc.

Levine, M. (2001). *Jarvis Clutch, Social Spy.* Cambridge, MA: Educators Publishers Service. (AS-AD)

Levine, M. (2002). *A mind at a time.* New York: Simon & Schuster.

LINKS Curriculum. Educational Performance Systems, Woburn, MA.

Maag, J.W. (2004). B*ehavior management: From theoretical implications to practical applications.* (2nd edition). Belmont, CA: Wadsworth/Thomson Learning.

Manassis, K., & Young, A. (2001). Adapting positive reinforcement systems to suit child temperament. *Journal of the American Academy of Child and Adolescent Psychiatry,* 40, 603–605.

McAfee, J. (2002). *Navigating the social world: A curriculum for individuals for Asperger's Syndrome, High Functioning Autism, and related disorders.* Arlington, TX: Future Horizons. (AS-AD)

Meyer, R.N. (2001). *Asperger's Syndrome employment workbook.* London: Jessica Kingsley Publishers. (AS-AD)

Moyes, R. A. (2001). I*ncorporating social goals in the classroom: A guide for teachers and parents of children with high-functioning autism and Asperger's Syndrome.* London: Jessica Kingsley Publishers. (AS-AD)

Myles, B.S., & Adreon, D. (2001). *Asperger's Syndrome and Adolescence: Practical solutions for school success.* Shawnee Mission, KS: Autism Asperger's Publishing Co. (AS-AD)

Newport, J., & Newport, M. (2002). *Autism-Asperger's & sexuality: Puberty and beyond.* Arlington, TX: Future Horizons. (AS-AD)

Nowicki, S., & Duke, M.P. (1992). *Helping the child who doesn't fit in.* Atlanta: Peachtree Publishers. (AS-AD)

Ozonoff, S., Dawson, G., & McPartland, J. (2002). *A parent's guide to Asperger's Syndrome and high-functioning autism.* New York: Guilford.

Packer, A.J. (1997). *How rude! The teenagers' guide to good manners, proper behavior, and not grossing people out.* Minneapolis, MN: Free Spirit Publishing. (AS-AD)

Prince-Hughes, D. (Ed.) (2002). *Aquamarine blue 5: Personal Stories of college students with autism.* Athens, OH: Swallow Press.

Rourke, B.P. (Ed.)(1995). *Syndrome of nonverbal learning disabilities*: Neuro-developmental manifestations. New York: Guilford Press.

Rosenn, D. (2002). Is it Asperger's or ADHD? *AANE News*, Issue 10.

Shore, S. (Ed.) (2004). *Ask and tell: Self-advocacy and disclosure for people on the autism spectrum.* Shawnee Mission, KS: Autism Asperger's Publishing Co.

Shore, S. (2001). *Beyond the wall.* Shawnee Mission, KS: Autism Asperger's Publishing Co.

Tanguay, P.B. (2002). *Nonverbal learning disabilities at school: Educating students with NLD, Asperger's Syndrome, and related conditions.* London: Jessica Kingsley Publishers.

Thompson, S. (1997). *The source for nonverbal learning disorders.* East Moline, IL: LinguiSystems. (AS-AD)

Tsai, L. (2002). *Taking the mystery out of medications in Autism/Asperger's Syndromes.* Arlington, TX: Future Horizons.

Volkmar, F.R., & Wiesner, L.A. (2004). *Healthcare for children on the autism spectrum: A guide to medical, nutritional, and behavioral issues.* Bethesda, MD: Woodbine House.

Wagner, S. (2002). *Inclusive programming for middle school students with autism/ Asperger's Syndrome.* Arlington, TX: Future Horizons. (AS-AD)

Whitman, T.L. (2004). *The development of autism: A self-regulatory perspective.* Philadelphia: Jessica Kingsley Publishers.

Willey, L.H. (1999). *Pretending to be normal.* London: Jessica Kingsley Publishers. (AS-AD) (and subsequent books)

Williams, M.S., & Shellenberger, S. (1996). *"How does your engine run?"* Albuquerque, NM: TherapyWorks, Inc. (AS-AD)

Winner, M.G. (2000). *Inside out: What makes a person with social cognitive deficits tick?* San Jose, CA: Michelle Garcia Winner, SLP.

www.socialthinking.com>(AS-AD)

Wrobel, M. (2003). *Taking care of myself: A hygiene, puberty, and personal curriculum for young people with autism.* Arlington, TX: Future Horizons.

Websites

www.udel.edu/bkirby/asperger/support.html (OASIS)

www.aane.org (Asperger's Association of New England)

www.tonyattwood.com.au/ (Tony Attwood's site)

www.aspie.com (Liane Holliday Willey's home page)

www.faaas.org (Families of Adults Affected with Asperger's Syndrome)

www.autism-society.org (Autism Society of America)

www.researchautism.org (Organization for Autism Research website— includes a downloadable version of "Parent's Guide to Research)

www.naar.org (National Alliance for Autism Research—another source re latest in biomedical research)

Contributing Author Teresa Bolick, Ph.D., Licensed Psychologist—Dr. Teresa Bolick is a licensed psychologist with a special interest in neurodevelopmental disorders, including autism, Asperger's Syndrome, and other autism spectrum disorders. Dr. Bolick graduated from the University of North Carolina at Chapel Hill with a B.A. in Psychology. She holds M.A. and Ph.D. degrees in psychology from Emory University. Dr. Bolick provides evaluation and treatment to children, adolescents, and their families. She consults frequently to schools in New Hampshire and Massachusetts. She is an enthusiastic speaker, presenting workshops for parents, paraprofessionals, and professionals across the United States. Dr. Bolick is the author of *Asperger's Syndrome and Adolescence: Helping Preteens and Teens Get Ready for the Real World* and *Asperger's Syndrome and Young Children: Building Skills for the Real World*.

HOW TO CHANGE THE DISMAL JOB MARKETS FOR THOSE WITH AUTISM

Note: This article is a compilation of articles written by Joanne Lara and Lyn Dunsavage Young, published in the Autism Asperger's Digest, 2016.

Prior to 1975, very few people were even thinking about how students with autism could be brought into the work force, because individuals with disabilities often were not allowed to be educated in the public schools in most states in the country before that time, where, assumedly, they would have been trained or prepared for a job or advanced education so they could subsequently obtain jobs, if they had been in public schools in that time period.

Once that barrier was broken through, most students on the autism spectrum were placed in special needs classrooms rather than inclusive classrooms, which generally took a toll on expanding their abilities beyond the basics, if that. The No Child Left Behind, 2001, had at least one impact on these children with autism, whether they were still in special needs classrooms or not at that time, which was that teachers got the message that all special needs students needed to be trained in the basics of test taking and information upon which they would be tested, like other students in the schools. That became critical because the overall rating of the tests was tied to funding to the school, so efforts for special needs students in this regard were accelerated.[1]

It wasn't until the late-1990s—within the last 20 years—that "secondary transition planning" became a federal mandate, first authorized in the 1997 Individuals with Disabilities Education Act (IDEA) and, subsequently, reauthorized in IDEA 2004, specifying that "transition services"—defined as "academic and functional achievement of the student with a disability to facilitate movement from school into post school life"[2]—were to begin by 16 years of age, instead of the 1997 mandate, which was the program was to be initiated at 14 years of age. IDEA mandated a "coordinated set of activities designed within a result-oriented process."

A full ten years later after this mandate, in June 2014, only 19.3 percent of people with all disabilities in the U.S. were participating in the labor force, either working or seeking work. Of those, 12.9 percent were unemployed, meaning only 6.4 percent of the population with disabilities were employed (Bureau of Labor Statistics, 2014). To look at these statistics another way, fully 93.6 percent of those with disabilities were either unemployed (because they were seeking work) or had given up on getting a job.

To appreciate the impact of that 92.9 percent, it's important to realize that those on the autism spectrum faced a double whammy, because, of the many disabilities, those on the autism spectrum—statistically—are the least likely to be employed, apparently because of their lack of social skills, which many executives expect of their employees or, certainly, require as a major component of an interview, which, commonly, those on the autism spectrum find to be extremely difficult. Worse, approximately 50,000 young people on the autism spectrum began turning 18 years old annually, the single largest category of those with disabilities (in fact, greater than all the other disabilities' groupings numerically). The sheer numbers of this huge and rapidly growing number of individuals with autism constitute the largest majority who couldn't land jobs, either at the 18-year-old age point or, subsequently, after a minority of them attempt to complete additional years of education.

The vast majority of those on the autism spectrum pack up their cell phones and computers after they "age out" of high school (with only a few states giving them additional years of education, the highest of which is 23 years), and, after attempting to get jobs, they return home to stay permanently, abandoning hopes of becoming independent and self-sufficient. Because most go home and end up staying there, this is known as the "School-to-Couch" model, a human tragedy that is growing exponentially.

The failure of the education, social, and political systems to provide training for this growing number of unemployed autistics is creating a tsunami that is rapidly moving to crash, possibly destroying our economic well-being in this country along with the toll it obviously is accumulating with those who have the capabilities and desire to work but are being excluded for a host of reasons. Because the primary reason for failure is in the educational system to train them for employment, they're left with their family members who harbor their most-common fear: "What will happen when we are gone?"

To address what can be done, one first has to look at why the present system is failing.

What Is the Individual Transition Plan (ITP) and Why Is It Critical for Students with Autism?

To ease the transition from high school into the adult world, teachers and school personnel, along with others (e.g., families, community agencies), are required by law to assist students with disabilities in middle school, well before they transition from high school. They're charged to select appropriate goals, so they can develop the requisite skills needed to achieve these goals.

Called the Individual Transition Plan (ITP), there are three main areas that should be addressed:

- *Work:* To identify a job the student wants and might be good at doing; *Living:* A location where the individual might like to live; and *Community involvement:* Activities he would like to undertake to become a part of the community after he finishes high school, which might continue throughout adulthood.

The process takes place generally at the age of 16, but in some states—like California, North Carolina, and Texas–it begins earlier, at age 14.

The ITP process requires that the student must be invited to the ITP meeting, because the plan should be put together to prepare the child for life. The student should be a part of the process because the transition services should be based on the individual's needs, which should also take into account the student's preferences and interests. More important, the student needs to learn self-advocacy at an earlier age, particularly if he plans to go to college, where he most likely will not have his parent(s) as an advocate.

How do we ensure that the ITP process is in compliance with the IDEA 2004 mandate? The student's annual IEP goals should be related to the student's transition services required for him to be successful, and they should align with his post-secondary goals."[3] To derive the goals, the student should be given an informal or formal transitioning assessment, using a tool like

WorkSmart, Transition Planning Inventory (TPI), YES!, Choicemaker Self-Determination Assessment and Self-Directed Employment Assessment, or COPs. The goals for the IEP should come directly out of the transition assessment tool results, so the team—including the student—knows where the student's strengths lie in work, living, and social skill sets. The "8 indicators of Compliance Checklist" indicates goals are measurable and indicates mastery of skills.

Why Is the IEP Not Working Effectively?

The IDEA 1997 and 2004 transition revisions were both well-meaning and direct descendants from the 1975 Public Law 94–142, but the program has to be viewed skeptically at best because of the after-high-school statistics in the job market, in which less than 20 percent of all graduating students on the autism spectrum have jobs—even inconsequential jobs after high school. Worse, the percentages become less over time.

Because of the hovering 80 percent unemployment for youth with autism, it is time that educators present a truthful idea of what the student is capable of doing for a living, which means that we might want to rethink all together the way that we are addressing/interpreting the ITP transitioning process, the jobs, and living accommodations after high school in this country.

Ironically, the very program that elevated the academic side of programs for those on the autism spectrum is also the reason for the failures that are mounting on the jobs' side of the equation. One of the reasons for these dismal statistics may be the lack of realism on the part of the IEP team members when they undertake the Person Centered Planning element. They focus on where the student's skill set in core reading and math actually lies and how this skill set can equate to a paying job.

IEP team members and, especially, parents often want to honor a student's dreams, but—when that student's case history indicates that he/she may not be a scientist, an astronaut, a veterinarian (because he hasn't evidenced that level of success in academics), or have a three-picture deal at Warner Brothers Studio in Hollywood (because writing scripts or research per se is not his forte)—they must ask themselves if they are really indeed serving the student well by entertaining these fantasy dreams of improbable employment. In reality, the student may be able to work in a vet's office or neighborhood shelter, gain employment on the Warner Brothers' lot, or work in a hospital, but the IEP team needs to be addressing practical job options for these students who are not going to transition into a four-year college or, even, a two-year community college, because they don't have the academic background to continue the academic route. The students should be directed down a path that will give them a realistic idea of job options when they transition out of the public school setting.

The downfall of not entertaining true options earlier is that, oftentimes, the student becomes attached to the fantasy job and has an impractical idea of where he might fit in. In the case of his visions of becoming a scientist, a vet, or an astronaut in the American job market, he becomes reluctant to seek jobs outside of these unlikely positions, even though other jobs could more likely meet his skill set and lifestyle. An unrealistic evaluation of the student's academic capabilities and skill set contributes to the existing 80 percent unemployment statistic. For the student who wants to be a scientist, why not have him/her research jobs that are available in a university science department? Or companies that do medical research? Or organizations where she can still be working in the area of her interest?

In the IEP team meetings, they need to begin to present a more realistic approach to job options for the student so he can fit into the work force. They stand a far better chance of getting the outside community employers' and stakeholders' support to help the youth to be successful if we are realistic using his past success in the academic institution as a barometer.

Parents Need To Realize That Vocation Programs Have Been Phased Out

Parents also need to understand that there is now a huge absence of vocational education in the high schools, which consists of programs that may well have been a route by which many children on the autism spectrum could have found great success and well-paying jobs after graduation.

The Smith-Hughes Act of 1917—the law that first authorized federal funding for vocational education in American schools—explicitly described vocational education as "preparation for careers not requiring a bachelor's degree." Vocational education was not designed to prepare students for college.

In the late-1990s and early-2000s, the standards and accountability movement in the school systems was taking hold, so the states had begun to write academic standards—or goals—for what students should learn (and, in the process, what wasn't critical), which was reflected in the elimination of many subjects that previously had been "core courses." Because the goals were tied to funding, many courses that could have been perfect for many of the students on the autism spectrum began to disappear from the schools' curriculum at the same time when autism diagnoses were expanding exponentially.

When Congress passed the "No Child Left Behind" Act In 2001—a law requiring states to test their students every year and to ensure that all students would eventually be proficient in math and reading in exchange for federal education funding—it substantially affected the end of vocational training in this country.

For one, the vocational programs in the schools didn't have the academic faculty to pass the law's requirements. They often had the skilled labor experts/ workers to teach skills, like metal working, wood working, horticulture, bakery and culinary arts, automobile mechanics, cosmetology, and so on; however, the instructors themselves were not considered "the academic piece" that would fulfill the "No Child Left Behind" Act's standards. So, the very skill sets that could benefit the youth of the autism spectrum the most—because what they learn in vocational training could be turned into meaningful jobs–were rapidly wiped out, no longer available in the public school setting.

Secondly, to understand why the ITP process is failing, those in the academic school setting (the ITP team) can assess and tell you what your child is good at or could be good at doing that would allow him to get a job once he graduates from high school—as per the 2004 IDEA ITP mandate—but they can't teach him many of those skills because the majority of the schools don't have the vocational programs any longer to do it. In addition, the programs for independent living skills (e.g., computer science, animation, art, home economics, shop, drafting, advertising/layout/design, photography, economics, banking, budgeting, cooking, sewing, cleaning, fixing, etc.) basically only exist in the Moderate/Severe Special Day Programs in most schools at a time when most children on the autism spectrum have been moved into inclusive classrooms. They're generally not available for the Asperger's and higher-functioning students with autism, who also could benefit from vocational knowledge and independent living skills, if they are to live self-determined lives independently after high school.

Suggestions of how the ITP could be more effective:

- The ITP must be started early in the schools—at 14 years of age—but parents really need to have a vision for their child from kindergarten and the early elementary school years. Temple Grandin's latest book, *The Loving Push*, not only explains how critical it is to begin at this age, but it also gives concrete suggestions on how to implement a job-oriented child at an early age. Everyone who is a member of that child's team, including the child, needs to be creating an idea of who he or she is and what capabilities are in the home, the community, and the world. It's being done for the neurotypical children. Why are we not doing it for our children with autism? Because we feel guilty? Because we ourselves are not certain that indeed there is a place for them in the community? In the job force? If this is the case, we must work harder to get our youth with autism to have realistic choices for employment, options for social activities and outings in the community, and alternatives to the "school-to-couch" living alternative, which must begin even before they attend school.

- If an opportunity exists to bring back vocational programs into the public schools—even if your child isn't oriented toward vocational education—support the effort because it will benefit jobs for thousands of individuals, whether or not they're on the autism spectrum. At as early a time as possible, while the child is still in high school, parents need to evaluate and consider vocational schools for their post-high school graduate, linking the child's interests and job skill sets to what is taught in vocational schools outside the public school program. Research before your child graduates, so he or she can go from one school into another.

- Many of the subjects that provide great jobs and incomes are taught in junior colleges, such as agriculture/plant management, cosmetology, nursing assistance/home health care, computer science, automobile mechanics, and restaurant/food services. If they don't exist in your community, consider other close-by communities because many junior colleges house specialty programs depending upon their locations (e.g., some of the best schools in cuisine/restaurant/food services are in major metropolitan areas).

- Look at specialty schools like the Art Institute, design schools, retail training and management programs, information technology schools, secretarial schools, bookkeeping programs, and electrical and plumbing schools, because they provide high-end salary possibilities and are vocations in great demand. Like vocational schools, check them out long before graduation!

- If your child is planning (realistically) to go to college, parents need to understand that these institutions are regulated by privacy laws and federal regulations. In other words, parents rarely can continue as the advocate for their child; the child must become his or her own advocate, so the child should use the ITP process to become that advocate. Also, while college and universities might state that they have programs conducive to and supporting those on the autism spectrum, it's important to know that the college and universities' support normally doesn't match the support systems your child had in high school. The levels of support and the programs have to be evaluated well before your child attends the college campus.

Colleges and Universities Are Governed by Laws Different in Support from High School

Universities—to be federally compliant—must have a Disabilities Support Services Center with which the student registers when enrolling in the college. The Disabilities Support Services Center assesses the student so that, together, the college and the student decide what accommodations are needed for the student to succeed in the college setting. Does the student require a sign language interpreter? A note taker? Extended time for assignments? Extended due dates for tests? Extra time to get to classes? Proximity to the instructor? All the very same modifications that were available to the student in the public school setting are also supposedly available in the college setting.

Typically, by this time, the student has reached the "age of majority," when a young person is considered to be an adult. Depending on state laws, this can happen between 18 and 21 years of age. At this juncture, the state may transfer to that child all (or some of) the educational rights that the parents have had up to the moment. Not all states transfer rights at the age of majority, but if your state does, then the rights and responsibilities that parents had under IDEA with respect to their child's education will belong to that child (http://www.parentcenterhub.org/repository/age-of-majority/).

This is a major difference in your child's life because—typically in the case of those with children on the autism spectrum—the parents have been the child's greatest advocate. Suddenly, the child has to become his or her own advocate, which many young people on the spectrum are not used to being. A book recently published about the difficulties of this change is written by J.D. Kraus, *The Aspie College, Work, and Survival Guide.*

If the student hasn't reached the age of majority, the state must establish procedures for appointing the parent of a child with a disability or, if the parent is not available, another appropriate individual to represent the educational interests of the child throughout the period of the child's eligibility. If under state law, a child who has reached the age of majority and has not been determined to be incompetent can be determined not to have the ability to provide informed consent with respect to the child's educational program, then that representative will make the decisions.

Some Basic Planning Strategies for College

- Parents should register their child with the college of their choice and provide all the required documentation for registration. To receive special accommodation as mandated by the Americas with Disabilities Act (ADA), it is important to register with the College Disability Services.

- Families should be familiar with the ADA, which mandates the laws as to how colleges must accommodate people with disabilities.
- Additionally, know if there is a special room in the dormitory or assigned location where your child can go during sensory meltdowns.
- Staff responsible for the dormitory should be trained and educated to accommodate special-needs students. They must be aware of the accommodations necessary to make the college experience a pleasant experience.

What Can You Do, If Your Child Isn't Ready for College on His or Her Own?

Paul Hippolitus, Director of Disabled Students Program, University of California Berkeley, developed a course called C2C+ or Bridging the Gap from College to Careers that is a university/community's 17-lesson model that includes internships, peer and career mentoring, and placement assistance for individuals with disabilities. The course is offered at UC Berkeley, Silicon Valley Business Leadership Network, Orange County Business Leadership Network, San Diego State University, and San Diego Business Leadership Network. More and more of these types of programs are becoming available to students with autism across the country, filling the void that is left when our students exit the public school setting at 18 to 22 years of age and transition into secondary education or the community setting to find that they are not prepared to compete in either arena.

Most important, check out programs that transition students after high school into the work force or into college. There, they can learn to keep a budget, take care of themselves, and live independently because these are the cornerstones of these programs. Parents really need to visit them and find out their success rates in their ultimate goal, which is obtaining jobs for their students and/or supporting them through the college experience. In most cases, their costs are not inconsequential, because it often requires housing, transportation, staffing, food, and many other support systems.

These growing numbers of structured residential or camp programs are specifically transitional, meaning they teach life skills like budgeting, transportation, living with others outside the home, and college-level preparation coursework. At the least, attending college requires students to develop self-determination skills, self-management, self-advocacy, and social skills, along with self-monitoring to excel and be successful.

We provide three examples of these programs—all very different in their structure and orientation—to show the many paths to success. These are just three in the California area, but numerous others are located in other states, including the granddaddy of them all, TEACCH in North Carolina.

Meristem

A central aspect of the MERISTEM method involves preparing students for life after graduation. Throughout the three-year program, students build skills to enter the workplace or higher education. Many will work independently, others with assistance, but each graduate leaves with a greater sense of self-reliance.

Meristem is a 13-acre residential transition program serving young adults who have graduated or transitioned from high school. The campus is in Fair Oaks, California, a small agriculture suburb outside Sacramento. Integrated with a teacher training college, it adopts the biodynamic approach to learning, a spiritual-ethical-ecological approach to agriculture, gardens, food production, and nutrition. In addition, Meristem offers movement education, digital media, independent living skills, woodworking, metal working, jewelry making, textiles, and the performing arts. Meristem President Oliver Cheney explains that "Meristem is a stepping-stone between school and employment."

Currently, the three-year program houses 18 residents from across the country, ranging from 18 to 28 years of age. The modern dormitories have the capacity to house up to 65 residents. Meristem currently has 35 students, and 12 of those students attend the Day Program from nearby communities. This private pay model is $73,000 a year, from September to June, for the full residential program and $45,000 for the day program. Managing Director Michael Mancini explains that Meristem is a regional center client, so it works alongside the California Department of Rehabilitation.

The Meristem residential school and vocational work training facilities are integrated with a teacher training college, with a farm apprenticeship program that follows a community-supported agriculture (CSA) model. The strong farm traineeship program curriculum involves the students caring for goats, sheep, and cattle; farming the land; and learning to work extensively with wood and metals. "Bronze, copper, and then iron," says instructor Keith Gelber, "because this is the order of the Ages of Metals, and we want the student to make the analogy or connection through working with metal to his world around him."

All the classes are conducted by highly successful model artisans, who use curriculum-based, task analysis-driven strategies and assessments designed to measure independence and real-world skill-based outcomes for the students. There is a student-run café, part of the students' "real-world work" experience curriculum, and a lovely bookstore on the campus, frequented by the locals. The bookstore and café provide the opportunity for students to develop increased social skills through community integration and inclusion. In addition, Meristem takes pride in incubating social skills enterprises for students and its graduates to run in the community.

The philosophy of the Meristem program is inspired by the well-known British model used throughout the United Kingdom, Ruskin Mill Trust (RMT), which has a 35-year history of successful employment in the UK. Ruskin Mill Trust was founded by Aonghus Gordon in 1989. The Meristem model, like the UK Ruskin Mill Trust model, is unique in that it has a strong body/brain component with the ideology that it is through working with the hands that the brain develops. Meristem's goal is to assist individuals with autism in transitioning to meaningful jobs and to increase self-image and self-esteem through practical applications of real-world skills. Managing Director Michael Mancini (mm@meristem.org) says, "We have a proven method to develop independence and self-determination for young adults with autism to be a part of their community and, at the same time, develop skill sets that will serve them in the future."

Advance LA

A personalized residential program designed to fill the "gap year" and located in Los Angeles is Advance LA. Its motto is "Preparing young adults facing unique challenges for a successful future." Advance LA is a post-high school residential program located in Los Angeles on the American Jewish University campus. It houses and supports seven adults with autism who attend nearby colleges: University of Southern California, California State University Northridge, Santa Monica College, Pierce Community College, and Valley College.

Director Holly Daniel feels that one reason the program has been so successful is that "it is designed and individually personalized so that each student can grow at his or her own pace." Holly explains that Advance LA is geared to the student who graduates from high school and wants to attend a secondary academic college but is not quite ready to go off on his or her own. Advance LA acts as the chaperone, so to speak, so the student gets the support that otherwise would not be available, unless the student lived at home with his or her parents.

At Advance LA, the student gets a feel for dorm life with enough adult support that allows him or her to experience college on an independent level but also provides the safety net that the student needs to be successful. The students are encouraged to become self-advocates and learn to handle their own cleaning, cooking, and banking while nurturing meaningful friendships in a dorm setting. The students also have access to the company van that transports them to and from classes and to all planned weekend social outings.

The three- to four-year program includes 18- to 30-year-olds and costs $4,200 a month, which includes room, board, meals, and transportation.

College Internship Program (CIP)

One of the oldest residential and, again, successful comprehensive transition programs for young adults on the autism spectrum and with learning disabilities is the College Internship Program (CIP), located in Berkeley, California, as well as five programs on the East Coast. CIP is a post-high school residential program that supports diploma track graduates who are both college and career bound. Sarah Williams (swilliams@cipworldwide.org), the National Communications Coordinator of the College Internship Program Berkeley, explained that there are six CIP campuses across the United States: in Amherst, NY; Berkshire, MA; Bloomington, IN; Brevard, FL; Berkeley,

CA; and Long Beach, CA. Founded in 1984—the first of its kind—CIP's president is Dr. Dan McManmon. A psych evaluation is required. The cost of the program is approximately $60,000 a year. CIP also offers several summer programs.

The 18- to 26-year-old students at Berkeley CIP live in apartments that are facilitated CIP sites with roommates in residences that are close to the secondary education colleges and campuses that they attend. In addition to supporting the students in their academic goals, CIP also provides them with a structured 30-hour-a-week life skills program aligned with a weekend mandatory recreational activities program that includes attending ball games, visiting art museums, and shopping at farmer's markets.

The CIP program promotes independent living as well as academic success for the candidates through a structured work/internship-driven program. Some of the internships that the Berkeley campus offer are with Berkeley Community Media, Alameda County Food Bank, Partnerships for Change, East Bay Humane Society, Berkeley Public Library, KPFA Radio Station, Spectrum School mentoring positions, Satellite Housing, World Institute on Disability, Alta Bates Hospital, The Bridge Church, Oakland Zoo, Hearts Leap Preschool assistant, St. Vincent de Paul—feeding the homeless, and the YMCA.

The CIP model is assessment driven and utilizes the person-centered planning approach, which promotes working with each student to develop his or her own goals, dreams, and hopes for a successful future.

Another Option for Jobs: Think Outside the Box of Traditional Interviews, Higher Education

If you haven't realized it yet, throw out any preconceptions you may have held about how a high school or college degree will result in your child getting a job. Statistically, it just doesn't compute. You need to face the reality that a young adult with autism—even those with an incredible knowledge about a particular subject or one who has great talent or amazing skills—has a very small chance of landing a job in the traditional way of submitting a résumé, attaining an interview, and being offered a job.

There is hope beyond the statistics, but you will have to open your mind to investigate some possibilities that offer something other than the traditional pack-up-your-kid to go to college route. To really shake things up, we'll begin with some of the newest and most innovative programs—purposely mind-bending—so you'll begin to put on your own creative thinking hat.

1. Consider becoming an entrepreneur yourself by creating a business purposely structured around the talents and/or interests of your child. Follow the footsteps of Thomas D'Eri, the COO and Cofounder of Rising Tide Car Wash in Florida.

Like yourself, Tom D'Eri has a family member—in this case, his brother Andrew—on the autism spectrum, whom he considered talented, detailed, and someone who hoped to be able to use his abilities in a job someday, but Tom and his father both believed that there wasn't even a slight possibility that someone would hire him.

Why? As D'Eri explains his fundamental position, "Autism is seen as a disability that requires sympathy instead of looking at it as a valuable diversity. We've been taught to feel sorry for people with autism, which creates a really challenging stigma to overcome. Why would someone hire someone who they feel sorry for? The thought of Andrew rotting away in his bedroom playing video games all day with no friends or sense of purpose propelled us to action."

Tom, who had just finished a business degree a year before, and his entrepreneurial father decided they needed to identify a business that would work well for his brother's attributes, so they began looking, ultimately coming up with a car wash, which everyone knows requires a lot of detail to produce the product that will bring people back in.

To acquire one they thought could be "turned around," they moved from New York to Florida and created the Rising Tide Car Wash. It is their means of creating a community for Andrew and to show the world just how capable people with autism are. The business employs 35 individuals with autism (80 percent of the staff), which they began in 2012. They average 500 cars daily and 150,000 cars annually. Their Facebook page has over 7,000 likes.

A critical component in its success is that he markets the business around its workers' strengths.

"They're detailed; they're really enthusiastic and proud of the work they accomplish. It's all about telling the story in a way that it's about empowerment and success and never about sympathy. We focus on the individual stories of our employees because they're better! They are our business advantage, because we view autism as one of our key competitive advantages, so people come back."

It's been so successful, they've already purchased another car wash about six miles away to expand. Tom also plans to travel and speak on how critical it is to develop "a massive number of entrepreneurial businesses that employ those on the autism spectrum because that's the only way to change people's perceptions about their capabilities."

He's not expecting everyone to become car wash owners. He recognizes there are many opportunities, but "to be successful as an "autism entrepreneur," you have to identify existing business models that already work in your community and, then, design a way to employ individuals with autism in them because of their special skill sets."

His position is that it's the skill sets—not just your child's interests—that are the critical turning point to success in creating a business. He's in the process of creating a program for parents and others who want to create jobs for those on the spectrum, so they, also, can join the movement for "entrepreneurial autism." He's willing to travel to talk to groups in a community that want to consider entrepreneurism as the way to go to get those on the autism spectrum into jobs for which they're suited. So, if you're overwhelmed by the thought of stepping out on your own—because you're not entrepreneurial—consider attending the Rising Tide U program or commissioning D'Eri to come to your community to teach you and others how to create a business for autistic employees.

Another entrepreneur, Dennis Mashue, has taken a different route by creating Tuck's Toques, a small company that sells hand-woven Himalayan (and very colorful) hats. He also has a vested interest in the business because his son, Tuck, is autistic but, as Tuck says, "It's just a small part of whom I am." He also loves kayaking, cycling, hiking, camping, music, road-tripping, bowling, and working out, according to his site.

Dennis considers the yak-wool woven hats as a way to develop the business skills and a long-term future for Tuck, while demonstrating to society "that all people can contribute to their communities."

Tuck plans to go to college, but the business is a way he can continue to grow vocationally, whatever the results may be in his college career.

Note: Dennis found a product he could retail to accomplish his goal. He didn't invent it. He matched his child's passion, which is to spend as much time as possible outdoors in the generally cold environment where he lives with a warm hat product that protects him from the cold. You may be able to do that as well, providing you know how to market it to make it a viable business.

2. A college degree is not necessarily the "end-all" for computer expertise, so, if you have a child who is a computer geek or hacker, begin by reconsidering college (unless he wants to teach or be a business major).

In the last several years, computer and other Internet companies are offering paid internships to those on the autism spectrum and actual, outright hires (particularly for those who have high hacking capabilities).

Why the turnaround from the traditional route for hiring? What is important to these companies is how an individual thinks, which computer companies now recognize is a significant asset that people on the autism spectrum have. They not only think differently, they often are more creative! They can see patterns others can't. They have prodigious memories in areas of their interest. They're detailed. Recognizing that their businesses depend presently and in the future on that single characteristic—being wired differently—a number of businesses have instituted programs to teach the necessary social skills so the computer "geek" can survive and thrive in their businesses.

One of the outstanding businesses in Europe, which is now in the U.S., is Thorkil Sonne's Specialisterne (www.specialisterne.com), which is harvesting that talent. Sonne, in Denmark—and, now, many major computer companies in the U.S.—have found a competitive advantage in the business market by assessing and training people with ASD.

Specialisterne provides software testing, quality control, and data conversion services for businesses in Denmark, in which 75 percent of his employees have a diagnosis within the autism spectrum. They use LEGO Mindstorms robot technology to help identify the strengths, motivation, and development possibilities of the individuals they hire.

In conjunction with SAP, Germany's largest software company, they are expanding—"not because of social responsibility or philanthropy," according the Jose Velasco, the head of SAP's U.S. initiative who spoke to Josephe Erbentraut of The Huffington Post, but because "SAP values the unique skills and abilities that people with autism bring to the workplace."

Another organization, Aspiritech out of Chicago, hires individuals on the autism spectrum as test engineers "with a combination of intensive training, structure, and support to mitigate potential workplace challenges." As a nonprofit organization, their delivery services enable them to serve clients throughout North America.

There are also recruitment and training programs now to help people on the autism spectrum into tech jobs, with companies like New Relic, which has partnered with a San Jose nonprofit, Expandability, which provides people with disabilities with access to career transition services in the tech industry.

Also, hopping onboard with Internship Programs (degree not required) are some of the megacomputer companies, like Microsoft, which is launching a small pilot program in conjunction with Specialisterne for ten full-time positions. If your high school graduate gets accepted, he will be paid while being trained.

If, per chance, you have a child who is a "hacker," that talent is highly prized. There are national "hacking competitions," which, if he wins (and, perhaps, even comes close to winning), businesses beyond your imagination are waiting in the wings to compete for such talent. Recently, a CEO of a major company confirmed on a PBS station that he awaits the results of the hacking competitions because the winners are one of his highest priorities for hire.

In late March, 2016, one of the largest consortia of businesses and organizations announced its goal to train and hire 5,000 people on the autism spectrum in the next four years! The backbone of this program is that AT&T has committed to most of the funding, with organizations offering staffing and additional funds to help pay the expenses of the training.

The program includes commitments for jobs from heavy hitters like AT&T, Canadian software consulting firm Meticulon, software company Ultra Testing, and technology service provider MindSparks Technologies, as well as many as 20+ other companies and organizations, also committed to make the program work.

LaunchAbility, a Texas job placement agency for people with cognitive disabilities and a member of the new consortium, has developed a training program in Dallas as a pilot phase of the program. Others in the consortium, such as MindSpark Technologies, will roll out training programs to help meet the 2020 goal also. The critical component will be to keep those who've been trained employed.

If your child is into computer animation, Yudi Bennett in Sherman Oaks, CA, has a program called Exceptional Minds in which the students' achievements and her contacts offer opportunities in the movie and television industries in that area for its graduates (see article in Feb/Mr/Ap 2016 issue of Autism Asperger's Digest, "Five Simple, Inexpensive Therapies the Scientists Say 'WORK'" p. 31).

Jobs fairs for companies who are interested in hiring those on the autism spectrum are starting to pop up. Look for them. In April, on both coasts—in North Carolina, sponsored by TEACCH, and in California, sponsored by CIP—a Jobs Program to hire those with ASD was held in 2016. Just some of the companies that came to the CIP program included 20 exhibitors including Microsoft and Project Search.

Contact Extraordinary Ventures, an organization in Chapel Hill, NC, in which they convened over 150 autism specialists and business leaders at a summit, in which they agreed that small businesses and entrepreneurs can meet the needs of their communities while providing a range of jobs that match the skills of autism. Applying the lessons learned from 15 model programs across the country (including some depicted here), the attendees identified the essentials for creating sustainable small business solutions to the autism employment gap. According to their press, these "must-haves" include "taking a business approach to developing quality products and services, empowering parents, building partnerships in the community and identifying skills in people across the spectrum." The 15 models were identified by Autism Speaks in a 2012 study. Lori Ireland, mother of a 23-year-old son with autism, who cofounded Extraordinary Ventures in 2007 with other parents in the Chapel Hill area, explained that "the answer is creating new self-sustaining businesses that will provide meaningful jobs for people with ASD and other developmental disabilities at the grassroots level."

3. As outrageous as this may sound, consider moving to a state that either has a strong program for transitioning into the workplace for those with ASD or one that has a higher level for support for those on the autism spectrum.
Actually, this makes economic sense, as strange as it may appear on the surface. As Temple Grandin explains, you either have to take affirmative action early to develop job training for your child, beginning with early childhood chores, or you must find additional support for most children on the spectrum when they get out of school so your child can get a job. If you don't do either, there's a high probability you'll spend the rest of your life financially supporting your child and worrying what will happen to him when you're no longer there to take care of him.

If your child is just getting out of high school and can't get a job, figure the cost of, perhaps, 20–30 years of dependence compared to a move to a location where support for finding a job is a primary consideration of an organization or institution. Also, consider your child's level of productivity, happiness, friends, and self-worth that a job can provide (all of which are intrinsically more important than the financial side of the equation). Below, we're skimming some of the best programs that offer hands-on assistance for those on the spectrum who obtain jobs, so they can keep them.

North Carolina has the "granddaddy" of all autism programs in the UNC TEACCH Autism Program, one of the original and longest ongoing programs that support those with autism, their families, and those who teach them. TEACCH is part of the North Carolina Area Health Education Centers (AHEC), under the School of Medicine at the University of North Carolina (UNC) for certain services and trainings. TEACCH has a much broader program than the one we're focusing on here, which is their work with students on job skills in secondary school programs and, thereafter, a focus on adaptive living and actually getting jobs. In all their programs, they emphasize family collaboration.

Their methods are evidence-based and assume most people with ASD are visual learners, so they emphasize and implement intervention strategies that focus on physical and visual structure, schedules, work systems and task organization. Individualized systems aim to address difficulties with communication, organization, generalization, concepts, sensory processing, change, and relating to others.

The TEACCH Supported Employment Program presently serves 320–340 people in two areas of the state, the Triad (Greensboro, Winston-Salem, and High Point regions) and the Triangle (Chapel Hill, Durham, and Raleigh), with 250 of their job seekers presently holding down jobs. They work both with developing job providers and the employers, as well as for however long it takes to support those with ASD.

Like the entrepreneurial autism advocate D'Eri, TEACCH "markets the attributes of the person with autism and markets what a great employee they will make, because they're capable and competent individuals," says Mike Chapman, current Director of the Supported Employment program, who has worked with the program since its beginning in 1989.

Their program is impressive in its numbers. They've worked with over 800 people transitioning into jobs. While the national survey of employment programs range in job success for those with ASD in the 37 percent level, TEACCH is in the 83 percent range. They're constantly reevaluating their work "in the trenches" to get and keep those with ASD on their jobs, because "we learned the traditional programs just didn't work for many of our clients who have autism," explained Glenna Osborne, Director of Special Projects for Employment and Adult Transition.

Most of the costs of the Supported Employment services are paid by Vocational Rehabilitation (VR), which is a federal and state-funded program. TEACCH is a vendor for VR, and they contract with the agency to provide vocational services. They also have a contract with several local management entities/managed care organizations in the state to provide vocational services. Although they take private pays, it's rare.

The brilliance of their program, however, is that they also train teachers and other professionals the TEACCH methods "all over the place," according to Osborne. They're teaching several programs including the T-Step Program and Supported Employment Trainings, which emphasize "successful adult outcomes, including employment or secondary education. They provide trainings in NC as well as around the US and the world.

Another state (among a number, fortunately) is Michigan, because, if nothing else, it supports educational programs for those with ASD up to age 26, the highest age in the country. They have numerous job-oriented programs for those on the spectrum. For example, if your child is a foodie, loves to cook, and/or appreciates a restaurant environment, there are several successful programs that are comprised of job training for those with ASD in every aspect of restaurant management, from cooks to waiters to book-keepers. In fact, there is a restaurant in Michigan called After 26, a project originally inspired by a restaurant called the Junction of Hope. The Junction was the first nonprofit 501 C-3 restaurant in the country. Their purpose was to employ special needs adults in Southern Saginaw County.

Following their example, the After 26 project filed for nonprofit status with the federal government and received tax-exempt status in the summer of 2008. Both restaurants have been successful based on their program to market around their employees with ASD.

Perhaps one of the most successful programs to train graduates in the food industry is Max's Positive Vibe Café in Richmond, VA. Since 2204, Positive Vibe Café has trained over 1,000 students, all with scholarships!

The training program prepares students for the work world by giving them hands-on training in basic food service skills such as cleaning and sanitizing, proper use of kitchen utensils, food safety, commercial dish washing, communication in the work place, interviewing, and job seeking. The program typically lasts four weeks and culminates with a graduation ceremony.

The concept of the café grew out of a father's desire to help his son with Duchenne Muscular Dystrophy to get a job after repeated attempts had failed. What started as a job for Max grew into a major industry of training others with challenges, so the company was set up as a nonprofit, turning to the community to help with their goals.

Since 2005, Garth Larcen, Max's father, has worked monthly to have a Guest Chef's dinner night and other community fund raisers to help train the restaurant's trainees. In an interview with Quest magazine (online) by Richard Senti on July 1, 2013, Garth said that "Probably the most important thing we teach our trainees is self-confidence. . . Most of the folks who go through our classes have never been recognized for having any real skills at all." By the time they complete the process, they not only have the skills, they have the self-confidence that they can effectuate them, and they've been trained as well in the program to make it through the interview process.

Other restaurant training programs have developed in Florida, California, and Texas, so—if your child is interested in a culinary job—check out the possibilities of getting him into the programs that have some great success ratios.

California, by the way, has numerous post-high school programs focused on getting jobs, one of the newest being Autism Works NOW! Joanne Lara, the executive director of the program, explains that "We are addressing employment too late in this country for individuals with autism," so they consider the program critical to helping a small percentage of the 50,000 18-to-22-year-olds with autism graduating from high schools annually looking for employment.

Lara and Director Susan Osborne have created a program that includes three class meetings and one field trip per month to local businesses, where participants meet hiring managers. They also act as a temporary job agency to help place individuals with autism in local businesses, so they function as advocates for the individuals as well as for the skills and talents of those with autism.

Because the eight-month program was funded partially with an Autism Speaks Community Grant and a fundraiser in LA in 2007 featuring Dr. Temple Grandin, the cost is minimal—$125 a month per student. Their site, www.autismworksnow.org, provides more detailed information.

New Jersey is a class act in itself, perhaps of necessity because it has one of the larger per capita numbers of autistics in the U.S. They have created a program where "helpmates" support and assist those on the spectrum not only to get jobs for those on the spectrum, but, once they've gotten jobs, they assist in various ways so they can keep their jobs. The problem is not a lack of capability, but, often, the perplexity associated with deviations from the routine.

4. Look into major corporations because they've begun to hire people with ASD, and some have actually discovered their businesses' productivity has gone up because those on the autism spectrum are such good employees, once trained.

Compared to the size of their operations, the numbers aren't huge, but their retention rates are high, so these few corporate pioneers are making a difference. Survey your large corporate neighbors and check in with their HR people to find out if they have a door to open for your child looking for a job.

Ken Langone, cofounder of Home Depot, created Ken's Krew in Philadelphia in 1997. Initially, they hired vocational coaches to train and monitor those with intellectual and developmental disabilities to successfully enter the workforce by providing access to good jobs. They provide professional training and support to prepare for and sustain employment. Initially, this took place in Home Depot. In 17 years, they've worked with 330 individuals, expanding into five states (DE, MD, NJ, NY, PA), which was significantly helped with a $1 million grant from Home Depot in 2008. They've added CVS Caremark in 19 states subsequently: Fairway Market in 2011; Outback Steakhouse and Wegmans in 2012; and, in 2013, Boscov's.

Trainees perform a variety of jobs, including stocking, unloading trucks, mixing paint, operating the cash register, cutting keys, customer service, stacking lumber, shelf maintenance, sweeping, dusting, collecting cardboard, bagging, cart maintenance, returns, rolling silverware, food portioning, product displays, and packaging.

Currently 184 participants are working at corporate partner locations. Their one-year retention rate is high, 74 percent, and 35 percent of the 80 participants who entered the program more than ten years ago still hold their jobs.

Walgreens, based in the Chicago suburb of Deerfield, is another corporate leader when it comes to this issue. The company employs a high number of individuals with autism and other disabilities at a distribution center in Anderson, South Carolina, which it opened in 2007. The pilot program in

Anderson had strong results because the facility turned out to be the company's most productive, so Walgreens expanded the model to other distribution centers. It's exemplary, bringing in more than 200 other companies in tours of the model.

The program was spearheaded by Randy Lewis, formerly a senior vice president of the company. Lewis's own son, Austin, has autism. Lewis told ABC News about the Anderson facility in 2008 that "people come to me and say, will this work in my environment? Yes, it will. This is not just a good thing to do, (it's) the right thing to do. This is better."

In addition, Walgreens has built a mock store in Evanston, Illinois, as part of a workplace training program for individuals with ASD and other disabilities. It established the program in partnership with the Have Dreams Academy. Walgreens intends to hire and train more people with autism to work in its stores.

Think beyond the obvious and traditional path of high school, college, job. The first two don't necessarily translate into the third category when you have a child on the autism spectrum. Susan Senator has written a book *Autism Adulthood: Strategies and Insights for a Fulfilling Life*, which is definitely worth checking out, as she identifies a number of entrepreneurial ways to create jobs for a young person on the autism spectrum. Temple Grandin has another new book out titled *Temple Talks About The Older Child*, which focuses on the job problem as well because she recognizes more than most how critically important it is to contribute to the betterment of society, in large or small ways. They "deserve lives of purpose and possibilities," according to Ron Suskind, author of *Life, Animated: A Story of Sidekicks, Heroes, and Autism*, a movie about his son.

Parents must research the variety of programs available after high school, based on their child's interests, skills, restrictions, and capabilities. If the job doesn't presently exist to fulfill their child's abilities, consider creating it.

References

1. American RadioWorks (2014). The troubled history of vocational education. Retrieved June 27, 2016 from http://www.americanradioworks. org/segments/the-troubled-history-of-vocational-education/

2. Brown, F., McDonnell, J., & Snell, M. E. (2016). Instruction of students with severe disabilities. (8th ed.). Boston, MA: Pearson.

3. Brown, F., & Snell, M. E. (2011). Instruction of students with severe disabilities. Upper Saddle River, New Jersey: Pearson Education, Inc.

H2C+ Bridging the Gap from College to Careers Retrieved 6/28/2016 online from http://interwork.sdsu.edu/c2c/collaborators

Parent Center Hub Retrieved 6/29/16 from http://www.parentcenterhub.org/repository/age-of-majority/

Special Education Advisor retrieved 6/19/2016 from http://www.specialeducationadvisor.com/special-education-laws/individuals-with-disabilities-education-act-idea/

Joanne Lara, MA, CTC M/S Education Specialist is the founder of Autism Movement Therapy and author of *Autism Movement Therapy Method: Waking up the Brain!* Joanne was the autism expert for the Fox show *Touch* and is core adjunct faculty at National University in Los Angeles. Joanne produced the documentary *Generation A: Portraits of Autism & the Arts* and is the executive director of Autism Works Now! For AMT certification, licensing, and online courses, visit www.autismmovementtherapy.org.

Lyn Dunsavage Young received the Sigma Delta Chi and Dallas Press Club Lifetime Achievement Award for her many journalistic accomplishments as the publisher of the Dallas Downtown News as well as the Southwest WICI Award as one of the three top journalists in Texas. She has written or coedited five books, including one published by the National Trust for Historic Preservation on Revitalizing the Inner City through Historic Preservation, co-authored by Virginia Talkington McAlester. She presently works for Future Horizons, Inc., as their national media coordinator and director of distributors.

ADVICE FOR PARENTS SEEKING EMPLOYMENT FOR THEIR CHILD WITH AUTISM

I was first motivated to become involved in employment of adults diagnosed with ASD in 2009 when *Wired* magazine published an article about a Danish company specifically focused on the good fit of this population with the Information and Technology (IT) sector. At the time I read the article, I had been a single mother for 10 years to my sons, both of whom are on the autism spectrum. And, coincidentally, the career I had left behind in order to meet the demands of single parenting was in IT.

As I read the magazine article, I was intrigued with the win-win success of this innovative IT company called Specialisterne not only for their employees with ASD, but for the unexpected benefits to their clients, as well. The Danish software testing company had reaped great benefits from hiring adults on the autism spectrum. Along with my own background in IT and as a parent of two children diagnosed with autism, the Danish project spoke loudly to me. I have the background and motivation to make this happen in Vancouver. My vision was set!

And so it came about that from September 2013 to September 2014, for one year, I volunteered for the Toronto-based team at Specialisterne to source, train, and onboard the first six Canadian ASD hires in Vancouver at a large multinational software business. Three years later, as I write this article, the six individuals I recruited are still employed with at the same company. A wonderful success.

During that volunteer year, I realized the great impact this could have to expose as many organizations to people with ASD as possible and in a larger variety of companies. And if it was set up as a for-profit business, we could have a better chance of providing the employees with a secure middle-class lifestyle and career. Once again, I followed my gut and took a leap of faith.

In October 2014, I incorporated Focus Professional Services Inc.("Focus"), and in the summer of 2015 it was operational. Within one year, we had 12 employees, nine of whom are on the autism spectrum. We provide services to the Vancouver business community in software testing and data quality. Our employees typically work at our client's sites. We promote and are a model of full-inclusion within the business community. We provide both the training and the on-site support necessary for successful inclusion.

In the future I want to broaden our client base, hire more employees, and branch out into data analysis, statistics, and security. Our first fully operational year was quite a fantastic journey through which I and my team learned many important things. I'd like to share some of these with you.

First, there was the development of a business model. We turned to Meticulon in Calgary, a similar organization to Focus, who had been operational for a couple years after adapting an open-source business model developed by Passwerks in Belgium. This business model has been implemented globally and proven by several companies.

It was an easy decision for Focus to adapt this same business model and become a part of an international community of transparency and sharing among companies who employ individuals with autism in the STEM (Science, Technology, Engineering, & Math) sectors. We learned that collaboration is invaluable and that there are many people and programs we can learn from and import to Canada to improve resources for the autism community very quickly, without having to reinvent the wheel.

Second, we needed start-up funding. I deliberately set the company up as a for-profit organization. Focus is not a charity nor are we a not-for-profit. We are a business. Government grants and funding were not available to us as a result, with the exception of wage subsidies, which are available to all Canadian companies. So, we secured funding through a traditional financial institution. We believe that by designing Focus as a business instead of as a charity, we instantly reframe the perception that many people hold that people with disabilities or differences need charity, volunteer hours, and donations. Instead, we want to highlight our staff's employable strengths and talents through paid employment in meaningful mainstream work.

When we hire new employees, we require no previous experience, education, or training in IT. We seek individuals who have natural aptitudes in logical reasoning, numerical abilities, pattern recognition, perseverance, and accuracy. We test for these essential IT aptitudes using a subset of the CEBIR assessments that universities in Europe use to qualify students for free tuition. We hire those applicants who show above average IT-related aptitudes.

We then train our new hires. During the 200 training hours that includes software testing, students learn how to work in a professional business environment while we assess their ability to cope with ambiguity, timed assignments, changing priorities, and working in teams. We assess each person's preferred work style to ensure our employees will be comfortable and at ease in the typical IT workplace environment. And, importantly, we assess their coachability.

However, while training our very first group of recruits, we discovered that we had two very distinct groups of interest and skills: one group was naturally aligned to data quality while the other group was much more aligned to software testing. As luck would have it, at that same time we landed our first contract, which required these same two distinct "specialist" teams. The lesson here was a reminder that there is a range of strengths and motivations within the autistic population. Contrary to many autism treatment and service programs designed around the stereotype of adherence to routine, our success has been in our ability to be customizable, adaptive, and flexible to accommodate this range of differences.

Before our employees start work at a client site, I present *Autism in the Workplace,* our one-hour training session to clients' employees. The intent of the presentation is to dispel myths about autism, to make the unknown known, and to replace fear and judgment with understanding and curiosity.

I find interesting the number of people who tell me after these presentations that they recognize some of the sensory-sensitivities and social behaviors associated with autism in themselves, amongst their coworkers, or their family members. I like to take the opportunity to suggest that higher-functioning autism is really just a point on the spectrum of the range of human traits that are part of our human neurodiversity. There's a tipping point where there are sufficient challenges that arise from these differences to warrant access to supports in this neurotypically-designed world. Unfortunately, to get access to special services, you need a label.

Through these training courses and the job placement, I've witnessed the transformative and positive personal impact that greater understanding about differences among people can have. Working with employees with special needs in a work place has cascading effects of promoting greater cooperation, reducing bullying, improving communication, and generally deepening empathy and caring in the workplace.

There have been a number of studies on happiness in the workplace, and there are two findings from all these studies that have truly resonated with me and are ingrained in everything we do at Focus. The first is to tap into a person's strengths. We can't all be good at everything. Too often we spend too much time dwelling on our weaknesses. My older son cannot tie shoelaces. The choice is to keep him practicing until he gets it or buy slip-on shoes. We chose the latter so he could succeed at his strengths: post-graduate studies and research in mathematics. It's been found that people who use their strengths in the workplace are happier in their lives and their relationships improve.

The second contributor to happiness is to feel that you belong. At Focus, we accept how autism presents in each of our employees. If someone doesn't make eye contact, for example, it is not an issue. There's a reason for the lack of eye contact, and that reason deserves understanding and respect. Our employees have experienced many changes and opportunities to learn and grow. We check in regularly with each Trainee to review performance, provide feedback, and ensure the fit is good for Focus and for the Trainee. Together, we have addressed various sources of anxiety associated with working, from traveling in crowded public transit to forgetting to do the laundry and having no clean clothes, to fretting about making a mistake on the job.

Remarkably, the personal development through work can generalize in positive ways to our employees' lives outside of work. For example, by becoming more flexible and adaptable at work, one of our employees traveled on his own for the first time from Canada to visit his girlfriend in the U.S.A. On his return trip, one of his connecting flights was canceled. He was able to handle the situation in stride. As an employer, it is rewarding and inspiring to see how our employees are growing and engaging in new life experiences.

As for their careers, all the software testers are now ISTQB certified, an internationally recognized software testing certification. Their examination marks ranged from 82 percent to 92 percent. Amazing results on what is considered a challenging certification exam. And our clients are beyond satisfied with the quality of our services and the value we add to their teams. But it is also the exposure to autism these clients are experiencing. They, too, are learning and growing personally from their experiences and telling others about it.

I feel that many changes need to occur in current hiring and retention practices. Employers miss hiring talent because of practices like rejecting résumés with no related experience or education, language-based interview processes that are biased toward extroverted and conversation-confident applicants, that are biased toward organizational "cultural fits" including extrovert socializing, and the expectation that everyone should want to be promoted. All these biases need to be challenged and reframed to be more inclusive of a broader spectrum of neurodiversity.

As for my two sons, the ones who opened my mind and my heart to autism, they are doing really well. My older son had been told by his high school that he should never expect to graduate, but he did, and with honors and scholarships that paid for his first two years of postsecondary tuition!

My younger son rehabilitates and socializes abused and abandoned animals. They seem to sense that they are safe with him. He can tell what clothes will look good on you just by looking at you, and he is becoming quite the chef in our home. He claims he is not ready to work at a paid job. Someday he may feel differently, but in his own time.

As a parent, I have had to learn to step aside and let my sons work things out for themselves and recognize when to gently step back in to guide and let them know that they are not alone. They can be amazingly creative, resilient, and insightful. With Focus, my employees, and my sons, I am filled with hope for a more inclusive and accepting neurodiverse world.

For more information, please contact info @ focusps.ca.

Carol Simpson is the founder and CEO of Focus Professional Services, devoted to training and placement of individuals on the autism spectrum in good-quality, full-time employment and careers. She started her career in Vancouver as a programmer at IBM Canada and moved on to operate her own software development shop. She has worked in the IT field for over 30 years, managing departments with 60+ IT professionals and project budgets of $50M. She has worked in the private and public sectors at senior and executive levels of management and has taught at the University of Toronto.

She recently completed a one-year volunteer assignment in which she successfully recruited, trained, and onboarded six individuals with autism for an international company's autism employment initiative. Carol is one of a handful of individuals in Canada who has successfully placed or hired individuals with autism into full-time careers that afford them solid, middle-class lifestyles.

Carol sees Focus Professional Services as a contributor to the normalization of employing individuals with autism in the workplace. She believes strongly in the equal rights of autistics to acceptance and inclusion in society's constructs of community, education, governance, and employment. She has two adult sons on the autism spectrum.

10

SUPPORTING SIGNIFICANT OTHERS EMOTIONALLY

MAINTAINING
A STRONG PARENT TEAM

Note: Selection from *Maintaining a Strong Parent Team.*

Ask any parents with experience in the autism world, and they are likely to tell you that the first rules of success are: don't go it alone, and don't wait for a crisis before taking steps. Simply stated, among the best things parents can do for themselves and their families is to get connected with support groups and services before they reach a point of desperation.

A proactive position begins with the recognition that having a child with special needs is going to add to the challenges a couple will face. However, many parents and researchers report that, handled correctly, the challenges associated with raising such children have actually strengthened and benefited families in many deep and meaningful ways. But going to bat without adequate preparation can only lower anyone's chances of success. Knowing what you're likely to be up against is half the battle won!

A little bit of research or a few books and articles will quickly bring into focus a handful of the challenges most commonly reported by parents. These include: avoiding blame, finding adequate child care, finding resources for support and guidance, maintaining effective communications, finding time alone and together, managing the extra expenses, and maintaining a positive outlook. Space does not permit exploring these issues in depth, but here are a few suggestions from those who have faced these challenges with success:

Finding time alone:

- Give yourselves permission to take time out for self.
- Make plans for weekly or monthly time alone (schedule it).
- Meet for lunch or arrange a regular hour before or after work.

Ask for support:

- Let it be known when you need help.
- Connect with other parents facing similar challenges.
- Join a support group right away and get involved in its activities.

Communicate effectively:

- Recognize how important this is and make an agreement to work on it.
- Use "I" statements and a tone of caring, as opposed to anger, blame, and frustration.
- Set aside time on a regular basis to talk; don't wait for a crisis.
- Be patient and sensitive to your partner's feelings and priorities; ask how best to approach him or her, when would be a good time to talk, and how he or she wants to be kept informed.
- Seek professional help if necessary.

Contributing Author Nicholas Martin, M.A., Clinical Practices, Psychology Department, University of Hartford—Mr. Martin is a conflict resolution consultant residing near Fort Worth, Texas. He is a very popular conference presenter with a background in clinical psychology and in court and postal service mediation. Among his published works are *An Operator's Manual for Successful Living, Strengthening Relationships When Our Children Have Special Needs*, and *A Guide to Collaboration for IEP Teams*.

HELPING OTHERS UNDERSTAND YOUR CHILD WITH ASD

You are walking through the shopping mall or buying groceries with your family. Suddenly you are approached by a stranger who either stares, pointedly looks away, or asks you a point-blank question: "What's wrong with your child?" The stranger's look and action show lack of understanding and tolerance.

How do you respond? With righteous anger or compassion? You will almost certainly feel anger on behalf of your child and family, but giving in to it will leave you drained and frustrated. And what if the person who doesn't understand is actually part of your immediate or extended family? This can cause even deeper emotional wounds.

I want to encourage you to do all that you can to respond with compassion in these situations. You have started on a journey, and so have they. They just don't know it yet! Make your goals (A) awareness, (E) education, and (AC) acceptance—usually in that order.

Disability awareness

Disability awareness or, in this case, autism awareness is about helping someone make the leap from confusion and fear to acceptance and understanding. Sometimes that leap can be made quickly and sometimes it only happens with lots of encouragement and persistence.

We will start at home and walk through ways you, your spouse, and your family can practice this process. Then we will move on to practical ways to move through this process with your child, your child's classmates or peers, and your community at large (including those aggravating strangers at the mall).

Although it may feel counterproductive to start at home when strangers on the street are the ones causing you sleepless nights, I do this because it gives you a chance to increase your personal circle of support, and it gives you lots of practice talking about your child's diagnosis, so that you can fine-tune your explanation and provide it in a way that is calm, clear, and concise.

Step 1 : Start with yourself

If your child has received his/her diagnosis recently, then the first person you need to escort through this process is yourself.

> **(A)** Listen to the stories of other parents raising children with autism spectrum disorders. Do you see yourself and your child? Try not to focus on the stories that scare you. Instead, tuck away helpful hints and jot down names of parents you may want to talk with more, down the road.
>
> **(E)** Do your homework. Do the symptoms ring true for your child? Do you believe that this is the correct diagnosis for your child? Do you understand the challenges that lie ahead as well as the resources that can offer hope and support to your family?
>
> **(AC)** Apply what you have learned. Begin to build the network of support that your special child needs (medical treatments, education strategies, personal support).

Step 2 : Support your spouse

Often the spouse not involved in primary childcare has more difficulty accepting a diagnosis of autism. This person may withdraw into roles outside the family or even withdraw from the family completely. It's important to do all you can to help your spouse reach acceptance. Your spouse's active participation will make your efforts as a parent, caregiver, and advocate much more effective. To get started, think about how your spouse makes decisions and help him/her find the kind of input needed to reach acceptance.

> **(A)** Share the realities of your day. Encourage your spouse to spend time alone with your child and experience his/her care first hand. If verbal discussions become highly charged, try writing a journal or a letter and sharing that.

(E) If your spouse responds to facts, have him/her complete a signs and symptoms checklist for your child. Seeing the results in black and white can be an eye-opening experience. If he/she gives greater weight to the voice of experts, find a parent book on autism for him/her to read or take them along to a therapy session.

Is there a need to process in private or in a group? Attending an autism conference where he/she can meet others living your reality can provide opportunities to connect with other spouses. Online options like teleclasses and multimedia presentations can provide all the information of a conference in a much more private forum. The key is to find what works for your spouse and connect him/her with the necessary information.

(AC) Involve your spouse as much as possible. Your advocacy efforts will be strongest if you attend school meetings and medical appointments together. This will allow both of you to help establish priorities, contribute to the "the plan of action," and take advantage of opportunities to ask questions. It also ensures that the support you offer your child at home will be a united effort.

Step 3. Support your extended family members

Loved ones who don't see your family frequently may find it easier to see your child's behavioral symptoms as a reflection of your parenting rather than the special needs of the child. *Accept that this is a coping mechanism,* an attempt to block out information these people don't want to receive.

(A) Let family members know about your child's diagnosis as soon as possible. Often writing a letter makes a more lasting impression than engaging in a conversation. Chances are this will be their first introduction to the subject of autism. So try to use your own homework to explain it as simply as possible in words that are familiar.

(E) Not every family member will be open to knowing more, but encourage any who show signs of interest. Loan them your resource books to read. Spend time together with your child or write out a typical day, so they can understand the reality of your child's needs.

Print and provide family-friendly information that you find online and let them learn a little at a time.

(AC) Talk about ways individual family members can support your family (coming with you to meetings, babysitting so you can go to a support group or out to dinner, spending time with a sibling who may be feeling overlooked, etc.). By letting them do just a few non-threatening tasks and showing your appreciation, you both benefit and your family bond is strengthened.

Step 4: Support your child

Parents go through a range of emotions when a child is diagnosed with autism. Your child also needs to be given information about the diagnosis and support for understanding and coping with this new information. Adults on the spectrum who are successful have learned who they are and accept and use that information to help themselves become the best they can be in life.

Does the idea of discussing autism or Asperger's Syndrome with your child seem scary or even silly? Lots of parents put this task off. They fear that the child won't understand or that hearing the information will make the child feel bad. Chances are your child won't understand what you have to say the first time, but a journey can't start without that first step. Your child's diagnosis will affect his/her entire life. Problems will occur and the road will have challenges, but correct information about the diagnosis and his/her differences offers the child a better chance of being successful.

Timing:

There is no exact age or "right time" to tell a child about the diagnosis. You know your child best, and you will need to make a decision based on his/her personality, abilities, and social awareness. Look for signs that the child is ready for information. Some children will actually ask: "What is wrong with me?"; "Why can't I be like everybody else?"; or, even, "What is wrong with everyone?" These types of questions are certainly a clear indication. Others, however, may have similar thoughts and not be able to express them. The bottom line: try to offer your explanation before your child has lots of negative experience related to his/her diagnosis. Just as early intervention is the key to effective treatment, early communication is the key to healthy self-esteem and self-acceptance.

So, when you're ready . . .

Set a positive tone and focus on uniqueness as the quality that makes each of us special. Talk about the qualities of different friends and family members, how each has their own likes and dislikes, strengths and weaknesses, and physical characteristics. This makes uniqueness just a matter of course. It also makes it easier to talk about differences related to your child's diagnosis.

Practical tools:

(A) When your child is young, read simple stories about autism or other children who have autism spectrum disorders. A book like *My Friend with Autism* by Beverly Bishop is a great choice. It is a coloring book designed to help children ages four to eight understand autism and Asperger's Syndrome. It was created by the mother of a young man with autism and is highly informative. Best of all, it is simple enough for young children to understand and short enough to keep a younger reader's attention. For an older child, try *Asperger's: What Does It Mean to Me?* by Catherine Faherty. It comes in a workbook format that provides activities that help explain an autism spectrum diagnosis and make the information more child-specific and concrete. The child and you, as the trusted adult partner, can complete the workbook together.

(E) Check with your state Parent Training & Information Center or your local autism support group. Many have a library of videos that can be checked out for viewing by your family.

(AC) Talk with your child one-on-one. If your child is very visual, videotape them and watch the video together as a conversation starter. Consider your child's ability to process information and try to decide on what and how to give them information. Remember, it doesn't all have to happen in one big session. A series of conversations may meet both your needs better.

Step 5: Inform your child 's classmates and teachers

Just as you come to rely on your coworkers as an extended family, so your child will see his/her classmates at school as a primary source of interaction and support. Time spent ensuring that this group is well informed and supportive when your child is young will make the road easier as your child grows.

(A) Volunteer to do an autism awareness presentation for your child's class as soon as school starts. Use strategies and conversations you have already developed with family and friends to explain this complex diagnosis in child-friendly language. The Center for Disease Control & Prevention has a Kids Quest of Kid-Friendly Fact that may be helpful. Be sure to personalize your information for your child and cover critical issues like communicating with your child and understanding his/her social signals.

(E) Work with your child's teacher to integrate autism awareness into the class's regular curriculum through stories, empathy building activities, and reports.

(AC) Discuss ways to encourage peer friendships for your child through the use of peer mentors or friendship groups, such as a Circle of Friends. Add these items to your child's individualized education program (IEP) to make them a priority. And be sure to focus attention on your child's social responses, as well. Utilizing techniques such as social stories, social circles, and software programs designed to help children with spectrum disorders recognize and interpret facial expressions can all help your child feel more comfortable and confident in social situations.

Step 6: Build awareness in your community

When it comes to the community at large, you may have great difficulty moving any particular individual through the entire process. Instead, focus on building awareness. Plant many seeds and hope for a beautiful garden of wildflowers.

- Volunteer to give presentations to community organizations. Talk about your family's experience and about your child's particular diagnosis. Most community members will have little or no experience with autism, and you can explain both the joys and the challenges in a uniquely personal way. If there is a way the organization can help, don't be shy about suggesting it. Most civic organizations are constantly looking for ways to improve the community and are very open to ideas.

- Take part in regular autism awareness events/activities with your support group. Frequently, a group of parents working together to raise public awareness will have a larger impact than an individual can have acting on his or her own. Globally, April is recognized as National Autism Awareness Month, but for a larger impact, consider working with your group to do small activities throughout the year. Whether you are sharing information or doing a fund-raising event for autism research, let your voice be heard in your community.

- Write letters to the editor giving your perspective on special needs issues. Many sectors in your community will affect your child with autism (childcare, healthcare, education, employment). A simple, personal letter can have great impact. Don't allow your child's options to be limited because you didn't speak out on issues that were close to your heart.

- Remember that calm, clear, concise message you've been working on? Consider that your "elevator speech" and have it polished and ready for anyone who approaches you on the street. Your goal: give your message within 30 seconds.

- Educational cards—If you aren't sure you can talk calmly when someone has spoken rudely to you or your child, create a set of educational cards. This allows you to "do your part" for raising awareness by simply handing the individual one card and walking away. Your local chapter of the Autism Society may have cards that you can purchase, or you can print your own with a personal message. They are usually about the size of a business card.

Now what about that stranger on the street? Try these quick solutions:

- For the person with the awkward question, use a snappy comeback, such as "Kids come in all shapes and sizes."
- If a stranger simply stares, walk away. But as you walk, focus on your child and count five of your child's small, amazing accomplishments. Genuine pride and delight will soon put the smile back on your face.

For more information, you can write to Ms. Simmons at lisa.simmon@cox.net.

Contributing Author Lisa Simmons is the creator of the Ideal Lives Online Advocacy & Inclusion Center and author of the special report, Disability Awareness: Special Kids Don't Have to Feel Left Out.

SIBLINGS OF CHILDREN WITH AUTISM

For most of us, life is in families. Every child on the autism spectrum has a powerful influence on parents, grandparents, siblings, and other caring people who surround the family. When we think about the needs of people on the autism spectrum, we must also think of the needs of the family as a whole. As a parent you have a responsibility to provide the best possible childhood for all of your children. However, you will not be able to meet this challenge unless you also ensure that your life and that of your family is one of substance and value.

Next to their child with autism, most parents worry most about the other children in the family. They worry about whether they are neglecting these children because they are trying to do their best for their child with autism. In any family it is always a balancing act to meet everyone's needs. We all have limited resources and many things to do. But children with autism have exceptional needs, and that heightens the stress for parents as they try to meet the needs of other children in the family.

Fortunately, there are things you can do to address your concerns about whether you are supporting all of your children appropriately. One thing is to remember that all of us have had jealous feelings about our brothers or sisters. As children we all felt competitive with our siblings, and there were times when we thought our parents were giving more to a sibling than to us. Those concerns are not unique to parents of children with autism. Remembering that may help you keep your typically developing child's feelings and needs in perspective.

It is also important to remember that children have different needs at different points in their development. The very young child needs a sense of security and safety. That means ensuring they are protected from the tantrums or aggression of an older sibling with autism. As they get older, children are more concerned about issues of fairness. You may not be able to devote exactly the same time or resources to each child, but you can try to ensure that each child has opportunities for your focused attention. Try to provide individual time and attention to each child. As your child grows up, she will be able to understand your explanations about why her sibling with autism needs more from you, but she still needs to know there are times during which she is the focus of your attention Many children take a page from their parent's book when it comes to understanding their sibling with autism. If you as a parent have achieved some comfort about such things as going into the community or dealing with your child's problematic behaviors, it is likely that your other children will model your behavior in these situations. That does not mean they will not have moments of embarrassment, especially when they are in their teens, or that they will never be unkind to their brother or sister on the autism spectrum. Most children, like most adults, say unkind things from time to time. But remember that you are your child's most important role model, and he or she will very likely come to share your perspective over time.

It is also important not to allow brothers or sisters to become auxiliary parents. Although everyone in the family needs to do his or her part in keeping the family afloat from day to day, children should not be asked to take on too much responsibility for the care or supervision of their brother or sister with autism. They should especially not be called on to deal with challenging, hard-to-manage behavior problems.

Finally, it is important to keep in mind that research shows that brothers and sisters of children with autism are pretty much like other people. Most of them cope well with the special demands created by their sibling and have good lives as adults, including an ongoing connection with their adult sibling.

References

Feiges, L. S. & Weiss, M. J. (2005). *Sibling stories: Reflections on life with a brother or sister with autism.* Shawnee Mission, KS: Autism Asperger's Publishing Co.

Harris, S. L. & Glasberg, B. (2003). *Siblings of Children with autism. A Guide for families.* 2nd ed. Bethesda MD: Woodbine House. You can write to Dr. Harris at sharris@rci.rutgers.edu.

Siegel, B. & Silverstein, S. (1994). *What about me? Growing up with a developmentally disabled sibling.* New York: Plenum Press.

Contributing Author Sandra L. Harris, Ph.D., Psychology, Rutgers, The State University of New Jersey—Dr. Sandra L. Harris is Board of Governors Distinguished Service Professor at Rutgers University and executive director of the Douglass Developmental Disabilities Center, a university-based program for the treatment of children with autism. Her research and clinical interests focus on children with autism and their families. She has written extensively in this area, including several books and dozens of journal articles and book chapters. Dr. Harris consults nationally to schools and organizations that serve people with autism and has served as an expert witness in legal cases concerning the rights of people with developmental disabilities. She is an associate editor of the Journal of Autism and Developmental Disorders, a fellow in the APA divisions of Clinical Psychology and Child and Youth Services, and a fellow in the American Psychological Society. Dr. Harris is a licensed practicing psychologist. Harris's book *Siblings of Children with Autism* received the 1995 Autism Society of America Award for Literary Achievement.

11

PLANNING FOR THE FUTURE

A LIFE MAP

For typical children, moving through the cognitive, emotional, and physical developmental stages of life is a natural progression. With the right people and experiences put in their path, they continue to move along. But if we want children with special needs to become responsible, capable, and happy adults, we need to chart a path from where they are today to where we—and they—hope they will end up.

To determine who you want to become and what you want to do in life, you need to know yourself, what you like and don't like, what you can and can't do. You also need a certain amount of social smarts—because, like it or not, the road of life is paved with relationships and interactions. How absolutely unfortunate, then, that some children with special needs have trouble in both of these areas—introspecting and relating to others. They don't think much about their inner selves at any given moment, never mind thinking ahead a month, a year, or a lifetime. And they pretty much live in the moment in a state of social confusion. Their hearts are in the right places, but their social senses are not.

If your child is going to make it in life, there is a greater chance that he will do so if there is a roadmap to guide him, one that draws on his strengths and minimizes his challenges. You will have to be intentional about his future. You will also need to teach him to be intentional, being mindful of what he needs to be successful and being able to access the tools to get there.

The Life Map can help define a vision and goals for your child's future and provide the tools to achieve them. Depending on your child's cognitive and emotional abilities, you will need to figure out how much he can participate in the Life Mapping process. As he matures, his role in this process should increase until he is eventually able to take the lead in creating his own Life Map.

The Life Map is a framework for helping a child reach his potential and become the best he can be. If it's a clerk at the local grocery store, let's help him become the one with the biggest smile and the largest helping hand. If it's a herpetologist, let's figure out how to teach him effective listening skills so that he can be part of a research team.

Supporting your child with the skills that he needs does not mean that you are defining his dreams for him. If your child is high functioning, he will have his own dreams. Your role is to look at the competencies he needs to achieve them and help him get there.

Competencies go beyond technical skills. In fact, technical skills are probably the least of your worries. If your child is succeeding in school, he will probably be able to get through the necessary technical training and education to reach his goals. You need to think about the social, relational, emotional, and practical skills he will need—defining what they are and creating opportunities to practice, practice, practice them so that they become competencies.

Following is an excerpt from a letter that we received from Jack's teacher and advisor several weeks after Jack began middle school:

> "Jack really is beginning to show his personality, and as we have a great abhorrence of cookie-cutter kids, we like the fact that he is so independent and outspoken. For instance, in class today I was explaining that academic competitiveness at the school is not really encouraged. That we judge each student by his or her individual progress, not by how they measure up to other students.
>
> "Having said that, I handed out the vocabulary workbooks, where each student works at his own level. Of course, they started comparing their levels immediately. I went through the explanation again. Jack raised his hand and said, 'I don't go for all that mind-control stuff. Of course, it is better to be in a higher book.' Inside I was chuckling (thinking, there's my little rationalist), but I tried to assure him that I don't play 'mind-control' games and am as honest as I can be, given the circumstances."

You've got to love a kid like that. Carving a path, being conscientious and careful to match your child's temperament and personality to the environment and culture, whether it is school, an activity, or the structure of your home, pays off. You'll see it the minute your child's tent starts unfolding.

What is Life Mapping?

Life Mapping is a process used to realize a person's fullest potential by drawing on his strengths and interests and working on his challenges. Companies go through processes like this all the time. They identify their competitive edge, take a look at what barriers are in the market, and come up with goals and a way of reaching them that will satisfy both consumers and stockholders.

This process can also work for individuals. In fact, maybe you've done Life Mapping (although you probably haven't called it that) for yourself—getting to know who you are and what you're good at, setting goals that relate to that, and then establishing a way to accomplish them. I'm not suggesting that you won't have a perfectly satisfactory and fulfilling life if you don't do Life Mapping. But for children with challenges, being intentional and thoughtful about who they are and what they need throughout their life will improve the odds that they will live a satisfying life.

Pretend that it is your friend's birthday and you have offered to throw her a party. You ask her who she would like you to invite and what she would like for dessert. Tossing Dr. Atkins to the wind, she says breathlessly, "Triple chocolate mousse cake with extra filling—and don't skimp on the frosting." Determining what you need to do to put the party together, from invitations to cake, is the plan.

Having your friend enjoy a wonderful party and that delicious cake is your ultimate goal, vision, dream, and desire. To make the cake, you look in your kitchen cabinets and see that you've got a couple of eggs and some vanilla. That's the starting point. You go to the grocery store and buy the rest of the ingredients and then proceed to make the cake. From finding out what ingredients were on hand to spreading the last of the butter cream frosting on the cake is process. In fact, all of the actions that you take between coming up with the party idea and holding the event are part of the process. The actual party is just the endpoint, the goal.

The people are everyone involved in the event, from the birthday girl to the clerks at the stores where you shop to the guests and yours truly. They are the ones who carry out the process.

The birthday party could be thought of as a mapping experience: making a plan, using a process that leads you toward the goal, and working with people in the process. These three things are at the heart of Life Mapping:

The three elements of Life Mapping

Let's take a closer look at the elements behind Life Mapping: the players, the process, and the plan.

The players

The child, the parents, and those who regularly work with your child make up the foundation of the Life Mapping model. At the center is the child. That probably seems obvious. You might even say to yourself, "Of course, it is all about him. I spend half of my waking minutes thinking, worrying, making calls, setting plans, and fussing about him." It is a full-time job, no doubt. But doing the work without understanding the child is not enough. Life Mapping will only be as strong as the foundation. And the foundation starts with the child. Understanding your child means more than knowing what the doctors have told you that he "has." It means knowing many different aspects of him. By the nature of his challenges, it is often hard to get close to or understand your exceptional child. But you need to keep trying, because the more you understand your child, the better you'll be able to develop a Life Map for him.

The next part of the foundation is the parent(s.) You're the one(s) who provide the overall support for your child. You might think this support focuses on how your child functions at home, but since you are his coach, mentor, and case manager, your influence extends into every part of his life. You have a huge impact on the success of your child's Life Map. So it's vital to understand yourself. The more you know yourself and are aware of how your behavior and attitudes impact your child, the more effective you can be.

The folks who support your child make up the final piece of the foundation. We have all been on teams that are effective and teams that are not. Effective teams can move mountains, let alone move toward goals. The dysfunctional team cannot. The better the team functions, the more your child will benefit.

The process

In Life Mapping, there are many factors that influence, impact, and drive the process. But for our children, the two primary factors are the parent(s) and the team that supports the child. These individuals work closely and on a regular basis with the child. Their interactions with the child may be positive, negative, or neutral, but they all have a huge impact.

The plan

Defining goals and having a plan to reach those goals provide a structure for helping you stay focused and mindful that what you are working on are the things that you should be working on; that is, those that will make the greatest impact and difference in your child's life.

It doesn't matter how good a job you do if you are doing the wrong job. And in the case of helping a child reach his potential, you have to know what specifics, when added together, constitute that potential. If you want your child to reach his highest potential, you need to define what that might look like and then develop the steps that are needed to achieve it.

Contributing Author Anne Addison, M.B.A. Kellogg School of Management, Northwestern University—Ms. Addison worked for nearly 10 years in marketing management at several Fortune 100 companies before she launched her own management consulting practice. When her son was diagnosed with Attention Deficit Hyperactivity Disorder at the age of three and, later, with Asperger's Syndrome, she made a life-changing decision to close her consulting company and turn her business skills toward managing her son's case.

Through her effective personal style and her ability to successfully manage a health care and education team, Ms. Addison helped her son navigate the last heart-wrenching, sometimes overwhelming, 10 years—through educational failures, medication disasters, and more. Today, her son is a strong student in a typical fourth-grade classroom. He's involved in outside sports, church choir, and music. Ms. Addison's book *One Small Starfish: A Mother's Everyday Advice, Survival Tactics & Wisdom for Raising a Special Needs Child* won the Publishers Marketing Association's Ben Franklin Award, which recognizes excellence in independent publishing.

PERSON-DIRECTED PLANNING

The Ontario Context

In September, 2004, the Ministry of Community and Social Services in Ontario, Canada (MCSS), announced a process to transform developmental services for adults with a developmental disability. The intent was to create a more equitable, accessible, and sustainable system of community-based supports. Over the past several years, there has been a growing emphasis on self-determination, community involvement, and overall quality of life. To this end, the fundamental goal is to enable people to live and participate in their communities as independently and fully as possible, and to make their own decisions to the fullest extent possible. Regulation 299/10 promotes the social inclusion of persons with a developmental disability and recognizes the critical importance of planning and support networks as essential components of this larger process.

Person-directed Planning

Person-directed planning is highly consistent with the emphasis on self-determination and the achievement of personal outcomes for people with developmental disabilities. Through an action-oriented approach to planning, people with disabilities are the architects and directors of their plan. Other people in their networks or circles of support participate in the planning and assist these people to think about dreams, goals, and supports needed.

There have been many approaches introduced over the past two decades that describe a person-centered and more recently a person-directed approach to planning. All approaches look at a person's place in the community and at his or her strengths and needs. A person-directed plan tells us about the person's hopes and dreams, the supports necessary for success, and the actions required for the desired outcomes. The person directs and owns the plan. Such an approach highlights the importance of the person taking the lead on the plan, deciding what is most important to the person, and what the future could look like.

Principles of Person-Directed Planning

The following principles underpin person-directed planning:

- Focuses on the talents and strengths of the person
- Remains a flexible, open-ended and ongoing process
- Respects individual rights. Embraces cultural diversity
- Builds relationships
- Promotes inclusion

Guiding Principles for Effective Facilitation

The term *facilitation* refers to a process of supporting others to achieve self-growth. Simply put, facilitation is the process of helping others engage, learn, and achieve. This is accomplished through attending to, responding to, and understanding how best to build upon a person's strengths and gifts. The facilitator invests in the outcomes and is knowledgeable about the process and content in person-directed planning. For example, the role of the facilitator is to support the person and establish, grow, and maintain a support network. The facilitator supports the person to direct planning to the greatest extent possible. An effective facilitator is an enabler and a connector who supports others in achieving goals. The facilitator supports others in doing their best thinking and practice by encouraging full participation, and by helping to define roles and responsibilities among the support network. The facilitator also provides structure and process to each meeting so that focused conversations and action planning can occur. The following principles underpin effective facilitation:

Person-Directed

- Accommodates the person's style of interaction and preferences in the planning process; focuses on what is important to the person; explores natural supports in the community; always respects the dignity and worth of the person

Effective Communication

- Active communication; open-ended questions; acknowledges and affirms all contributions through frequent feedback; cultivates trust, cohesion, and acceptance among participants

Embraces Diversity

- Recognizes and values person's cultural background in the planning and decision-making process; sensitive to the needs, fears, and goals of the person

Fosters Connections

- Facilitates connections and the development of healthy relationships in the community; connects to natural and more formal services to support desired outcomes

Effectiveness in Coordination

- Ensures plan remains current as SMART goals and preferences evolve; organizes time and resources, and administrative tasks; monitors and tracks progress

Culturally Responsive Practice

Being culturally aware during the planning process involves enhancing the facilitators' knowledge and skills to effectively work with people who are different from them. It is important to be familiar with the cultural characteristics, history, values, belief systems, and practices of the person at the center of the plan. A good facilitator engages in various learning opportunities to gain this knowledge. Self-reflection and dialogue with others may help facilitators confront their own biases and assumptions about how someone else sees the world around them. Becoming culturally competent or proficient involves building capacity in self-assessment and managing the dynamics of difference.

Considerations for Persons on the Autism Spectrum

In planning with persons on the autism spectrum, special attention needs to be paid to challenges often associated with executive functioning, language and communication, social interaction, transitions, emotional self-regulation, behavior, sensory needs, and often accompanying anxiety. It is essential to fully integrate a person's communication system into the process. Developing an understanding of how a person communicates his or her likes, dislikes, agreement, disagreement, interests, and preferences during choice making is key to a successful planning session. To be sure, literal interpretations of language often occur and need addressing. Furthermore, additional time often needs to be provided for processing information and inviting responses. Using a lot of visual information also may support the person with more fully understanding his or her plan. Moreover, significant attention to context often enhances opportunities to discuss social understanding, set social rules for the group, and explore coping strategies for intense situations. Developing a deep understanding of what the environment needs to look like during person-directed planning is essential for successful inclusion of the person on the autism spectrum. For many individuals, anxiety is an issue that needs to be addressed when designing meetings and encouraging participation. Exploring and understanding the areas that contribute to a person's anxiety will be important in supporting them throughout the planning phases. Finally, much attention must be paid to their passions and special interests!

Elements of Practice

A facilitator will be focusing on different elements of practice while engaged with a person and his/her support network. The outcomes of those interactions will inform and drive what elements of practice the facilitator applies to the next session. The elements of practice are meant to be used in an iterative, not linear way. They are as follows:

- Preparing for the Process
- Getting to Know the Person
- Learning What Is Important to the Person
- Mediating Differences of Opinion
- Exploring Cultural Identity
- Building Relationships
- Exploring Natural Community Supports
- Accessing Disability Supports and Services
- Facilitating a Planning Meeting
- Setting SMART Goals
- Developing Strategies

- Aligning Resources with Priorities
- Determining Outcomes

Preparing for the Process

In the beginning, the facilitator guides the planning process and is then guided by the person and his/her network. Through this preparation, the facilitator will also learn how the person responds to the path the process is taking and makes any necessary adjustments. The facilitator wants the person and his/her network to participate in the process and must be skilled at posing questions to encourage creative problem solving and collaboration. A facilitator must repeatedly check that he/she is not imposing his/her own interpretations on what's being communicated. For individuals with autism, the facilitator will need to spend considerable time building context and understanding of the process.

Getting to Know the Person

There may be one or several sessions devoted to Getting to Know You depending on the person and his/her directions in the planning process. For many individuals with autism, it is essential to spend time understanding how their interests and passions can sometimes serve as a powerful motivator for planning or in fact as an impediment to planning. Developing deeper understanding around sensory and/or anxiety concerns also needs much attention in order to set the person and the planning up for success.

Learning What Is Important to the Person

For the facilitator to learn what is important to a person, an exploration of the experiences that the person enjoys may be necessary. For example, the facilitator might explore engagement in social activities of interest linked to developing friendships. Exploring things of importance to the person is a key component of person directed planning and forms the basis for setting meaningful goals linked directly to desired outcomes.

Mediating Differences of Opinion

Family members or others in a person's support network may not always agree on all goals or activities identified by the person. They may see a potential health or safety risk, or identify a conflict with their own beliefs or practices. The facilitator may need to mediate some of these conflicting views about what the person should or should not do. The role of the facilitator is to support the person and his/her support network to work through these differences of opinion and arrive at some solutions. For individuals with limited communication skills, providing ways to facilitate choice and demonstrate preference are key to ensure their voice is heard in the process.

Exploring Cultural Identity

It is important for the facilitator to understand the person and the identity of the person as it relates to ethnicity, race, nationality, language, faith, disability, sexual orientation, etc. Recognizing and incorporating the diversity of that identity into the planning process is critical to the formation of a person-directed plan. Moreover, including any cultural support networks is an essential part of assisting the person with supports to enhance meaningful and inclusive participation in communities.

Building Relationships

Many people with disabilities have a significant imbalance in terms of paid and nonpaid relationships. It is important to work toward a better balance. Relationships are critical to our health and well-being. The role of the facilitator is to assist the person in thinking about with whom he/she spends time, how much time he/she would like to spend with them, and ways in which they can strengthen and expand the number of relationships. For many individuals with autism, building the context around relationships and establishing an understanding of whom he/she would like to be involved in their planning is critical to its ongoing success.

Exploring Natural Community Supports

Person-directed planning focuses on building informal supports and networks in addition to formal supports when appropriate. Natural supports can be identified through collaborative brainstorming and problem solving. Members of the support network look to what is available through family, coworkers, neighbors, and other community members. The overarching goal here is to assist the person in becoming better connected to his/her own community. Some people enter the planning process with a strong support network or circle of support already in place. Others have very few people as part of his/her support structure. For individuals with autism, this is an area that may need considerable strengthening, as issues of isolation often accompany the social and communication challenges.

Accessing Disability Supports and Services

Some people may want access to more formal disability supports and services. The role of the facilitator is to assist the person and the network to explore and access such services. This may be achieved through referral processes, and by connecting the person to a particular service provider. There are a variety of pathways to supports and services that a facilitator would explore with the person. The facilitator can also assist in brainstorming some new and creative opportunities for supports. It is important to make sure that the resources that are accessed are the most appropriate ways to achieve a goal.

Facilitating a Planning Meeting

The facilitator supports the person to lead or direct the planning process to the greatest extent possible at each meeting. All invited participants are encouraged to fully engage in the process. The facilitator also assists everyone in arriving at an agreement about how the meeting will be conducted, how long the meeting will run, and what they hope to achieve within that time frame. Some find it helpful if the group develops some "ground rules" to keep the meeting respectful and person-directed.

The plan of action includes the development of goals and strategies prioritized by the person, identifying the resources required, and the people responsible for assisting with the implementation of the plan. Time lines for completion are also important to set out in a plan.

Setting SMART Goals

The facilitator assists the person, family, and network in setting goals that emphasize what is most important to the person. The language of the goal must capture what it is the person wants to have in his/her life now and into the future. It is important to understand that goals should never be restricted to what is currently available in both informal and formal supports. This thinking does not encourage creativity and innovation about what is possible for future growth and achievements. A good balance should be achieved in exploring both present and future resources and opportunities. This thinking will influence the setting of both short-term and long-term goals.

Setting goals involves creating a written plan that includes reasonable and measurable long-term and short-term objectives. The best goals are smart goals. SMART is an acronym for the five characteristics of well-designed goals. SMART goals are Specific, Measurable, Achievable, Relevant, and Time Bound. Start with some long-term objectives that the person might want to accomplish by the end of the year. Next, establish some shorter-term goals so that you can help set the person and the process up for success. There should be plenty of opportunities for celebration of short-term goal attainment as the individual and others work toward the longer-term goals. Short-term goals can include monthly, weekly, or even daily targets that help move the person toward his/her long-term objectives. The goals become the roadmap!

Developing Strategies

Strategies are specific actions that help the person achieve the goal. There may be a number of strategies required to achieve a single goal. Even within a particular strategy, there may be a need to break it into smaller steps. The number of strategies and how much rehearsal time is needed to achieve a particular goal is uniquely dependent upon the person and his/her support network. Strategies build upon a person's strengths, level of independence, current relationships, and other connections.

Aligning Resources with Priorities

Both human and material resources need to be identified at this stage in the planning process. The facilitator encourages the person and others to think beyond what is accessible today. Together the group engages in creative thinking about other supports that might change in even a small way what resources are actually needed at any given time. This might include an environmental accommodation or a piece of equipment that would enhance a person's independence and quality of life over a particular period of time. During this stage, the facilitator also assists in identifying who will be responsible for finding a particular resource. The person identifies any preferences for the ways they wish to be supported. For example, a person may want to be accompanied by a peer to a social event, yet be fine with having an older adult act as a reading tutor.

Determining Outcomes

An outcome describes the change that is likely to take place for the person as a result of implementing strategies to achieve a goal. Discussing outcomes right at the beginning of the planning process enables all members to develop a better understanding about what achievements and success actually look like for the person. Outcomes also assist with assigning roles and responsibilities for tracking, monitoring, and reviewing the plan on a regular basis.

Sustaining Commitment to Action

It is important that the facilitator model a commitment to sustaining the person-directed planning process with the person and his/her support network. Some planning circles might need to meet more frequently than others to keep the momentum going. The facilitator may also need to check in with the network members to ensure follow-through with assigned actions and possible outcomes in between meeting times. The role of the facilitator is to support the person and his/her family/network in staying invested and engaged in the planning process. In order to do this, the focus must always remain on helping others make connections to the ways in which their actions are enriching the quality of life of the person and enriching the contributions the person can make to his/her community. Celebrating and building upon short-term successes is critically important for sustaining commitment. Person-directed planning should be viewed as an organic journey. Such a perspective allows for some inevitable ups and downs and ins and outs with all participants who have invested their time and efforts to the planning process. Yet this also invites the integration of new experiences and fresh perspectives and ideas, which can further motivate everyone and help sustain their commitment to the individual and the PDP process.

Debbie Irish—Striving to ensure full acceptance and equitable opportunities for all, Debbie Irish has over 25 years of experience supporting individuals with autism and/or developmental disabilities in a wide variety of roles from front line support to training and awareness building to operational and leadership activities including most recently the role of Chief Executive Officer of Geneva Centre for Autism.

Debbie has a broad understanding of systems and services for children and adults in the developmental sector. She brings a solution-focused approach to her work and believes strongly in collaboration, creativity, and teamwork.

Lindy Zaretsky—Holds a Ph.D. degree in Education Administration, Theory and Policy Studies from the University of Toronto. Her research, publications, presentations, teaching, and advocacy practices focus on leadership for social justice, values and ethics, inclusion, parent and self-advocacy, and person-directed-planning. Lindy has served in a variety of executive leadership positions in the education sector and not-for profit social service sector. She is also a human rights mediator focused on disability and accessible/inclusive practices. Lindy is currently President of Reaching Education Resolutions Inc. consulting to organizations who aspire to operationalize inclusive practices for children, youth, and adults with disabilities. She also serves as Board President of the South Asian Autism Awareness Centre (SAAAC).

PLANNING FOR THE FUTURE
By Sharon A. Mitchell, B.A. B.Ed., M.A. (Writer on the ASD spectrum)

Why think about the future now? It comes up on us fast, this future thing. Often we are so busy trying to make it through the day-to-day events of our lives that we give little heed to what's down the road. But think about the length of time it takes for your child to acquire a new skill. How quickly does he adapt to a new teacher, a new classroom, or to other of life's transition?

Now is the time to begin thinking long term. What skills might he or she need? How do you begin to teach them? And how will you find the time to even think about such things?

Where do you want your child to be in five years? Ten years?

To know how to begin, you need some idea of where you might see your child in five, 10, or 15 years. What is the life you'd hope for him? What are his interests? His talents? Can these be turned into useable skills out in the world? Where might he live? With you?

With family? Independently? Sharing an apartment with a friend? In a group home setting? Will he be spending his days in a special class at school, in an integrated classroom, in post-secondary school or at a job placement?

Habits—start early with changes and preparations

It's likely that your child does not take readily to change. He needs time to adjust to the change and to acquire any new skills the situation requires. Life can be going along fine, when a change is foisted on us. We have to move for a new job. Your child's age requires that he move on to the next classroom or school. A beloved teacher assistant is transferred.

While such change can be hard on all of us, for the person with an ASD, such transitions can be especially upsetting. Yet, do we do the child a favor by not introducing change into his life? To help him prepare for change, try bringing in smaller changes while things are going well for him. I know it's hard to think about upsetting the apple cart when you think you are going through a peaceful spell, but it's as necessary to "teach" change as it is any other skill.

Being smart is not good enough

Sometimes we watch our children with Asperger's Syndrome struggle with life. While so much seems hard for them, they do have one strength—they're smart. As parents, it's tempting to focus on the positive. Yes, he's having trouble with this and this and this, but look at his science marks.

While those marks are nice, keep in mind that being smart isn't good enough. There are many very bright ASD people who are unemployed or seriously underemployed because their lack of social skills keeps them from holding down fulfilling occupations.

Overhelping

In our desire to assist and protect, sometimes we "overhelp." This occurs when we do for a child what he could do for himself. Yes, we can do it better ourselves or the child can do it better with our help, but is this what we want? It's faster to do Johnny's coat up for him, true, but in doing so we deny him the pride of learning to do for himself.

Be reasonable in your expectations, but pick a skill you would like him to have. Break the task into parts by walking yourself through it first, step by step. What does he need to be able to do before he can tackle the task? Demonstrate, practice, and hone that skill. Build it in increments until he can handle it first with assistance, then on his own. Then build on that success with another skill. Determine the level of assistance that your child must have and offer no more than that. Reevaluate this level often and wean off when possible.

There are many ASD children who graduate from high school only to bomb in postsecondary or the world of work. Might they have become too reliant on the assistance of a teacher aide? In schools we adapt and accommodate to meet a child's needs and help them achieve success. The world rarely proffers such understanding, and the transition can be daunting for the young person.

Yes, with TA assistance, your child with ASD might be a straight-A student. But are the marks the important thing or is learning how to handle yourself in class the key? It might be better for the student to take those steps toward managing on his own while under the shelter and guidance of his school rather than at college or in the work place.

What is realistic?

While we know that everyone grows and changes, just how much do you realistically think your child will change between childhood and adulthood? It might surprise you. Many of us think of those toddler years and wonder how we survived. Looking back, our children grew and prospered, albeit at their own pace, but they did learn and mature.

Be hopeful but realistic in your plans. Keep in mind the child's talents, special interests, and the things he or she will find hard in life. Listen to the opinions of others, but know in your heart that you know your child best. Read what adults with ASD have to say about their years growing up and how life is for them now. We can learn much from their willingness to share the commonalities that make up autism spectrum disorders.

Askanaspie.com (no longer in use) was a site run by students from the University of Chicago who have autism. Although it is no longer online, here is part of what they have to say: "When it comes to information about autism, there are a lot of resources written by professionals for parents. There are a lot of support groups by parents for parents. But how much information out there aimed at parents was written by autistics? It can be hard for a neuro-typical parent to understand how an autistic child sees the world, especially when that child has trouble communicating. It can be useful to read books by people on the spectrum and to speak with adults on the ASD spectrum if you can to gain some insight into how to plan for the future."

Build on your child's interests

Having special interests is a feature of ASD. These interests may change over time, but chances are your child will always have a special interest. Rather than trying to fight the preoccupation, go with it. Use it to your advantage. Build lessons around it. Practice "First . . ., then . . .," where your child must first complete the assigned task before spending time on his area of interest. Allow time for him to indulge his interest, but you will likely need to limit the where, when, and how long. Ask yourself: Can this interest or talent be used as a teaching tool? Is there a way to turn it into a life skill? Can he engage in his interest while performing a service to or with others?

Life is a group process

We know that social skills are a troublesome area in ASD. We know how Theory of Mindblindness explains that it is harder for these children to put themselves in someone else's place. The sensory sensitivities and tendency toward rigidity can make being with others difficult.

But life is a group affair. Almost anyplace we go, we have to interact with others. And, for the most part, like it or not, the world does not bend for us; we need to fit into the world to the degree that we are able.

If you foresee your child remaining at home with you always, then your adult child will need to be able to function within the parameters of family encounters within your home. If your child will be in a work situation, he will need to tolerate the proximity of others and abide by rules and imposed time-lines. If he goes to college, again, handling proximity and time, along with a host of other features, will be paramount to success.

No matter what level your child functions, he will spend large portions of his life as part of a group. Work on the skills he'll need to survive and survive well with other people.

Quality of life goals

There are things we want out of the good life, and these same things we want for our children:

- We want to be happy.
- We want to have friends.
- We want to love and be loved.
- We want to feel useful.
- We want work we enjoy.
- We want variety.

- We want to laugh.
- We want to have fun.
- We want a safe and stable place to live.

Which skills can you begin teaching now so that down the road your child can enjoy "the good life"?

Contributing Author Sharon A. Mitchell, BA, B.Ed., MA, McMaster University, University of Saskatchewan, San Diego State University—Ms. Mitchell has been involved in the field of special education for over twenty- five years as a Resource Room teacher, counsellor and consultant. She's also worked in a hospital setting doing neuropsychological assessments. Her current position is as a Special Ed Consultant and Coordinator in an amalgamated school district. As well, she is seconded by the provincial department of education to present workshops on working students with autism spectrum disorders. Parents, school personnel, social workers, day care staff, occupational therapists, speech/ language pathologists, psychologists, and counsellors attend these workshops.

12

BY AND FOR PEOPLE ON THE AUTISM SPECTRUM

MY MOTHER NEARLY DIED FROM GERMAN MEASLES

My mother nearly died from German measles, in Chicago, when she was three months pregnant with me, hoping to end an untimely conception. I was born with Infantile Autism. She told me, and I remember, screaming, wailing without consolation, from an onslaught of environmental offenses, clothing, light, noise, touch, and her mother's milk. You may not believe that I could remember, but I do, especially the white cap of the nurse who peered over the portable basket, lifting my tightly swaddled body, cooing into my face, nose-to-nose in an effort to calm me, her face devoid of features, the sounds emulating from the triangular hat.

My mother sought a neighbor's advice, a squarely built woman who knew how to raise farm animals. "Wrap her up real tight in a flannel blanket, then keep her warm in a cardboard shoe box, and don't disturb her for three hours at a time." My mother placed me in the kitchen next to the oven door, then did as she suggested, drip fresh goat's milk down my throat from a glass bottle with a hard rubble nipple. "She's just like the dear little animals that aren't quite finished developing their nervous system," she told my mother. Thanks to her, I survived, but my nervous system remains sensitive, overloading when I receive too much stimuli, such as riding a tram, eating in noisy restaurants, attending sporting events, and at celebratory parties, causing my arms to ache, nausea, and a disorientation of time and space.

High Functioning Autism, a category, niche, diagnosis that gives me a mailbox for many of my defining characteristics, some positive, even extraordinary, my sense of color and smell, awareness of environmental emotions, like the visceral awareness of angry, happy, or, sad energy permeating a space, even when no one else is present in the room. And then, other, challenging aspects of my being: my tactile defensiveness, when someone approaches me from behind, with a highjack response to plant my elbow in their solar plexus. I have a photogenic recall of spaces with a keen observation of changes in the decor, any changes, mentally editing the film that replays in my head from the previous time that I was there. Then, there are my problems with sensory overload from fluorescent lights, noisy fans, obnoxious odors, which are painful and distracting. I scan the room to locate a safe space from the offensive elements, allowing me to calm my sensory system enough to process visual and auditory information again. And, the biggest challenge, hiding my discomfort, if I am with strangers. Appearing calm, moving my body gracefully, responding appropriately to social overtures.

The friends I have, today, are understanding, perhaps even cherishing, my unusualness, allowing me transition time, even helping me find my comfort zone in social situations. Maybe, it is my playful nature and oblique sense of humor that I share, when I am relaxed, that help maintain our relationship. I see and experience the world from a unique perspective, as you may say, as *all* of us do. I believe that this is a major communication gap between those of us who are aspies and those who are considered to be neurotypical. What I mean to convey is the *degree* of uniqueness that we experience. I agree with the father of a son who is diagnosed with Aspergers, who said, "Differences for my son are more like ten thousand times normal." He said ten thousand, not ten or one hundred times. It is the difference between carrying an empty backpack on the hike of life and one filled with boulders.

When asked, "Would you like to get rid of your autism," I said, "No." I am who I am and accept myself. However, I am willing to change. I continue to modulate sensory overload, avoiding some situations altogether, and learn to ask for accommodations in a friendly way. I value the fresh approach and unique perspective that defines my autism. Like adjusting a camera angle, I celebrate the differences between my view and others. Vive la différence! Ultimately, we are all part of the great human condition, and in the magnificent scheme of all things, we are interconnected and the *same*.

Hi Stephen, how do you do?

Here is my first essay that I am sending you and hopefully it is OK.

If I need to make changes to it, please let me know. I do have one request only. I would not want my real name to be place in the link.

I have chosen Serendip as my pen name, if it could be use I will certainly appreciate it.

Please let me know if this is possible or not.

I have two more letters—as I call them—that I would like to post if they fit what they (Autism Today) are looking for.

One talks about ways of communicating between two people in the spectrum and outside the spectrum too. The other one talks about what I feel the experts are missing about us and how their labels bring a shadow to many lives.

Send my regards to your wife and will pray for you and your trip to Lincoln, Nebraska.

Autism and I

I am a female with Asperger's Syndrome, I was born and raised abroad and now live in the USA.

My diagnosis was given to me when I was 37 years old, opening the doors for me to harmoniously try to channelize my autistic journey which began so long ago. I wanted to bring the fragmented part of me to a whole, and in the process I have learn to recognize my weakness, my strength and part of me that links both.

Autism, my weaknesses, and I

Control of oneself and the emotions I feel are perhaps one of my biggest challenges in my life with autism. I did not know—*before I was diagnosed that*—what I felt at times could be an obstacle in my life.

I did not know how some of my flaws could impair my interaction with others.

There are times in which it is hard for me to control emotions of frustration and of sadness, and they both pose a threat to the way I communicate with others.

Ambiguities are not my forte, and when I have no control of what goes on around myself I feel anger, and frustrations that show. If at times I have plans and they do not go my way, I have a hard time adapting to what is to happen next. I worry, I get confused, I might withdraw, and I wish I could shut off and retreat into my world to find peace in my secure refuge.

Those are things that I have to combat in my daily life. Things that I have leaned to recognized and I am trying to understand. Life is not easy for me, having to constantly battle the way I feel, trying to gain a more even control of me. Molding myself to a more assertive being in order to interact with others in better ways and be able to achieve a simple dream.

Autism, my strengths, and I

One of the biggest strengths I have is that I persevere in what I believe and that I never cease to try to achieve a better way to communicate and a better way to adapt to the world.

Even though I am an Aspie and naturally resist change, I have a brain with the capability of reasoning and of learning new ways. I learn from my failures more than from anything else, so every time I have failed, at the end I fight to transform it into gain. I have read many books in search for new ways to help myself understand the mechanics of what is called Emotional Intelligence; and I have learned to *rethink* a previously *set thought.*

Changes are not easy for anyone in the spectrum, but they can be achieved; especially if there is a third person who could guide us more to learn to interpret the outside world. I was raised in an extended family setting, and in a way that helped, I was guided by family all the time in the things I should do or say.

The social world was a lot more complex than what I thought and I failed a lot, but with the passage of time I gained knowledge by practicing—*role play*—and at the end I was able to adapt better to change.

Life continues to be a challenge in the social world, but it is not an impossible task anymore. It takes time, it takes energy, and it takes a lot of prayers from me to be able to go out there and relate.

I thank my upbringing for the way I have turned out to be, but most of all I thank God for helping me.

I am still having many problems communicating with others in the outside world, especially when people behave in unconventional manners.

However, I do no longer try to impose my orthodox ways, I just try to understand the mechanics of their thought so that I can help bring down the barrier and thus communicate. I believe in self-improvement, perseverance, and progress; every time I am out there I think of better ways to help myself and my Aspie friends to overcome the fears and ambiguities of the social world. In time all will fall into place, but until then I continue in the search for ways to communicate.

Linking my weakness and my strength

When I am in the outside world, I have to control and channelize my emotions and my belief in order to be able to communicate effectively with people in different types of settings.

I have to remember that my orthodox ways are not the rule and that I have to adapt to what is the norm. It is then when I have to make a great effort to change from my true self to my pretend self.

I have to come to terms with the fact that in order for me to better communicate I must learn to decipher others people's ways. I am scared in a way—*after failing so many times*—of the ambiguities that I might find when I am among others; however, I am mostly prepared to face them with the knowledge that using less emotions and more logic is the way to go.

Emotional intelligence plays a great role in how I communicate with others as much as thinking of me in a third person does—*my pretend self*—and not my true me.

When I link past experiences, knowledge, and self-control of my emotions and beliefs I am better prepared to have a more successful way of dealing with social situations of any type. Knowing my weaknesses and my strengths is a plus, since I can use both of them to make life easier for me and for others around me as well.

Communicating effectively will always be a challenging task for me, but it is achieved by means of perseverance, control of emotions, knowledge, and practice.

I was 37 when I discovered why a part of me was fragmented, I cried, I raged, I calmed down, and I learned to understand my weakness and strength; so that I could try to rebuild my fragmented self and turn it into a whole.

The journey has been long, at times I leave pieces of my heart on the road, at times I pick a rose; but throughout it all I know that I am not alone, that there are many fellow Aspies like me on the road . . . And so I continue to persevere in ways to learn to communicate so that others can hear my inner voice.

Contributing Author Veronica York is a female with Asperger's Syndrome. She was born and raised abroad and now lives in the USA. Her diagnosis was given to her when she was 37 years old, opening the doors for her to harmoniously try to channel her autistic journey that began so long ago. She wanted to bring the fragmented part of herself to a whole and in the process had to learn to recognize her weaknesses, her strengths, and the part of her that links both.

AND THEN, THEY'LL SEE MY MOTHER

Autism: the word once rang of despair for a lot of mothers who only hoped that their children's actions would be controlled by, perhaps, a behavioral medication. The word once rang of loneliness, for the children on the spectrum had become lost to their own void, their own world, and the mothers and children who had become outcasts to the society to which the mothers once belonged. The word also once rang of defeat, for the mothers broke down, losing all hopes that their lives would ever be the same again, and sometimes leaving their children to try to fight the darkness alone, only to fail and lead a life with no purpose whatsoever. This was the word's definition 11 years ago, when I and many like me had no hope. This was its definition before my mother, Lynley Summers, came and inspired a different meaning behind my once-terrible world.

True, I was only four years of age in 1994, but that didn't stop the doctors from trying to trap my mother in the same kind of depression that had ensnared the other mothers of autistic children. They ran diagnostics and IQ tests, among other things. But what they were telling my mother was so much worse: "Your daughter has an IQ of 50. Normally, that is considered "mental retardation."; "Your daughter will probably never be able to speak English."; "Here's how it works: when Jessica gets a little older, she will have to start wearing a helmet. There is always the option of a group home, full of other people like her (and other misfits to society). Any questions?"

Had I understood what the doctors were saying of me at the time, I most likely would have broken down and gone even further into my own void. My diagnostics had clearly explained to my mother why other people labeled me as a "freak," and why our own family—YES! OUR OWN family—had abandoned us as though I had the plague and like Mom caught it. My autism was something that neither of us could control at the time. However, if my mother had been like the other moms out there at the time, I would not have turned out the way I ended up. And, lucky for me, my mother still isn't the type to give up without a fight.

We went through therapy after painstaking therapy, and sure enough, one year later, I was able to walk into the world again. They had considered me a genius for my age, though I do not remember how high my IQ was after that one year of therapy. I still acted autistic, but I was still getting some more of my mother's Chaos Theory Therapy in the meanwhile, to help me "act" normal. There were major setbacks at times. After all, kids will still be kids.

I was still acting sort of "funny" when I entered kindergarten, and so the other kids harassed me. They framed me for almost everything, and the teacher believed every single one of the kids but me—just because I was different. She didn't know what autism was and didn't seem to care what it was. Before I knew it, that lady put me in a remedial class part-time, and the kids made fun of me there, as well. My mother tried to set things straight after she caught one of the kids framing me again. Guess what the lady said: "I've been around your kid more than you have and I can tell that she's nothing but trouble . . ."

Mom was madder than I'd ever seen in my life.

Not only did she move me away from that school, she started doubling our therapy sessions, making sure that I'd never have to deal with anything like that ever again. Before I knew it, after school I was coming to the college where Mom worked and practicing what we had learned in therapy. Sometimes, Mom was interviewing college students while I was in the other room, practicing what I had learned by myself. Other times, my mom and I hung out together with some of her friends while we practiced some more therapy.

Most of the friends that I had in first, second, and third grade were my mom's friends: adults. They understood me; I understood them; all was right with the world, and we could have had a party celebrating our friendship. That's how happy I was, despite the fact that I was still in therapy. And my adult friends liked me so much that I was recruited as the first Junior Member of Alpha Psi Omega, the college's drama fraternity. Even when I went to Japan with Mom for two years, most of my friends were adults, and a lot of them even hung out with me during my therapy.

By the time I went into junior high and high school, when I came back to America, you could hardly tell that I was autistic at all. My mother's love had already brought me out of the void that I was in. And people just didn't care anymore. Autism had become just another condition, just another bump in the road, so to speak—much like nearsightedness. I found friends who were my peers. Sure, I was teased every once in a while, but that's just what it was: teasing. So it wasn't a big deal to me. However, every once in a while I end up wishing that I could tell the world some very major points that could probably turn their lives around.

Mothers, please: DO NOT GIVE UP ON YOUR CHILDREN! Although the world might be sunny and bright outside, the void is a dark, lonely place to be, filled with your children's fears, anger, and sadness. I know because I've been in that horrible place. If anything besides my mother's therapy regimen can bring your children out of the void, it is your love, faith, understanding, and guidance. You have to believe in them. That's all it will take to bring them out of the void.

It's always easier to be lazy about it. It's always easier to think that all is lost or that nothing can be done. You'd probably hear a person after the diagnostics, crying, "Oh, no! He has autism! All is lost! Alas!"

But that's the thing: all is not lost. That is the mistake that some parents with autistic children make. They give up on them and allow them to sink deeper and deeper into the void. Most of them expect their kids to learn all they need to know at school. What a joke. Parents leave their kids alone too much. They don't get involved. They let their kids be raised by the television or by the Internet, or they expect everyone else to do it for them. Then, they blame it all on the autism. And one of these days, they're going to sit on a chair, missing their precious children, wondering where they are now. And then they'll realize they're right where they left them: lost in the void, some of them perhaps in a home where they have few opportunities.

I shudder to think of my "self," left shackled by a "disability," helpless. Some parents may say to themselves, "What have I done? What have I done that made my child deserve this treatment? Why should he have to suffer for the fact that I abandoned him in his time of need? Why didn't I fight for him? He was my child. Why did I have to give up on him?"

And then, they'll see my mother: not the woman who defeated autism, but rather embraced it and formed it to her liking. I was only the clay to the potter, and I was shaped into person I am today not only by experience but by love itself. My mother had so much faith in me that it helped me to carry on in life. Yes, there are times when I feel desperate and weak and as though I might falter to the mission in which I must succeed, but my mother is the one who gets me back up on my feet with her faith and love, as she tells me, "You can do it, Jazz; I know you can . . . ."

Every once in a while, at Mills University Studies High School, the school I go to now, when I tell people about Autism, some people already know about it or know someone with it. That, I believe, is progress on our part. However, some of the other people I tell do not know about it or make fun of it afterward. Like I mentioned before, that's just how kids are.

One of the more infamous, but hurtful, jokes goes something like this:

"Why did the Autistic girl cross the road?" "Well, I don't know. Why?"
"I don't know, either. Why wasn't she in the asylum?"

Like I said: hurtful. It sounded a lot like they were laughing at me, but the truth of it is that they had no clue what it was really about. They didn't even know I was autistic, and when I told them that I was they automatically kept their mouths shut about the "autistic girl joke." I also meet people who have absolutely no clue what autism is. I tell them a little about it, and usually I get: "Autism? What is it, like mental retardation?" People should learn that being autistic just means you're a little bit more special than some of the normal kids.

To be perfectly honest, I really don't think that anyone is truly "normal." The only people who really are "normal" are the really boring adults and the really mean kids. Other than that, everyone has their own special qualities. Just like there are special shapes and sizes; everyone is going to be different from you. Different is a good thing; America is a land of diversity, after all.

My point is that you shouldn't shun people just because they're different. According to a song in Schoolhouse Rock, we are said to be the Great American Melting Pot. The way I see it, we, the autistic, are just one more ingredient to this delicious country that we call America. Just because we're different doesn't mean we're defective. It just means that we make America all the more unique.

Contributing Author Jessica "Jazz" Summers was born in Arkansas in 1990. Diagnosed as mentally retarded at age three and autistic at four, she is the daughter of Lynley Summers. Jazz is the youngest member of Bobbi McKenna's Write Your Own Book Club, a club intended for adults, and will release a book next year.

She speaks in her community to increase autism awareness. Having skipped 6th grade, she is an honor student at Mills University Studies High, ranked #20 in the nation by Newsweek.

MY STORY

The journey begins.

It was one of the last things my Dad said to me in our final conversation prior to his death last December, at the age of 82. "You know, I never did understand why you were always so different from other kids. You were just different, is all I know how to put it. No one else in my (extended) family ever had that problem learning how to talk." He went on to tell me how it was both a surprise and a mystery for him. I seem to recall my Mom, prior to her succumbing to Alzheimer's, telling me the same kind of thing. I took it was a mystery to her as well, though she did tell me she was immensely relieved when the doctor said that whatever was causing my speech delay, it was definitely not due to any kind of cancerous tumor on my vocal chords. According to the doctor, in that respect, I was completely healthy.

You see, all my life I've been on a journey, even before I realized I was on one. Even in college, others realized it before I did. One acquaintance remarked, "My goodness! I just realized the truth about you. You're in a search for yourself and you're lost in the woods." Then he shook his head some more and walked away. Now, after so many years, I finally understand what he meant. Truly, I was different from other people, had compulsions and habits others did not have. The same sporting events that others seemed to enjoy so much, complete with all the crowd noise, repelled me. What especially bothered me was how my level of functioning kept changing for no apparent reason. Some, with contempt in their voice, openly labeled me "retarded"; others, with an unmistakable air of amazement, expressed how much they admired my intellect. An enigma indeed.

My journey toward self-discovery began in earnest in the spring of 1995 with work at a local print shop. The work, being fairly routine, suited me well. One day, I went to the break room as usual, but this time I noticed a religious newsletter on the table. I put my bologna and cheese sandwich aside and picked up the colorful magazine. A front page article titled "What is

Autism?" captured my attention. I had heard the term before but was not quite sure what it meant, if anything. Inside the brochure, I found the various identifying traits of the condition.

I gasped in shock. It was like looking in a mirror.

It was me, all me—the delayed speech, the rituals, the rigid thinking, the difficulty grasping abstract concepts. A storm of mixed emotions stirred inside me. I felt elated, and yet I also felt violated. I was elated because now, for the first time in my life, my sensory related difficulties felt real. I could now grasp them in ways I couldn't before. I felt justified in believing they were real. Yet at the same time I was shocked that the whole article of information redeeming my belief system came from a person or people whom I had never met, who didn't know me. They somehow knew my deepest secrets, things I'd never told anyone. I threw the offending paper back onto the table and rushed out of the break room, resolved not to ever research the subject. It was too disturbing.

Late that evening, I went to the grocery to attempt to shop. As I entered the store, I noticed that few other shoppers were around and the Muzak heard over the intercom was even soothing. I took a deep, satisfying breath; I could shop with little or no torture this time. I grabbed a cart, careful not to make any more noise than necessary. As I glanced up, a child in another shopping cart caught my attention. Though I had never seen this boy before, he seemed so strangely familiar. The boy had a fixed stare at the wall, almost like a statue. The mother, standing to his side, raised her hands and began speaking through sign language. Without ever turning around, he signed in response.

My hands felt cold and clammy. Chills ran down my back. I tried to get a breath and couldn't. An image began to form from the distant, intentionally forgotten memories of my childhood. This boy was like me as a child. Then a storm of memories flooded my psyche. I drew back, unsure what to do next, or how to assess what had just happened. Slowly, I looked back at where the boy and his mother had been. They were gone.

Some days later, my professor told us to research a list or newsgroup. After a quickly prepared, tasteless supper, I went to the local computer lab to do the assignment. After a while, I glanced up at the clock and rubbed my aching eyes. It was 2:00 a.m., and I sat alone in the campus computer lab—except for a lab technician who was busy running programs. Bleary-eyed and tired, my only thoughts were of how I should be in bed instead of torturing myself at this computer station. After all, it was only worth 10 points.

Yet, I felt compelled to continue. Though having seemingly accomplished little, I still felt unable to quit for the night, unable to fathom such a change in gears. I just couldn't decide on which article to print.

There were so many. Moments later, I came across a list that included an autism discussion group. My heart pounded. I couldn't sit still. I was convinced that if I didn't open this door right then, the matter would forever haunt my nightly dreams. I closed my eyes and took a deep breath. No matter what I might find, I knew I had to know more. What about the condition I had read about in that newsletter? Could there really be other people out there like me? I felt compelled to know one way or the other.

I rushed home, too excited to sleep. I poured myself some hot tea and thought about my discovery.

Could I really be autistic? What does it mean to be autistic, anyway? In the days and weeks that followed, I spent countless hours at the university library delving into the matter, and taking meticulous notes about what I found. A few months later, after rigorous testing and a seemingly endless number of interviews, I received my diagnosis. For me, the diagnosis was a relief. I was finally on the verge on understanding myself.

In the process of this journey, I've learned many things about myself. Autism is not just something I have, in the sense that one may have high blood pressure. It is something that I am, in that it affects every facet of my life. It affects the way I think, the way I perceive the world, and the way I respond to it.

2) The basic traits

One way the autism affects me is that I tend to think in much more tangible terms than do most people. In order to grasp abstract terms, I think of them in terms of what I can see, hear, touch. I think in illustrations and analogies, a trait medical experts often think of as mental rigidity.

To an autistic individual, mental rigidity is more than mere words printed on the pages of some psychiatric journal; it is the source of much of his being and who he is. It determines, to a great extent, how he learns about and responds to his environment. It is the reason autistic individuals tend to be so literal in their thinking and why figures of speech often confuse them.

To someone within the spectrum, abstract concepts of any kind are learned only with great difficulty, and realness is a constant issue. It has also been my experience that things I have not seen or touched in a while tend to lose their realness to me. For that reason, I have always had this affinity for nouns, and a certain dislike for verbs. Especially as a child, I had to go around the classroom touching the walls in order to feel comfortable being there. Things have to be tangible to me to seem real. The problem is that if they don't seem real, my mind tends to automatically reject them. Concepts that I reject, I soon forget, as well.

For the autistic, learning must relate to something tangible. For myself, the actual learning is not as important as the learning how to learn. So much of what I was expected to learn was abstract, and yet this was the very thing I had trouble grasping. I was puzzled when, in my senior year of high school, my fellow classmates voted me "most studious." I figured it surely could not be true because I didn't even know what that meant, exactly. Being studious was just another concept that I had difficulty grasping.

Thus, I had my own way of learning how to learn. For instance, the word "running" would conjure up for me an image, a memory of someone hurrying to the bus stop to catch the bus, breathing heavily, with me cheering them on.

Doing this not only made it more tangible, but easier to remember as well. Why visual imagery? I think perhaps so many people within the autistic spectrum are visually oriented because the other senses are even more vulnerable and thus more problematic.

I also discovered that the best time to learn was while I considered myself at play. I would make the learning situation into a game. I would be relaxed and comfortable, and learning became much easier. Experience has shown me that concept learning is best done when the child is relaxed, especially while the individual is at play—not during periods of high-pressure drills.

It is my belief that such drills produce masses of memorized statements, but little more.

Another aspect of mental rigidity involves the need for routines and rituals. Everyone has at least some need for a sense of order and, with it, daily routines. Just imagine how hectic life would be without those daily routines, if one had to decide every morning how to get out of bed, what to eat for breakfast, what route to use to get to work, and so forth. Indeed, our lives are filled with enough stress as it is, without making it exponentially more so with constant decision making, as would be the case if one had no daily routines.

Thus, we all need at least some sense of routine and purpose, but children especially need it, and autistic children need it most of all—simply because of the mental rigidity that comes with the disorder.

That mental rigidity is a major trait of autism that has been known for a long time. One of the implications of this is that autistic children, living in a chaotic world as everyone does, must find ways to impose on their environment a sense of order. Life never comes completely scripted, so far as I know, anyway. As much as I might like sameness, life still goes on. Since none of us live on a desert island, there are always changes in the way we go about our lives from day to day. I have found that if I know in advance what to expect and that there is a valid, important reason for this change, then I can usually accept the change on an emotional and cognitive basis. But if the change is a total surprise, and seems arbitrary at that, then I have difficulty mentally accepting its realness.

For the autistic individual, virtually everything about life is not only frustrating, but is so in the extreme. The rituals serve a useful purpose in that they impose a sense of order for those who need it. Otherwise, they are forced to cope with the continuously high level of frustration in other, less appropriate ways. Thus, a ritual is a vital technique for coping with a confusing, often disorderly world.

Especially during childhood, all the time I feel either very comfortable and secure, or else very uncomfortable and insecure. Back then, it was always either one extreme or the other. I recall many times things during childhood that when things were not exactly explained to me, and especially not in tangible terms, it caused me to feel mentally frustrated and quite insecure.

Thus, as one might expect, I found ways to cope, including rituals. Some of my rituals were common, such as not stepping on cracks in the sidewalk. But I also felt compelled to tap my teeth together a certain number of times and in a certain manner. Or tap my thumbs with my forefinger in perfect geometric patterns.

During meals, I ate in "rounds." That is, I would take one bite of everything on my plate, then start again. If I disliked an item on the tray, I simply removed it. Since it no longer belonged with my meal, I felt no obligation to eat it—and the sense of order that my psyche required was maintained. My drinks had to be placed on the tray so that they could be included in the meal.

Another ritual involved the way I walked the half mile home from the bus stop. I had a compulsion to walk with my right foot on the road and my left foot on the grass. Any deviation from this and I had to walk it over. Also, I could not enter a bathtub without first rubbing my feet three times each. At the front door, I would knock three times, turn around three times, and shuffle my feet three times before entering. At school, I had to go to my desk, shuffle my books, go touch the teacher's desk, then return to take my seat.

In time, as I developed and as I learned to cope in other ways, my need for rituals decreased.

Truly one of the beautiful aspects of classic autism is the sense of innocence. Autistic individuals tend to be playful, optimistic, and a bit mischievous. We tend to want to project good feelings toward others and expect that in return.

Out of this sense of innocence comes a sense of wonder that pervades every day. No matter how often I have experienced it before, it is always as if it were the first time. I am amazed at the way honeysuckles manage to fill a whole neighborhood with their fragrance. I look up at trees reaching up to the sky and marvel at their magnificence. I see streams bubbling and wonder about that, too.

3) Sensory difficulties

For all the inherent difficulties affecting those within the autism spectrum, I would have to say that, by far, the one that causes the most suffering and torture is the tendency toward Sensory Dysfunction, also called Sensory Integrative Disorder.

There are several sensory-related issues that, for someone who is autistic, cause the disorder to be much more troublesome than need be. Indeed, it is the tendency toward sensory difficulties that makes autism so difficult to deal with. Also called sensory defensiveness, the worst part is that it tends to go in an unending cycle and worsens as it continues—until abated. Parents and teachers may observe it as negative behaviors or as an extreme reluctance to do certain things. But what is really going on is that the child is suffering from sensory distress. Being unable to talk, as is the case so often in classic autism, the child is unable to express what it is that is torturing him or her.

The sensory dysfunction and overload tend to lead to a heightened level of frustration and anxiety. As the nervous system becomes increasingly stressed, the sensory dysfunction worsens, causing harsh sounds and rough textures to become even more irritating than ever. The sensory dysfunction, as it worsens, leads to yet more anxiety and frustration. The cycle continues until interrupted. As one can see, the well of sensory-related suffering goes deep.

Nature intended us, for our own survival, to have sensory defensiveness. A certain amount of touch sensitivity is necessary to warn us of dangers. Have you ever been out in the yard or in the garden and felt this spider crawling up your arm? Or tried to read with a fly annoy you? When a sensory system dysfunctions so greatly, as it frequently does in autism, the tactile system is especially affected. The skin itself becomes hypersensitive.

So, what does a light touch feel like? The best way I can describe a light touch from the point of view of someone with sensory problems is that it is like having bugs crawling all over you. Believe me, it is quite annoying. This can be anything with a rough, abrasive texture, like certain foods. This would especially apply to polyester-based clothing. Stiff, roughly textured blankets can be just as annoying. I often wonder why manufacturers ever make blankets scratchy like that. Tactile sensitivity is one of the main reasons individuals with autism so often have trouble sleeping through the night. After all, who can sleep with that kind of stuff going on? No wonder I had so much difficulty sleeping through the night for most of my life.

A second way this hypersensitivity affects is me visually. I often have to keep my computer screen dim to avoid high contrast and the brightly colored, animated advertisements that decorate most web pages. Such harsh glare tends to make me instantly nauseated. On my really bad days, even ordinary fluorescent lights seem to resemble strobe-like floodlights. I may not see the flickering, but I can certainly feel it.

For me, the worst part of going to the dentist was never the shots or the drilling; it was the glare from the lamp. More than once, I wanted to tell the dentist what he could do with his evil lamp. Unfortunately, I couldn't talk for having to hold my mouth wide open.

Noise can be a problem. Hearing sensitivity is especially troublesome for me because it is difficult to protect myself from. Unlike visual distress, it doesn't help just to turn the other way. Actually, turning my head so that one ear is facing away from the noise just makes the pain worse. It seems that both ears must hear the sounds to a similar degree for my brain to process it adequately. The two types of noise that bother me most, though in vastly differently ways, are sharp, explosive sounds and crowd noise.

Sharp or sudden noises may include such things as metal banging on metal, pencils tapping against a desk, chalk squeaking along a chalkboard, tires squealing, metal forks touching ceramic dishes, as happens at mealtime, car horns blowing, and car doors shutting. Leaf blowers, sirens, and vacuum cleaners are also major offenders.

What's worse is that the sound does not even have to be loud to be irritating. Water coming out of a faucet, a toilet flushing, the hum of a dishwasher or an air conditioning system all bothered me. It feels like electrical shock waves beginning at my ear, and being especially bad there, but also traveling along every nerve fiber of my body.

The other type is crowd noise. Our senses are like windows to the world. Information is uploaded to the brain for processing. Nature knew that our brains' processing ability needed protecting. Thus, during periods of loud crowd noise and such, most people are able to block out irrelevant noise. As noted earlier, it's the specialized cells known as Purkinje that do the magic. Unfortunately, without them in sufficient quantity, sensory information overload becomes a big problem for those of us who are autistic. Without this protection, we remain so vulnerable.

Crowd noise can be found everywhere, and even a small amount hurts me. So most of my life has been filled with torture. All too often I find myself in a social setting, filled with people innocently talking—and I am totally unprepared for the unwelcome bombardment of meaningful noise on my senses.

Unable to simply ignore it, I find myself forced to listen in on and try to make sense of every single conversation going on in the room. At such times, I feel as if I were a fortress under siege from both meaningful and meaningless sensory data. Mentally, I may know what noise is relevant and what isn't, but my senses don't know. So my senses pick up every bit of available information. Because speech is meaningful noise, my mind wants to somehow grasp it all, to somehow comprehend everything being said.

For the first few seconds, I feel my head filling up, as it were, and being overwhelmed by all the sensory data coming my way, and I cannot ignore it. At first I am acutely aware of the neural pressure, like one feels the pressure of the water when diving into several feet of water. I am also acutely aware of how uncomfortable it is, how much it hurts. I feel the shock waves start at the ears and travel through every nerve fiber in my body. It feels like an electrical jolt surging through my entire nervous system.

Then, as the sensory overload sets in, I become dazed and have difficulty functioning. I can't focus my thoughts. My brain gets overwhelmed to the point that conscious thought is difficult. Mental fog sets in. I begin to feel mentally and physically numbed and disoriented. If I stay there long enough, I feel an aura coming on, leading to yet another seizure. Later, after some rest, mentally I may feel I have recovered somewhat, but physically I feel bruised. I ache and sting all over as if my entire nervous system were in rebellion.

After repeated assaults, my senses would indeed become confused. I would get dazed and numb. I could have an ache without grasping where I feel the ache, or even whether I feel, hear, or see it. At times my senses have gotten so confused and all I have known is that it was torment of some kind and it was real. As anyone who has ever been to a dentist can verify, after being numb a while one begins to crave a sense of feeling in the anesthetized area. Now imagine if one's entire body remained numb over a long period of time. For most, the craving would be unbearable, and so it often is for the autistic individual. Thus, the level of frustration remains high and the quality of life low.

As a child, and even now at times, I have had a continuous feeling that my arms and legs were no longer attached. I have felt compelled throughout the night to continuously rub my joints and wiggle my toes, without ever actually gratifying the strange need I had to touch, to feel something, anything at all. It has caused me a lot of insomnia.

I once fell off the cab of a truck and completely broke my wrist but felt no pain or other discomfort at all from it. My body was that numb. As I looked down, the sight of my limp hand looked odd, but it did not hurt. I could not feel any physical sensation at all. I realize now I was fortunate not to have gotten hurt more than I did throughout my childhood, as things for me could have been much worse without my realizing it.

But there is a craving that often goes along with this kind of numbness. If one has ever been to a dentist and had one's gums and jaw numbed so the dentist could do a root canal, one may understand just how annoying numbness can be, no matter what the cause. After a period of such numbness, one starts craving some kind of physical sensation in the area that got numbed. Now imagine if one felt that same numbness all over one's body. Imagine, too, that this numbness is not only continuous but lasts for an indefinite length of time. This could be months, even years. After a while, one gets desperate to feel something, anything at all, even if the means to that end is inappropriate.

4) Some final thoughts

Do I feel cheated not to be like other people? Not at all. I like and accept who I am, and I have a passion for life. I am who I am and would not want to be anyone else, even if I could.

The difficulties of my life have made me more appreciative of the beauties of life and tend to make me appreciate the value of friendships I have made along the way.

For more information, Daniel Hawthorne may be contacted through his website: www.autismguidelines.com.

Contributing Author—Daniel Hawthorne is a diagnosed High Functioning Autistic. He is the author of *Child of the Forest* and *Guidelines to Intervention in Autism* and webmaster and author of the award-winning site www.autismguidelines.com. He has degrees in Communication and Business Administration, most recently through the University of Arkansas. He does numerous speaking engagements to autism support groups and to special schools, in addition to managing an online résumé posting business.

THE MAKING OF *NORMAL*

Making our film, *Normal People Scare Me Too*, with a cast and crew of autistic people was challenging, both during filming and editing. But when we finished our film in April, the rewards were worth it. We had about 75 percent of cast, crew, art, animation, and music done by autistic people. Beyond the cast and crew, though, making our film as mother and son was really hard at times—especially for me as an adult, and for my mom in the roles of both a director and a mother.

If you are a parent, you might relate to asking yourself this important question: "When do I back off, and when do I keep doing things in my kid's life—especially when they are adults?" If you are like me, you might ask yourself this about your parent a lot! We had to deal with this question—over and over—for an entire year while making our film, and it was definitely not always easy. We know lots of parents around the world who work as their adult child's "manager" to support and promote their futures and miro-enterprise-like businesses. This sometimes creates breakdowns and hopeful breakthroughs.

I worked on this article, at first by myself, and then side-by-side with my mom. When we made our first film, *Normal People Scare Me*, a decade ago, I was 15 years old. Today, I am 27 and live independently with supports. Mostly, these are my words with a bit of my mom's suggestions to help me word things that are hard for me to get out. She asked me basic questions to help get me started.

Mom: Taylor, what motivated you to make this film?

Me: OK, I'm laughing at myself right now. I'm sitting in front of my laptop, inside of a Chipotle, finding it difficult to find the motivation to write an opening paragraph that's almost all about motivation and how I sometimes have trouble with it. It's laughably ironic.

Mom: Is that a common theme for you, trying to find motivation for things you want or need to do in your life?

Me: Yes, it can be very hard. It is often the process steps that confuse or stall me. What does any of this have to do with my experiences filming *Normal People Scare Me Too*? A lot. It's about how I decided that I needed to get back on the proverbial horse so that I could lead a life that I'm more than happy with, and the journey it will take to get there, and the amount of effort it would take for me to get there.

I got involved with NSMP2 very early on in preproduction, when (you) asked me if I want to do the film. I accepted almost immediately. However, I was not heavily involved with the main production of the film behind the scenes. My primary responsibility during the filmmaking process of NPSM2 could be summed up fairly easily. I was essentially the lead actor who helped guide the other actors to better serve their parts on camera. I asked the questions that were in the script, and I went off-script to ask even more questions that were related to the people I interviewed. Some of the better recorded moments were even tangents that couldn't be helped because they showed the struggles some people as a whole go through on a day-to-day basis, and that's not even factoring in the autism. Those are the ones that I remember the most.

Mom: What were the highlights for you in the interviews you had with old and new cast members?

Me: For me, the things that I remember the most are some of the most emotionally intense in the film. However, they are intense for the same reason stated above, it's just some of the struggles and horrors people go through every day. I remember those moments because they serve as a strong reminder that people will not believe that things are going to be OK just because someone says so, but because they will believe things are going to be OK because they want to get help and will move their butts to obtain said help. Also, it makes the more inspirational moments shown in the film all the more special to me.

As an example, one of my childhood friends, Vince, got involved with wrestling—something he was passionate about since he was a kid. I was excited for him when he told me about that on camera. However, it also got me to think about where I was going in my life, because he showed that his passions have made him a much more emotionally healthy person. I wanted the same thing he had. So I reevaluated everything about myself. My likes, my dislikes, and my overall skill set. That got me on the path to going back to school, getting job development, and the support needed to succeed at both.

There were also points where I got to chat with some of the people from the first NPSM, like Vince, Ben, Kyle, Rick, and others who are now 10 years older and have gained more real world experience in between the two films. Some have become really cool people that I would totally hang out with if we lived in the same area code. With others, I just went and quickly put them in the "best kept as acquaintances" folder of my mind's file cabinet. We all have those, you know.

Mom: What are you doing now to help you with motivation?

Me: I have new and better staff in place now. My current staff, James, who is employed to work with me through a program called FADE, is on the autism spectrum. He is close to my age, and he gets me. Last semester, he attended an English class with me at community college. After failing college classes in the past, I finally got my first B. That was highly motivating.

I have fallen down a lot since I made the first *Normal People Scare Me* film. I graduated a Transitions to Independent Living (TIL) program through the ARC of Ventura County. Three years ago, I moved into my apartment supported by Social Security and support staff. People often ask me why I can't "just" follow through? Or say to me, "Taylor, if you would 'just' . . ." I seem capable, yet executive and administrative functioning are hard for me. Sometimes it is hard to say the right words or share my thoughts. It's just hard to get them all out. Sometimes, when I am interviewed for my film work, though, I get my words out OK.

Mom: Sometimes you wanted to drop out of the film. Why was that?

Me: During the filming of *Normal People Scare Me Too* this past year, I almost dropped out of the project. I just didn't know where I fit in to *Normal* and making my real dream of becoming a gaming reviewer happen. At one point I told you (Mom) and Joey Travolta (our producer) to just finish the film without me, because I felt no value to me in completing the project.

After I took some time to think about it and realized that I needed to form the skills that would be required of me to do what I really wanted to do, finishing this film made more sense to be a foundation for the eventual goal of being a good writer. So here we are. Needless to say, I completed the film because along the way I found inspiration among the people I interviewed in *Normal People Scare Me Too* to get back on the horse I mentioned so that I could lead a life I'm more than happy with and the journey it would take to get there. I am beginning to see I have to do many things that take a lot of effort if I want to reach my other goals.

Mom: What would you say to young autistic boys/girls, men/women about following their dreams?

Me: Well, now I feel motivated to go after what I truly want in life outside of this film (which was a lot of fun to do), and I will go to great lengths to get it. I hope that my thoughts on how *Normal People Scare Me Too* affected me on a personal level will inspire people to get either themselves or others to be motivated to live life to the fullest. Doing the hard thing eventually inspired me. It is not easy, but hey, who said life would be?

And now that the film is done, I look forward to speaking engagements and to sharing our film all over the world. And even though I like to travel with my mom to speak, if my staff, James, can come, I would really like that.

About the Film:

A decade after the award-winning film Normal People Scare Me *was released, Taylor Cross, the film's cocreator, is at it again with* Normal People Scare Me Too. *In the new* Normal, *he interviews former and new cast members and family about attitudes and first-person perspectives in autism today.*

Created by a film crew comprised of 75 percent autistic students and graduates of Joey Travolta's Inclusion Films, with music and art created and performed by 65 percent autistic musicians/composers/artists, the new Normal *is pleased to be a more inclusive production this time around.* Normal People Scare Me Too *is driven by Taylor Cross, directed and coproduced by Keri Bowers (Taylor's mom), and produced by Joey Travolta. Keri is the cofounder of The Art of Autism, a key supporter behind the scenes of the film, and has created four films in autism and other disabilities. The new* Normal *can be ordered through our website.*

Taylor Cross has worked on four documentary films, including *Normal People Scare Me, The Sandwich Kid, ARTS*, and *Normal People Scare Me Too*. These films have taken him all over the world to speak at conferences—with supports. Taylor lives in his own apartment in Ventura, California, and is currently taking a few classes at community college. He works with his support staff to improve the skills necessary to help him find gainful employment or micro-enterprise opportunities as a gaming reviewer and public speaker. Recently, he's begun booking his own speaking gigs and film screenings.

LIGHT AT THE END OF THE TUNNEL

I debated with myself during the writing of this as to when (in the course of the article) to disclose that I have Asperger's Syndrome. Should I come right out with it or should I build the suspense until the end. Needless to say I came right out with it (a very special coworker suggested I fill you in at the beginning).

I have spent most of my life wondering what was wrong with me and why I was so different. For the longest time I didn't have any answers and neither did anybody else. Not that many people wanted to know. It seemed that no one wanted to get to know me or understand me. But I must say I didn't know or understand myself, either. I didn't have any friends. Sometimes that really hurt, yet at other times it didn't bother me at all. I was quite content to do my own thing. What a strange contradiction.

There were many issues with family members. I remember my aunt telling me (within the last few years) that she would have her version of a pep talk with my cousins before we went for a visit. It went something like this: Okay boys, your Auntie Marilyn and the kids are coming for a visit. We all know how Terri can be, so we need to tread lightly. This isn't an exact quote, but you get the gist of it. I'm still amazed that even in my late-'30s these words had the power to devastate me. At times they still do.

There were good things about me, special gifts if you will, yet not many seemed to notice. I excelled at academics, music, and sports, but people only seemed to see my "obnoxious and socially unacceptable" behaviors. I wanted to shout, "there is a fun and enjoyable person in here," but I couldn't because more often than not I wasn't even aware of it myself. I was ostracized and bullied in school even though I was bigger than most of my peers. It wasn't "easy being green."

So I did my own thing and got in trouble a lot because I didn't conform to the norm. Just what is the "norm" anyway? It took me many years to develop coping skills and techniques to be able to do the things I wanted and knew

I was capable of doing. Yet there were two or three people who loved me unconditionally. For that I feel very blessed.

My music and my love of reading helped through the tough times (of which there were many). When I was playing my trumpet, and later the euphonium, I was able to put all the hurt, anguish, and joy into my music and no one was intimidated or repulsed. What an experience. There was joy in my life; I just wasn't able to realize it then.

My diagnosis of Asperger's Syndrome came late in my life; well, at the time I thought it was late. I was in my early thirties. Initially the diagnosis was ADHD, yet that didn't ever seem to fit. My spouse and friends didn't agree with the diagnosis because I met very few of the criteria. However, that's all I had so I went with it. A few years later my psychiatrist mentioned Asperger's Syndrome, and he believed I should be the recipient of such a delightful diagnosis. Lucky me, I'm an Aspie!!

Actually, he was bang on. As I started reading more and more literature, I realized I could have been (and still should be) the poster child for Asperger's Syndrome. What an incredible relief. I finally had something to hang my hat on. For those of you who are reluctant to label your child (or yourself), I encourage you to go for it. There was a reason I did all those strange and wonderful things as I was growing up. I wasn't just a big freak who didn't fit in anywhere and nobody liked. Now I'm a big freak with a label and I love it.

I have come to a place in my life where I love and respect who I have become and who I am. I still don't always fit in, but that's okay because I have my own space. I don't always say the right thing in public, but when my family and friends need my support I somehow figure it out. I'm honest to a fault and I'll be there for you through thick and thin. Once you've climbed my walls and seen through my behaviors and mannerisms that offend, you will have a very special place in my heart and I in yours. Love me for who I am and the rewards are tremendous (so are some the challenges, but hey, that goes with the territory).

Take the journey with your child, family member, or friend as you both grow and learn. Remember, there is light at the end of the tunnel. I have found mine.

Contributing Author Terri Robson is an adult with Asperger's Syndrome. She is the controller at Autism Today. She has a Bachelor of Education with a Music Major and an English Minor. As well, she has a Music Merchandising Diploma and is a Certified Journeyman Partsman. She is pursuing a designation as a professional accountant. She loves great music, good wine, reading, camping, and spending time with her partner of 10 years, family, and friends. She has two purebred dogs (one of which is a Canadian and American Champion) that she calls her children. Terri loves being an "Aspie" and wouldn't want to be any other way.

SELF-ESTEEM ON THE HIGH END
OF THE SPECTRUM

My name is Mary DeMauro, and I have Asperger's Syndrome. I am also a social media manager. My job involves managing professional social media accounts with the goal of broadening their reach and encouraging a certain action from the audience, such as buying a product, signing up for a program, or simply clicking the "follow" button. I schedule posts ahead of time for an optimal reach, search for and create new content to share, and use analytical programs to study my outreach. Social media is not just for sharing vacation pictures or telling people what you had for lunch. It is a vital part of the modern professional world. If you have any sort of business or organization, it is essential to have a strong presence online. But managing Twitter and Facebook profiles can be time-consuming. This is why you bring in someone like me.

I began this job a few months after I graduated from George Mason University. I had a bachelor's degree in art, specializing in graphic design. I also had a revived interest in writing and was working on several manuscript ideas while looking for a job. My mother put me in touch with Dr. Dixiane Hallaj of S & H Publishing, who gave me feedback on my work. She also asked me if I would be interested in helping build S & H's presence on social media, as well as doing some graphic design work. This happened in October 2015, and I have now been working for S & H over two years. In early 2016, Dr. Hallaj introduced me to Ms. Karen Simmons, and I began running several campaigns for her, including the social media pages for her company Gem Gallerie and her organization Autism Today.

This opportunity has been an exciting one. I never thought that only a few months out of college I would begin a job that I enjoy so much. I've learned a lot about social media marketing over the past year, and Dr. Hallaj has been an excellent mentor. I've had a fantastic year gaining experience in a job I've come to love.

This job has been a gift, not just because I love it, but because it works well with my Asperger's. I get to work from home, which means I can set up a workspace that meets my personal requirements, and a schedule that won't be badly compromised by problems such as anxiety.

I was diagnosed with Asperger's syndrome when I was a teenager, about sixteen. I also have Obsessive Compulsive Disorder, which is commonly seen in tandem with a spectrum diagnosis. It was originally suggested that I might be autistic when I was in preschool, but my parents, who had not heard of the high-functioning variant of Asperger's syndrome, were skeptical. However, in high school I was diagnosed with OCD, and this was followed with an Asperger's diagnosis.

Learning that I have Asperger's has explained a lot about me, such as why I feel bursts of energy that cause me to walk randomly around my house, why I'm obsessed with housing floor plans, and why I find denim to be so uncomfortable. Asperger's, especially the attached OCD, has been challenging, but it's also made me who I am. Because I have Asperger's, I was fascinated with dinosaurs as a kid, I have a close connection with my parents, and I have a deep empathy for others. The idea that people on the spectrum are not empathetic is profoundly untrue; I feel for others so deeply that it is hard to just go about my life when others are suffering. I have also bonded with my parents, both because they are so supportive and because I am more comfortable with them than with strangers my own age. Meanwhile, the "special interests" I've had over the years, from my love of dinosaurs to my fascination with UFOs, has kickstarted my love of storytelling. In addition to my social media work, I am also trying to start a writing career, and many of my novel ideas revolve around my Asperger's-fueled curiosities.

Nevertheless, Asperger's still brings challenges. Possibly the biggest difficulty has been my OCD, which forced me to live by nonsensical rules I set for myself. This severely impacted my quality of life and kept me from enjoying things that should have been fun. This struggle has also led to depression, which made school difficult. Unfortunately, there wasn't much help from school officials. In high school, my family requested academic assistance for me, but it was refused because, supposedly, my grades were too good. College was also a challenge, partially because my OCD issues reached a peak during that time, as did my depression. I was able to receive some help with test taking, but there was no help for my anxiety. When a professor callously told me she could not give me extensions unless I reported an issue more than twenty-four hours in advance—not possible with my anxiety attacks—the department supported her decision. However, with a few extra semesters, I was able to graduate college. My ability to graduate is a continued source of self-esteem for me.

Another self-esteem boost was learning that there were jobs compatible with me. As a social media manager, I get to work from home, which means I can work in a way that's comfortable for me. I'm grateful I was able to find a job that is so well suited to me, and I look forward to a bright future. I've experienced challenges, but I've come through them stronger for the experience.

Mary DeMauro is twenty-four years old and lives on the East Coast of the United States. She was diagnosed with Asperger's Syndrome as a teenager and has since embraced it as part of her identity. She holds a Bachelor's Degree in graphic design from George Mason University and currently works as a social media manager.

THE FUTURE IS BRIGHT

It's a long haul . . . but we are getting there . . . and yes, there's much more. However, inklings of making fulfilling and productive lives for individuals on the autism spectrum the rule rather than the exception is taking a turn towards reality as we transition from a model based on deficit, disorder, and disability to one of ability.

There are three steps to reaching the light at the end of the tunnel that every individual, organization—for profit or not—and all the way up to entire country makes: awareness, acceptance, and appreciation. For years, many have devoted themselves to making others aware of individuals on the autism spectrum. The Autism Speaks Light It Up Blue campaign is one of many such examples.

As awareness of the strengths and challenges the autism spectrum brings, a sense that autism is something that can be worked with develops as educators devise strategies for teaching to individuals strong points. Now, and growing ever brighter, are glimmers of appreciation where individuals with autism are valued for who they are. Perhaps the clearest example of appreciation can be found in Information Technology companies such as MicroSoft and SAP that have vowed to make 1 percent of their workforce be individuals with autism. These and other business recognize the extreme strengths people with autism can bring to the workplace realizing that hiring these individuals are good business decisions rather than being a form of charity.

Addressing the question of providing employment to everyone else who are not IT geeks, www.autismworksnow.org matches people more significantly affected by autism and/or skilled in other areas to meaningful employment, as well. Whether it's the parent of a child going through the steps of awareness of autism in their child before transitioning to acceptance and finally appreciation, or entire countries such as the Russian Federation and Bangladesh reaching out to experts to build their capacities for education of children with autism. Rather than staring at the closed door of disability, disorder, and deficit, let's walk through the tunnel together toward the light and ask what the person with autism can do.

Contributing Author Stephen Shore, M.Ed., Boston University—Diagnosed with "Atypical Development with strong autistic tendencies," Mr. Shore was viewed as "too sick" to be treated on an outpatient basis and recommended for institutionalization. Nonverbal until four, and with much help from his parents, teachers and others, he is now completing his doctoral degree in special education at Boston University with a focus on helping people on the autism spectrum develop their capacities to the fullest extent possible. In addition to working with children and talking about life on the autism spectrum, Mr. Shore presents and consults internationally on adult issues pertinent to education, relationships, employment, advocacy and disclosure, as discussed in his book *Beyond the Wall: Personal Experiences with Autism and Asperger's Syndrome*, the recently released *Ask and Tell: Self-advocacy and Disclosure for People on the Autism Spectrum*, and numerous other writings. A board member of the Autism Society of America, he serves as board president of the Asperger's Association of New England as well as for the Board of Directors for Unlocking Autism, the Autism Services Association of Massachusetts, MAAP, and the College Internship Program.

—